ENGAGE, ENERGISE, ENRICH, EVALUATE – a practical guide to medical education

Avril Danczak

This edition published by Consultation Skills Ltd 2026

First Published by Royal College of General Practitioners in 2015

ISBN 978-1-0369-5082-8

DEDICATION

This book is dedicated to all the many medical educators who spend so much time trying to help others learn. Theirs is an act of great generosity; even professional educators spend far more hours than they are paid for preparing pondering and evaluating. Those who educate as an "add on" to their main job, often do so for no pay at all, yet may spend hours at weekends or in the evening preparing educational sessions for their learners. In that same spirit I offer this modest contribution; a recipe book of tried and tested methods that can be used to improve the effectiveness and value of education in health care settings.

ACKNOWLEDGEMENTS

I would like to thank Rebecca Baron for her encouragement to embark on this project and Bob Kirk for supporting it at HEENW. I would like to thank Sally Howorth for helping to disseminate it, make it available to all North West Educators, and for all the meticulous work she has put in behind the scenes to enable us to work effectively as educators.

I would also like to thank my family for encouragement and for tolerating my absence to write and for their cheerful interest in what I am doing.

Finally, but most importantly I would like to thank two groups of people.

Firstly, my fellow GP educators who have taught me so much about how to be an effective educator in many contexts, from one to one in tutorials, through to small group and large group sessions and even helped me understand how to present in very large groups. At every encounter with another educator I have learned something valuable. This makes you as a group far too numerous to name; please know I have learned from you all.

Secondly, I would like to thank the participants who I have worked with over many years, who probably now number hundreds if not thousands. You have tolerated my experiments, given positive (and brutally negative) feedback, which has helped me learn so much. You have been a delight to get to know as individuals, as well as participants in groups. Nothing makes me happier than to see previous participants becoming effective educators themselves, or to hear that other educators are developing techniques even further.

To all of you, MANY THANKS and HAPPY EDUCATING!

NHS
Health Education England

INTRODUCTION

This manual came about because I am interested in the development of the next generation of medical educators, especially those training in the context of General Practice.

While new educators are better trained than ever, there is the potential for good ideas and techniques to be "reinvented" and useful techniques and ideas to be lost when older educators hand over to new ones.

I would like to share some of the methods I have found most valuable, to make them easily available to anyone embarking on any kind of educational event in a health related context. This could be training professionals, such as doctors or nurses, it could be training staff in a general practice or Primary Care Team. There is no one size fits all, the techniques and methods are like the raw ingredients in a recipe. When cooking you need to know how ingredients work and what they are for. The methods in the ENGAGE, ENERGISE and ENRICH sections are like a cooks ingredients. The EXAMPLES and EVENTS sections give a few examples of how these "ingredients" are combined to make a nourishing educational "meals". Creative cooks/ educators can have free reign here!

My urge to write this all down emerged after reading several textbooks on medical education which said things like, "interactive methods are better for this" (Reference 3), without actually spelling out what such a method might actually consist of, or what skills would be necessary to carry it out successfully.

In medical education circles, Education 101 goes like this; there is a thing called the educational triangle and when planning education, you can basically start at any point and work round to help you ensure all bases are covered in your plan.

Educational triangle

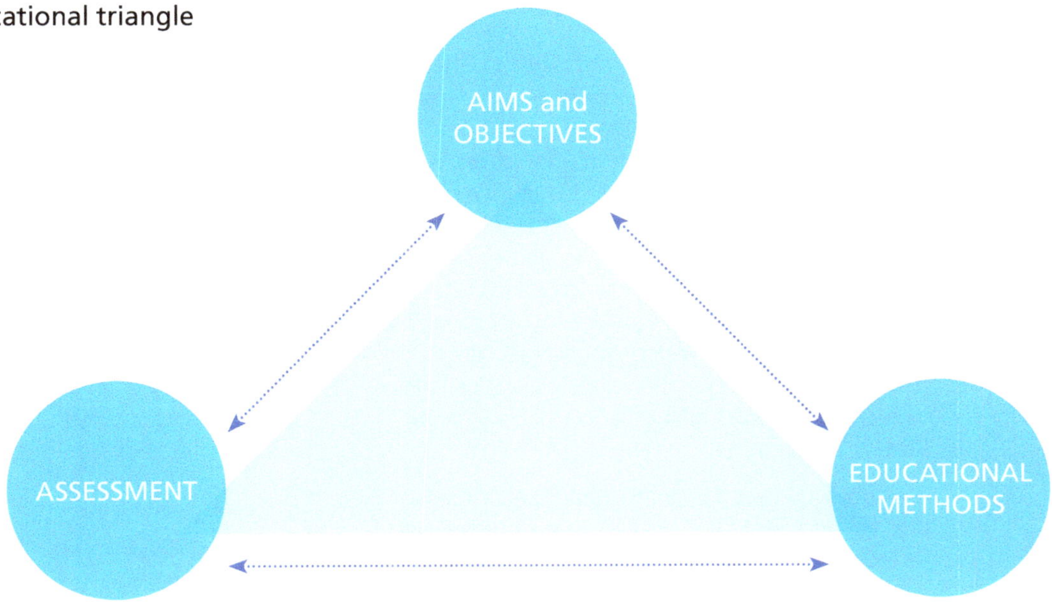

The **AIMS and OBJECTIVES** of medical education are really defined by the curriculum for that area of work; for a given educational session or for an educational programme, the subject matter is likely to in some way derive from this curriculum. Of course a curriculum is a tricksy thing. The formal curriculum is usually clear and open to all to see. The website of any Royal College has a myriad of relevant documents. However, the aims and objectives of any training become less clear cut when two other curricula are considered; the informal curriculum and the hidden curriculum.

The **informal curriculum** includes all those things which are understood to be important to learn, but which are not necessarily written down formally. This includes all the behaviours that reinforce and transmit the attitudes, norms and beliefs about what being a clinician is all about, and how that should be demonstrated in how we speak, dress and behave.

For example, there may be no formal teaching or curriculum about what to wear or how to speak to fellow clinicians, especially in between formal events such as break times or in the canteen. This type of curriculum is *imbibed* rather than taught. Although the informal curriculum is not necessarily explicitly taught it may be transmitted by role modelling by seniors, via peer pressure, and via the implicit expectations that educators have of participants. For example, the manner in which a clinician speaks and works with fellow clinicians and team members will be observed by learners and the overall style and approach absorbed without much explicit instruction. Observing seniors responding to requests for help, or examining patients sensitively, are examples of where an informal curriculum is coming into play.

The **hidden curriculum** is not overtly stated, but expresses the priorities, deeper beliefs and practices of the environment or institution. The aims of the hidden curriculum are not explicitly articulated and yet are woven through all the practical and educational experiences that participants have during their training. For example, a hidden curriculum could include the expectation that learners strive for, and that they are capable of, excellence. In contrast, the expectation could be that clinical practice is too difficult to do well and that "getting by" is all that is reasonable.

It is obvious that those contrasting attitudes in the hidden curriculum will have very different effects on participants' views of themselves and what their training is *for*. The hidden curriculum is *felt* rather than expressed and can have a variety of effects. If participants do not have a sense of belonging or of being valued in their working environment, their commitment and learning will be adversely affected. This can happen without anyone needing to state anything openly. If women are groped in their medical school (yes it does happen) the implicit message is that "you do not matter much". If all informal events involve alcohol, the implicit message can be read as "you need to be like us to succeed", or "non-drinkers are not really welcome".

When we plan educational events, we take account of the formal curriculum requirements as a matter of course. When we choose our *learning methods*, (the subject of this book), we are often expressing the informal and hidden curricula, the priorities, attitudes, beliefs and values we are signing up to educationally. The subject matter we prioritise (clinical knowledge or skills development? Ethical understanding or regulatory compliance?), the educational methods we choose, (lecture or interactive small group work?) will both *imply* the curriculum and become part of the way in which it is delivered to participants. The formal curriculum of the Royal College of Surgeons includes aspects of communications skills, including the need to communicate effectively with relatives and other team members; if these matters do not appear on surgical training programmes the hidden curriculum is "this is not so important" and "you do not need training for this, you will pick it up somehow".

General Practitioners may have other "hidden curricula" such as "the main thing is to finish on time" or "patients do not really want shared decision making", or "we have to follow the guidelines all the time".

Thus, while the nature of what is to be taught is often very clear from the formal curriculum, how we teach and how we choose priorities, must take into account our desired and intended informal and hidden curricula when planning our educational events. In the main, this book does not cover the content of the education; that is outside my scope here. The methods can be mixed and matched to teach subjects as disparate as consultation skills, the surgical treatment of appendicitis, sepsis, professionalism, fitness to practice or the biochemistry of antihypertensive drugs. Having decided the content, the educator can then choose appropriate methods to enable effective learning.

In order to create effective education, **ASSESSMENT** clearly plays a large role. The level that any given teaching experience aims at is determined by assessment of the level of attainment the participants are *currently* achieving. Clearly, the approach for a medical student in their first week needs to be different to that used in providing education for a senior and highly qualified Advanced Nurse Practitioner. Deciding how to work out whether your learners have reached the right standard is covered by assessment processes specific to the context. In General Practice, for example, examinations (Applied Knowledge Test, Clinical Skills Assessment), competency based Work Place Based Assessments (using Consultation Observation Tools, Case Based Discussions) and portfolios which log learning and reflection, are all used for assessment. Many participants are also subject to other assessments such as 360 degree or multi-source feedback. If things go a bit pear shaped, patients are more willing than ever to make complaints and give feedback. Most educators should have a pretty good idea of the level to which training should be pitched.

However, at Post Graduate level, participants often vary in their specific learning needs; a matter which seems easy for one participant (for example helping a person change their drinking habits), might seem daunting to another. For this reason, the techniques described in the ENGAGE section help educators assess the specific learning needs of the group of participants they expect to be working with.

If AIMS and OBJECTIVES and ASSESSMENTS are generally well covered and familiar, the choice of **EDUCATIONAL METHODS** can sometimes be given rather less attention. Instead of a robust educational triangle we sometimes experience something more like a broken three-legged stool, where the wobbly third leg represents the EDUCATIONAL METHODS most appropriate to the tasks of Assessment and delivery of educational objectives.

If the third leg, the METHODS leg is unstable, it will be hard to create robust education that delivers its objectives. Why does this matter? After all most trainees/learners pass their exams eventually and become employable in their professional role. I think the delivery of education, using the best and most appropriate educational methods, matters for the following reasons:

- **Training time is limited** – effective teaching methods make better use of this limited time, i.e. effective methods achieve larger effects.
- **Effective methods are quicker** to use than some conventional techniques such as the PowerPoint accompanied lecture.
- **Effective methods are easily acquired by learners themselves** – the result is that participants become more effective life-long learners. This can help to maintain professional development over their careers.
- **Effective techniques can be used across the board** – the effectiveness of learning in multidisciplinary teams, professional partnerships and working with patients groups van all benefit from the use of effective educational methods.
- **Effective methods deliver better informal and hidden curriculum objectives** – effective methods support rather than undermining desirable informal and hidden curricula.

Broken three-legged stool

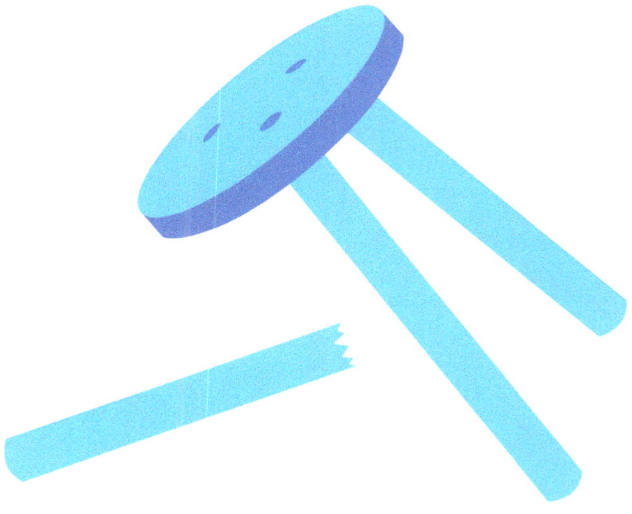

The educational methods described in the sections of this manual have a close relationship to the skills that are used in the consultation. Building a rapport with a patient, listening and really hearing what a patient has to say, working with their agenda and using skills for explaining and helping patients retain information, have a lot in common with the skills of required for an educational encounter. Furthermore, many of the skills that make for effective education are the same skills that make for effective teamwork. This is another example of the synergy between educational skills and the skills needed in clinical practice.

Just as training for effective Consultation Skills draws on a systematic approach to teaching, learning and assessing skills, the techniques described here are presented in a systematic way. However, in this manual, the skills are those needed when a medical educator works with groups of participants. Many skills needed in consultations (listening, summarising, and being patient centred) are similar to the skills needed when running education for groups (and indeed individuals). Doctors with skills in the consultation will find that these skills are transferable to an educational context. This has the potential to make acquiring educational skills easier and quicker – a big bonus. The educator will also find that the skills acquired in education will be useful in their local teams.

How do the skills of the consultation relate to those used in education?

ENGAGE

In the consultation we need to establish rapport and understand why the patient has come to see us. In a similar process, at the start of any education session, we need to ENGAGE with the learners, developing a rapport with them, and assessing what it is they are able and willing to learn that day. These methods encourage participants and educators to work together, create interest and motivation for learning, via the exploration of common agendas.

ENERGISE

As a consultation develops we have to constantly be aware of what the patient is concerned about, so as to maintain and develop the relationship in an effective way. As education sessions develop we need to maintain interest and commitment by using techniques that ENERGISE participants. These techniques maintain motivation and interest throughout training sessions and present information in ways that generate energy (and even excitement). This keeps participants on track. The benefits of educational time are maximised if everyone is awake throughout, everyone participates and no one loses interest during the session.

ENRICH

As the relationship deepens with a patient, our understanding of their predicament becomes more complex and we need to explain things, exploring the realistic application of our proposed management plans. Similarly, as teaching sessions develop, we can use techniques to ENRICH the content, to enable it to go deeper and work at different levels. This is especially valuable when there are learners at different stages in a group (for example a Primary Health Care Team, or a learning group with participants at different stages of training). Identifying ways to engage with formal knowledge and attitudes and values, deepens the range of possible learning from a session. Using hierarchies of learning when planning, can engage learners at different levels, while still creating education that benefits all. Using a wider range of methods avoids death by PowerPoint. Enrichment techniques can also promote reflection on participant's experiences and reinforce learning.

EVALUATE

Finally, after every consultation there will be at least a moment of reflection ("that went well" or "that was not my best moment"). This corresponds to the EVALUATE process of education; there are many different ways to do this effectively. Going beyond the tick box "Did you have a good time?" or "Did they pass the exams?" can enable educators to make sure that their work is linked to the reality of clinical practice, is fully absorbed by participants and can lead to important improvements in subsequent training interventions.

There are two tasks that run throughout any educational session; developing **relationships** with participants and attending to the **structure** of the session.

Throughout consultations and throughout education sessions we are always creating inter-personal relationships. In a consultation it is the one to one relationship that is the key. In education sessions it is more complex, as there are two tasks; we are constantly developing and monitoring the relationships between the *educator and the participants*, and the *relationships amongst the participants themselves.*

These relationships are a key way to support and enrich the learning process. Healthy relationships create a sense of belonging, encourage commitment to learning and to the learning of others and can enable learning to go to higher and more complex levels. All educators need to develop relationships with participants of appropriate intensity, to build the attention, rapport and commitment necessary for effective learning. This includes role modelling, showing genuine interest in participants as individuals, and working to promote learning in all participants. Participants can tell if you don't really care; nothing puts them off more. Poor relationships in the training session results in poor educational outputs.

Tuckman described the stages of team or group work as being "Forming, Storming, Norming and Performing" (see Reference 5). Tuckman later added "Adjourning/Mourning "which is the stage when a team or group break up having completed their task, (see ENRICH Endings). Although the term "team" is used by Tuckman, the same processes occur in educational groups that meet over time. Successfully "Performing" educational groups pay greater attention to the relevant tasks and provide effective support to the learning of all participants. This creates the potential for greatly improved outcomes. Methods to improve group work in education can be very profitably used in practice and other teams too. This is another example of the synergy between professional skills used in clinical work and the educational skills acquired by educators.

In a consultation, we are constantly attending to timing and structure, using signposting and nudges to help us make best use of the time available, for example, saying, "before I examine you is there anything else I need to know?" or "before you go, can we just go over the plan?". Education sessions also benefit from having the structure overt and signalled to participants; this helps participants to:

- **anticipate** when new things are going to happen
- **understand** the purpose of any practical exercises
- **ensure** that the material will be covered in a timely way
- **experience** an atmosphere in which they are "held", with a clear sense of direction.

Educators need to be skilful in knowing when to spend time on an important issue raised unexpectedly, and when not to get bogged down. Dealing with difficult participants needs skill; if left unchecked the learning of others can be compromised.

I have summarised these processes in Table 1, see below.

Table 1

	Stage of the educational intervention	
Develop the relationship with the participants	ENGAGE at the start to get learners and teachers working together and to establish the relevant agenda for the process.	Attend to the structure of the educational programme and make this explicit to participants
	ENERGISE throughout the intervention using techniques that maintain interest.	
	ENRICH the experience by using varied techniques that enable working at different levels, exploring knowledge skills and attitudes.	
	EVALUATE effectiveness during the intervention and afterwards using techniques to promote reflection and improvement.	

This manual is arranged in sections, each one with a brief introduction to the general principles, and then detailed descriptions of specific techniques to ENGAGE, and ENERGISE participants and to ENRICH and EVALUATE sessions. There are additional sections describing how to combine educational methods together to make whole sessions in the EXAMPLES AND EVENTS section. Finally, there is a list of handy resources.

The individual chapters in each section are laid out as below:

- Name of method
- What it is for?
- When to use it
- The set up: how to use this method
- Explanations/timings
- The debrief: maximising the benefits
- Equipment/resources needed
- Skills to make this work even better
- Pitfalls/when NOT to use this method
- Applications in other areas of the session
- How does this help to build relationships?
- How does this help to structure the education?

Part of the skill of effective postgraduate education is to be able to combine clear and structured aims, objectives and processes which still allow for unpredictable and spontaneous outcomes; the educator facilitating the group to work effectively towards clear educational goals. If this sounds a bit puzzling, all will become clear when you read about the potential activities in this manual and start trying them out for yourself.

Part of the art of education is developing a knowledge of different methods, knowing when to select a particular technique, how to vary it according to circumstances and when to avoid it. Preparation and planning are essential; on the day even the best laid plans may get waylaid by circumstances, such as participants distressed by a painful incident on their team, the imminence of exams, a change in official guidance that alters what you want to convey. In these situations the educator is like a musician – well prepared after practicing scales, technical exercises and also full musical pieces, who is also like a jazz musician, who is able to improvise within a formal and well prepared structure.

Style plays a part here too; some educators, like some musicians or some cooks, are more comfortable with pre prepared plans and scripts (like scores or recipes), which they bring to life with their own interpretation and input. Others can improvise from whatever material is available. The skills involved are the same but used differently. Educators can be very flexible about how they approach their work, as long as there is an underlying understanding of WHERE they want to go (the aims and objectives, the curriculum), HOW they are going to get there (the educational methods they will employ) and HOW they will know whether they have arrived (evaluation and assessment).

Does this matter? Do educators need all these special skills? Isn't enthusiasm and a passion for teaching enough?

Educational skills make education more effective for learners, and undoubtedly more interesting for educators, as they develop a range of educational methods. Using methods appropriately opens up educational riches, mobilising the energy and resources of the participants in ways that stay in the memory and enrich the experience of educator and learner alike.

One of the most gratifying things that a patient can say is "thank you for listening". As educators we could be aiming not simply for our participants to listen but also to remember, to be inspired and to acquire the tools to ensure their own continuing professional development. I hope these methods in a very small way will help to make education more interesting and more effective. The payback for this is sometimes long delayed, but nothing is more gratifying to an educator when someone says:

"I was in your sessions years ago when you got me thinking … and I have not stopped thinking ever since."

Glossary

Educator – the person responsible for planning, organising, supervising and facilitating educational events of any kind.

Participant – the people who come to the educational events.

Group – all the participants present.

Sub group – a smaller number of participants, when the main group is divided into smaller units.

Facilitate – what an educator does to promote learning in participants.

Time budget – the (strictly limited) time available for the education, whether in one session or over a period of training.

Session – a single educational event such as a one hour event, half or full day training event.

Programme – a series of educational sessions, combined over time to deliver a curriculum. For example, a Study Release Training Programme, or a postgraduate training programme delivered in several modules over time.

Resources and references

Formal, Informal and Hidden Curricula; some perspectives.

http://student.bmj.com/student/view-article.html?id=sbmj.j3287

The risks of following the informal and hidden curriculums

How following the unwritten rules of medicine can cause professionalism dilemmas and emotional distress. Marika Davies

http://website.aub.edu.lb/fm/shbpp/Documents/The-Not-so-hidden-curriculum.pdf
Thalia Arawi

Teaching Made Easy; Mohanna et al; Radcliffe, Oxford 2014

Skills for Communicating with Patients; Silverman et al; Radcliffe, Oxford 2005

There is a quick summary of Tuckman's ideas about Forming, Storming, Norming and Performing here:

https://www.mindtools.com/pages/article/newLDR_86.htm

and a useful Wikipedia section here:

https://en.wikipedia.org/wiki/Tuckman%27s_stages_of_group_development

ENGAGE

INTRODUCTION

This section is about methods that help to **engage** learners in sessions. The introduction considers the "Why, what and when" issues and then the sections that follow are detailed descriptions of different **methods** ("how" issues).

What does "engage" actually mean? Here are some definitions.

1. To occupy or attract (someone's interest or attention). "He ploughed on, trying to outline his plans and engage Sutton's attention." Also having ideas of capture, catch, arrest, grab, seize, draw, attract, gain, win, captivate, hold, engross, absorb, occupy. "The tasks must engage the participants' interest"
2. To participate or become involved in: "Organisations engage in a variety of activities." Also having the idea of participating in, taking part in, joining in, becoming involved with, "going in for", partaking of, occupying oneself with, or throwing oneself into.

Sometimes we only realise the importance of something when it is not there. We have all had personal experiences of learning events that were boring, when our minds wandered, when we fell asleep or when the clouds outside the window were far more interesting than the geography lesson about rainfall happening inside the classroom.

Educators sometimes complain about lack of learner engagement in post graduate training situations as if disengagement is a property of the learner, i.e. as if the learner creates the disengagement by being a lazy or uninterested student. While clearly, learners have a responsibility to learn when they get the opportunity, Educators have a responsibility to deploy skills which will increase learner engagement and make learning more likely to happen. Moreover, if we think that disengagement is a property of the learner, this hardly explains why those same learners who yawn and look bored during the session talk animatedly to each other during the breaks, and who have non work lives full of incident and drama. If we just say "well do not be boring and then engagement will improve" that's a bit like saying "be a better person", or, "make your jokes funnier"…it does not describe the "what, when, where and how" of what is to be done.

Many of the methods to increase engagement might seem superficially simple or to have nothing to do with clinical education at all. However, time spent getting to know participants and helping them to get to know each other, is an investment in better engagement and better learning.

The key to engaging learners is to invest in the beginning of the session, just as in the consultation we invest in the opening minutes, to ensure success later on.

What does "invest in the beginning" actually mean and why is it important? Kaiser Permanente, a large, not for profit, healthcare organisation in the US, educates all its clinicians regularly with something called the "Four Habits" model of the consultation. They spend a lot of money training people to do this, because it reduces patient dissatisfaction and reduces expensive litigation.

One crucial habit is to "Invest in the Beginning" (see http://www.ucdenver.edu/academics/colleges/medicalschool/education/graduatemedicaleducation/GMEDocuments/Documents/4%20Habits%20Model.pdf for details). This means building a good rapport, finding out what the main concerns are for that day and planning what is going to happen during the time available. The payoff for this is that a welcoming atmosphere is established, there is faster access to real reason for the visit, diagnostic accuracy is increased with less work, negotiating an agenda is facilitated and the potential for conflict is minimised. This is exactly what we need at the start of any teaching session; to create a good atmosphere, get to grips with what really matters to the learners, negotiating an agenda and timings for the day. This is an example of how consultation skills and teaching skills have a big overlap.

Does this matter? Learners know they have come for teaching so can't we just "get on with it"? Learning, like the consultation, is a complex business, and learning with groups of participants even more so. Attention paid to the larger context of the learning of the group will pay dividends. The methods described in this manual can also be applied to work with any team, for example a practice team, a Multidisciplinary team or a team working on a task for a CCG (Clinical Commissioning Group). While consultation skills help educators with groups, group skills will help educators in their daily team work. When training clinicians in any setting, attending to the whole environment and atmosphere we create on the day will help to ensure that:

- **Learners feel that they belong**. Research in education shows that a sense of belonging is crucial for learners to do their best. Lack of this factor may be one contributor to differential attainment in our learners). This happens best if…
- **Learners know each other and the educator and have a good rapport**. Rapport is like money; if you do not have any it causes a lot of problems; when you have plenty of rapport, (or money!) then many opportunities can be realised.
- **Learners' agendas and needs are taken into account**. This matters because what participants are ready, able and needing learn next, is more important than what the Educator wants to teach next.
- **Learners participate in a community of practice**. This is a group of people brought together by a learning need, whose collective learning becomes a bond amongst them, and whose interactions affect their clinical practice in ways that vary with individual. Their learning experience helps them in a variety of ways: individuals are able to develop in the direction that is necessary for them.

Engagement is influenced by how we start things … how we start training at induction, how we develop bonds for example on residential courses or away days and how we start each and every session.

The methods outlined in this section can be used at the start of any session, or combined together for participants to get to know each other in greater depth (for example, on a residential or in a practice team). This ensures that rapport is built and that the learning agendas are negotiated and suitable for the needs of participants. Choose the methods/techniques that seem most relevant to your situation. However, I would recommend that most, if not all, sessions start with some attempt to find out the hopes and fears of those present (corresponding to the ideas and concerns of patients in a consultation) and that participants' expressed learning needs are brought out into the open at the start, so that a realistic agenda can be negotiated (just as finding out what a patients expectations are helps in negotiating what can realistically be achieved). Some techniques for increasing engagement can be used in the middle of sessions to reignite engagement if it seems to be flagging.

Spending time at the start of things is an investment in success. It may seem that pausing for everyone to introduce themselves, or taking time to enrich and deepen introductions is wasting valuable training or education time. Far from it. Good introductions create warmth, commitment and energy in the room and also draw participants into the process. This makes them much more likely to participate fully in any learning activity as well as making the learning more convivial and hence more enjoyable. Appropriate introductions set the tone of welcome to all, can demonstrate that all participants are valued, that all are here to learn and that participants also learn from each other. Including elements beyond our professional roles, demonstrates that participants can be themselves, and be respected and accepted. This builds the "community of practice" which engages participants more fully and also enriches their learning from each other.

Carefully managed introductions also help to demonstrate the *informal* or *hidden curriculum* of the event or course. The *informal* curriculum is stuff that is not written down. For example, a course may have as its curriculum "the care of patients with cardiovascular diseases". However there will be informal things learned too; for example, the ways we talk to each other about

CVS (Cardiovascular Disease) disease, the types of things we say to patients about CVS disease, which aspects of disease are prioritised (the diagnostic tests or helping patients and families to adapt?). There may also be a *hidden* or *covert* curriculum. This may be entirely covert, "we do not want women in this specialty", or expressed indirectly via statements such as "its often impossible help people lose weight/give up smoking", or "the NICE guidelines should always be followed to avoid litigation". The hidden curriculum here is that some tasks are too difficult and therefore a waste of time, or that using guidelines will "cover your back".

Educators can use introductory exercises to set the tone and enhance the informal and hidden curricula; is this a serious and heavy session? Can it be playful and light hearted? Or both? Will the creativity and individuality of the participants be encouraged and valued? Or is the aim to get a uniform approach at the end where consistency and reliability are more important goals? Getting participants to talk about psychological problems in their patients may benefit from an introduction that emphasises the participants own feelings ("say your name and how you felt at the end of your last clinic"). The end point of a Basic Life Support training course may benefit from a more cut and dried approach ("say your name and the main element of resuscitation you would like to get better at").

So much can be said in a "simple introduction". Planning this part of the session carefully can have a big impact on the engagement and interest of participants, while also using time very effectively. An effective introduction can help a group to the point of working and active learning very quickly. If people just sit with their friends and never interact, the group may remain rather detached and uninvolved. In adult education, people will nearly always communicate better, learn more actively and engage more fully if they know the people they are learning with. Introductions help to orientate and relax everyone. Many participants are likely to be socially anxious when they come to training, asking themselves questions such as:

- Will I be accepted?
- Will I be asked to do things that reveal my weaknesses or failings?
- Will I learn anything useful?

Creating an accepting atmosphere helps people to be relaxed and less anxious. Anxiety interferes with learning. Being relaxed is not the same as being sloppy; punctual start and finish times, attention to preparation and structure within the session, responding to issues that arise and having effective arrangements for IT, handouts, group tasks and so on, make a containing, organising structure within which participants can feel held and therefore less anxious.

The **ENGAGE** section of this manual describes engagement techniques that Educators can use with their audiences, whether in a one to one session, a small group or even an auditorium sized set of participants. Each technique is described in detail, with the rationale and explanation. In most Postgraduate medical training sessions, the key to success lies in the set up (explaining to everyone what is going to happen) and the subsequent debrief (discussing and reflecting on what actually did happen).

Getting to know the participants to a level appropriate for the context (perhaps superficially in a one hour one off session, deeply at the start of a yearlong programme) starts the process of building the relationships on which effective education is based. In Postgraduate education the starting points and learning needs of groups can be diverse and not easily predictable.

Understanding where participants are coming from and working with that, enables suitable prioritisation during the session. When participants understand that the education is focused around their needs, their engagement increases.

In many postgraduate contexts interactive methods for education are taken for granted (for example, in General Practice), but participants still report "Death by PowerPoint" as the preferred option for many educators. This is the "fill up the bucket" model; tell people things, show them some pictures and they will learn the material. In practice, lectures may simply mean that participants are exposed to material. Understanding the material, applying new learning to daily practice and being able to take a critical approach to knowledge, require that participants interact: with the material, with the educator and with each other.

To this end, the precious time available in postgraduate education must be used effectively and with purpose. That purpose should be crystal clear to the educator and transmitted concisely to the participants; when participants know that their needs are understood and that the learning offered has a clear purpose in relation to those needs, full engagement will follow.

Meticulous planning of how any session, exercise or activity is set up will help to ensure that the expected benefits materialise. If each activity is debriefed skilfully, (again usually best when planned ahead), the educator uses the experiences of participants to draw out reflections on what has been learned. This results in maximum educational benefit. The debrief time is often not given the same emphasis as the exercise itself; this limits the benefits of the activity. Effective debrief encourages participants to think more deeply, to share the experiences and reflections of others.

This does not mean that all spontaneity and flexibility have to be removed during your planning stage; quite the opposite. An effective set up is like lighting the blue touch paper on a rocket … you know it is going up but not necessarily where it is going to land. Educators must avoid missing the blue touch paper and start trying to set fire to the stick, or the explosive at the top end of the rocket … you get the picture. The debrief process is like looking at the place the rocket ended up and saying "what happened here? How did we get here? What else do we need to do now?"

The techniques in the ENERGISE and ENRICH sections will help educators to take learning to the next level and maintain engagement throughout the session.

The different methods that could be used are summarised under these headings:

Techniques to establish rapport

Especially at the beginning of courses and the start of most sessions if you are not the regular educator, or if you are a visiting speaker.

1. Build your own classroom
2. Simple introductions
3. Picture cards introduction
4. An introduction using pairs interviewing each other
5. Shield introduction exercise
6. Walk around introduction
7. Broken card introduction
8. Using pictures as a starting activity
9. Ice breakers
10. Geographical introduction
11. Large group introductions for formal presentations

Techniques to establish and negotiate a learning agenda.

12. Buzz groups
13. Hopes,fears and dreads
14. Establishing learning needs at the outset

Techniques to encourage a community of shared practice.

15. Everything with a purpose (EWAP)
16. The sweep discussion method
17. Talking sticks
18. Preparing an educational brief

A worked example

The Title, Aims and Objectives and Intended Learning Outcomes are planned before the session, together with relevant, prepared didactic teaching and practical exercises to help participants embed what they have learned

Example

A one day session on Basic Life Support with assessment of competence suitable to certificate participants to the standard required for their continued training (or revalidation) which includes the relevant theory and practical hands on exercises to improve skills.

Begin the session with an introduction exercise of suitable length, depending on the number of participants and how well they already know each other/know you.

Example

A simple introduction if they all know each other, perhaps enhancing the introduction by asking "what setting do you work in and how does BLS feature there?"

Then assess the participants learning needs.

Example

Ask them for hopes and fears for the session and what they are most keen to learn about.

Negotiate the agenda for the session highlighting the identified needs you will be covering, dealing positively with any expressed fears, explaining why other issues will be best dealt with elsewhere. After this has happened it could summarised back to participants like this;

Example

Today we will cover Basic Life Support, the theory and practice. The ethical issues participants raised concerning allowing a natural death, avoiding resuscitation, and the skills needed to negotiate a Do Not Attempt Resuscitate decision, will be covered in the session on ethics later this month.

This need only take a few minutes, yet will get every participants attention, will enable some degree of participation from every member and will ensure that the session prioritises the things important to the audience. Trainers/Teachers can of course add in their own agendas just as doctors add their own agendas to a consultation.

Finally, summarise the session using the "Everything With a Purpose approach"; **today we will cover the knowledge and skills needed for you to be competent at Basic Life Support so that you will be confident in a life support situation and so that you will have the certification necessary to get your qualifications.**

By this point, all participants should be alert, fully engaged and confident that their own needs and concerns have been identified and taken seriously.

Resources

There is more Information available at:

https://insight.typepad.co.uk/40_icebreakers_for_small_groups.pdf

https://www.icebreakers.ws/small-group

http://www.socialworkerstoolbox.com/40-icebreakers-for-small-groups/

http://www.dvrcv.org.au/sites/thelookout.sites.go1.com.au/files/Games%20manual%20FINAL.pdf

https://www.mindtools.com/pages/article/newLDR_76.htm

1// BUILD YOUR OWN CLASSROOM

Paolo Freire, a famous South American educator, famously thought that if adult education participants literally built their own classrooms, then their engagement in learning was much greater.

What it is for?

He knew a thing or two about getting people engaged in education as he worked with people with very low levels of education and who were uncertain of its benefits. Freire considered that group formation through the planning and organisation, then working together on a practical and complicated task had a massive impact on the commitment learners would have. So, he began education, by asking participants to build their own classroom. Clearly, it is not likely that your participants will get to "build their own classroom", but we can harness some of the benefits of this approach by considering how rooms are arranged for learning.

Education takes place in many different environments; sometimes two people are crammed into a corner of an open plan office, discussing a difficult case while secretaries wander in and out, the cleaner empties the bins, and the fire alarm is tested. Other events take place in huge auditoria with hundreds, if not thousands of participants and all the mod cons that a conference centre can offer; simultaneous broadcast on gigantic screens, microphones, video, PowerPoint, background music and a pantomime horse. (Well I made the pantomime horse bit up, but I bet any decent conference centre would get you one if you need it … for a price of course!)

For most education, most of the time, size is somewhere in between … two to 12 participants for a small group, maybe up to 40 or 50 for a medium sized group. The chairs are usually laid out by the staff who manage the room who have no clue what, or how, you are going to be teaching and so they arrange chairs in tidy rows, like a cinema audience.

My first advice to any intending educator is to move the chairs in the room they are going to work in. Even better, if feasible, get the participants to arrange the chairs themselves into an arrangement facilitated or even mandated by you … this is not quite "build your own classroom", however, as you explain the layout you want and why, it starts to orientate the audience to what is going to happen next.

When to use it.

Unless the room is already arranged exactly as you need it, get the participants to arrange the chairs themselves, after an initial introduction exercise. In small group or one to one meetings for learning, ensure attention is paid to reducing hierarchy…everyone should have a similar chair and be sitting at the same distance from each other. Ideally, there should be no desks in the way (two people can sit round the corner of a desk with benefit).

The set up: how to use this method

Explain that you would like to ask the participants for their help in rearranging the chairs and explain why this is: because you want to facilitate discussion, so that everyone can see each other, so that everyone is welcome in the group, and so that everyone can see and hear everyone else easily.

Explanations/timings

A few minutes maximum is needed for this task.

The debrief: maximising the benefits

A brief, "good we can all see each other now" maybe all that is required.

Equipment/resources needed;

Enough chairs for everyone, but not so many that there are a lot of empty seats. Empty seats create a feeling of incompleteness in the room. Move spare chairs well out of the way and only leave chairs for late comers if you are absolutely sure someone is coming.

Skills to make this work even better

- Think about the arrangement you need ahead of time, so that you can give clear instructions to participants when they arrive.
- For small groups (ideally up to about 12 to 15, in practice up to 20), usually a tight circle works best or a U-shape if it is necessary for people to be able to see a screen. Bear in mind that didactic presentations to small groups should be very short and used as triggers to interaction, rather than lectures taking up the whole time.
- For medium sized groups (20 to 40) arrange two rows in a shallow U shape. Try and have the same number in each row. This facilitates use of Buzz groups when people talk to others near them/in the row behind, and means that people do not bunch up on the back row (making for distant communication) or in the front row, (when those further behind can feel a bit edged out). Encourage everyone to sit together … if latecomers arrive, try to get them into an existing row … having a few people scattered at the back means they often do not get to participate fully.

Pitfalls/when NOT to use this method

If you are visiting speaker as part of a longer day and the leaders of the session have arranged things, it may be meddlesome to change things around. I would still consider it though, even if it is not always possible.

Applications in other areas of the session

Rearranging the chairs can get people on to their feet and have an invigorating effect. Moving larger groups into smaller subgroups for discussions can really liven up a session, increase engagement and allow things to be tackled at deeper levels. See ENERGISE Group sorting methods, for information on how best to do this.

How does this help to build relationships?

Doing a task together helps to link people together. If the leader and the group are negotiating about how to do this task it can start to build rapport and relationships, if gently done.

How does this help to structure the education?

Learning is influenced by the "Hidden curriculum". The arrangement of the chairs can signal hierarchy: are we all equally important, in a circle, or does "God" sit at the front and all the minions at the back? The arrangements can signal whether active participation is expected, rather than the opportunity to snooze at the back and moving chairs to change group sizes during the session can help to break it up, signal a change of tack or mood or task.

2// SIMPLE INTRODUCTIONS

Introducing the participants to the speaker, and vice versa, is a crucial step for effective learning and should only be omitted when there are good reasons for doing so.

What it is for?

This step can be omitted if participants are part of a continuing group that has already invested time to getting to know each other well. The method described here is a straightforward one, acting as a simple ice breaker. Introductions orientate the speaker/educator and the group to each other, and to their roles and likely or possible preoccupations.

For sessions with participants who do not know each other and may not meet again, simple introductions followed by ENGAGE Hopes and fears and ENGAGE Establishing educational needs at the outset, will usually be enough to get the participants fully engaged and the session off to a good start. When participants do already know each other it can be fine to proceed straight to ENGAGE Hopes and fears and ENGAGE Establishing educational needs at the outset.

If participants will be working together over time (e.g. in a Specialty Training Programme, a Practice Team) a simple introduction should be followed with in depth introduction exercises (there are several in the ENGAGE section) to develop and deepen the interpersonal relationships within the group.

When to use it

This is a technique to use at the start of a session if participants do not work together regularly. Even if the participants know most of the people in the room, a brief introduction will enable new members of the group or those who are not good at remembering names to get to know their colleagues and improve their engagement in the proceedings. Introduce yourself and the nature of the session/programme.

Anticipate and adjust for the size and purpose of the group; will a simple introduction be enough, or, should it be followed up with more in depth introductions, or some kind of ice breaker method to engage participants' interest and involvement? (See ENGAGE Ice Breakers.)

The set up: how to use this method

The educator should explain that in starting the session there is going to a brief round of introductions to help everyone get to know each other and work together effectively.

The educator should model the nature of the introduction required as to content and length. If the educator just says "introduce yourself", people may say little or talk for 10 minutes, wasting session time.

Say something like "tell us your name and where you work" and model it yourself saying …
My name is … I work in X place …

At the start of the session participants may feel uncertain as to how the session will go. Giving clear instructions about the information you want will make people feel more comfortable and avoid any participants feeling embarrassed because they give the wrong info or are not sure what is expected of them.

See the ICE BREAKERS section for various ways to follow this up or make this introduction more light hearted/relaxing/tension reducing. Some participants can be so shy that they feel overwhelmed by having to speak in front of others even a relatively small group. Keeping it simple lets them off the hook.

Explanations/timings;

Ensure your explanation/instruction is simple, clear and brief. You need to allow about 15 seconds for each member of the group, as obviously it takes longer if there is a larger group. Overall aim to allow about five minutes. If the group is so large it will take longer, use an alternative method (for example ENGAGE Walk around introduction) so that energy is retained rather than being lost waiting for a large number of people to have a turn.

The debrief: maximising the benefits

Smile, look around the room, make eye contact with the participants, summarise what you have heard in one sentence ("people have come from far and wide today" or "its lovely to have you all here today") and reiterate your welcome. If you reach out and engage positively with the participants they will be more engaged in return and learn more.

Equipment/resources needed

None

Skills to make this work even better

Waiting in turn to introduce yourself can be a bit dull, especially if the group is on the big side. Give the person speaking some kind of token (see also ENGAGE Talking stick) and ask them to pass it to someone they are NOT sitting next to, signalling it is now their turn to speak. This means everyone has to stay engaged as they don't know who is going to be called upon to speak next.

Pitfalls/when NOT to use this method

Occasionally even with good instructions one participant will start on a long description of their roles and interests, even when there is not really time for it and others have modelled something more direct. Learn from this … that participant will need careful handling to avoid them dominating the group, while at the same time keeping them on board. Have some tactful ways to stop them and move on to the next person.

In a very large group (say over about 25) or a lecture to 100s of people this is not a suitable method of introduction. See ENGAGE Large group introduction instead.

Applications in other areas of the session

It can be useful to do similar "rounds" of all participants at other points in the session. (See ENRICH Making rounds effective.)

How does this help to build relationships?

Knowing who is in the room immediately creates relationships; between participants as they get to know each other, and between participants and the educator. A sense of belongingness and being a welcomed and valued participant creates an appropriate "learning identity" and promotes effective learning.

How does this help to structure the education?

When the educator explains the purpose of the process they are using, in this case the introduction, it helps participants to understand the structure of the session, and how they will be involved. This helps to focus attention.

3// PICTURE CARDS INTRODUCTION

This is a method of starting a group off which is a more intriguing, and therefore engaging, introduction than is achieved using speech alone.

What this is for

By using illustrations it adds to the aesthetic qualities of the education, which is also appealing and engages the "right brain", as people are curious about the picture cards. Choosing the questions carefully, according to the nature of the session can make this very effective.

Varying the questions used across the group, makes for a less repetitive introduction round, and can serve to introduce the material for the session, orientating the group to what is to follow.

When to use it

To introduce a new group, or to introduce a group that knows each other already to a new speaker. This helps the speaker orientate to what the group is like and what their learning needs are.

The set up: how to use this method;

Each participant is invited to choose a card from a selection which have a PICTURE showing upwards and to look at that picture for a few moments until everyone has one. People can choose any card they like.

When ready, the participants turn the card over and there is a statement on the back – "my name is" … followed by a statement or question that they have to complete.

Each card can have a different question, or there may be a selection of questions repeated randomly through the group (as people choose their own cards by the picture not by the question).

The statements could be neutral personal introductory information:

- my name is …
- my usual breakfast is …
- my last holiday was spent …
- my favourite Sunday dinner is …

Alternatively the questions may refer to and orientate the group to material to follow. For example in a session about palliative care the statement may be:

- my name is … I came here today to learn palliative care aspects of …
- my name is … my role in palliative care has been to …
- my name is … the most difficult aspect of Palliative care is …

If it feels necessary to break things up a bit, one or two of the statements can be of the form:

- if I was not here today I would prefer to be … (or, just now I would rather be …)
- what I am hoping for regarding the lunch break is …

Such less serious statements can bring some humour in, lightening the atmosphere around very serious subjects (such as palliative care).

Explanations/timings;

When everyone has a card ask them to turn over and consider the question or statement on the reverse. The educator can model the introduction as to length and complexity.

Ask the group to take turns to say:

- my name is … and then complete the statement or question"

Depending on the complexity of the question (best kept simple) allow about 30 seconds per participant.

The debrief: maximising the benefits

The debrief depends on the purpose of the picture round. If being used as a general introduction it can be followed with welcoming remarks, explicitly thanking everyone for their contribution, leading into setting the agenda for the session.

When everyone gets an equal chance to participate, the engagement in the group will start off on a stronger footing. If the statements link more explicitly to the material of the session, then some summarising and empathic comments will lead easily into a more formal agenda setting process. (See ENGAGE Hopes and Fears and ENGAGE Establishing learning needs at the outset.) Emphasising the contribution that everyone has made to the group increases a sense of belonging and engagement.

Equipment/resources needed

A simple approach is to use clean index cards or similar. Using picture postcards or the picture parts of old Christmas or birthday cards costs little and creates a more interesting start.

People sometimes think they are going to asked to justify their choice of card; while avoiding any attempt at psychologising or trickery, one reasonable question for the back could be "I was attracted by the picture on this card because …"

Choose the questions/statements on the reverse carefully, according to how you want the exercise to be used. Ensure that writing is legible and large enough to read easily.

Skills to make this work even better

An alternate approach is to have the card put message downwards on the seat for people to look at as they assemble, or to put the cards pictures showing upwards, underneath the seats and call participants attention to them at the start of the session. It all depends on the group. In a new group simply putting the cards on chairs or handing them out will usually be enough to engage; if a group has been going for a while and getting stale, then starting by putting the cards under the chairs can increase energy as people look for them (or lose them, cover them with their bags, etc.).

Using pictures orientated to the subject matter (for example, pictures of different sports if the session is going to about teamwork) can increase the interest. Movement is engaging, so it is also possible to stick the cards on the walls (picture showing) and invite participants to go and get one they like the look of before starting the introduction.

Pitfalls/when NOT to use this method

This method is not suitable if time is short, or the session is extremely formal e.g. a presentation at a conference. Avoid asking potentially difficult or embarrassing questions that may make people feel exposed or less knowledgeable than others. The aim is to bring people together and help them feel comfortable in the learning environment.

Applications in other areas of the session

Cards with specific questions or quotations can be numbered and spread through the audience by placing them on seats at the start. When the appropriate moment comes the educator can say "someone has card number … Can you read out what it says?" For example, in a session on feedback someone could get the quote: "Practice makes permanent; FEEDBACK makes perfect."

This allows suitable material to be presented in an interesting way, and engages attention as participants wonder who will be next … the cards called do not have to be in sequence. It's a good way of punctuating the session as a sort of summary at the end of one part or as an opening way into the next section of the session.

How does this help to build relationships?

This method builds relationships within the group as participants get to know each other and get to listen to everyone, and also builds relationships with the educator, as there is dialogue/interaction.

How does this help to structure the education?

Used at the start, this method can be used to begin to signpost the content and method of the session. If used during the session, quotations or prepared comments about the subject matter can act as a summary at the end of one section, or as an introduction to the next. This is a useful and efficient sign posting method and helps to keep the session flowing well.

4// AN INTRODUCTION USING PAIRS INTERVIEWING EACH OTHER

This method can be used as part of a one-to-one introduction (e.g. a trainer and trainee getting to know each other) or as part of the introduction to a small group.

What it is for?

When people get to know each other using an introductions exercise they can feel more at ease, it helps them to bond personally with at least one other member of the group and this creates an atmosphere of safety. This encourages discussions that are freer, deeper and more effective.

When to use it

At the start of something, for example, a new trainer/trainee relationship, the beginning of a new small group, the start of a residential or Study Release Course.

This method can be very helpful to use with established teams to help people get to know each other better. For example if training events are set up for Multidisciplinary Teams, Practice or unit Team meetings.

The questions can be altered to suit the situation, to be more or less personally revealing according to what is likely to be needed.

The set up: how to use this method

Give everyone the introduction sheet as an aid memoire (appended at the end of this section). Ask the group to get into pairs. With a new group pairings may not matter too much; in an established team ask people to talk to someone they know less well, or use a group sorting method (see ENERGISE Group sorting). Explain that the purpose of the task is to help group members get to know each other, to facilitate the work of the group afterwards. Explain that after the task each participant will introduce their partner to the group (see also ENGAGE Shield exercise for another variant of this).

Explanations/timings

- Explain the prompt sheet and ask them to spend 20 minutes on the task – 10 for each person.
- The participants take turns to interview their partner using the prompts on the sheet, i.e. tell me something concerning a where/what/how/why/who about their partner.
- Tell the participants that at the end of the interview process they will introduce their partner to the whole group afterwards. Stress that the prompts are there to facilitate understanding and that no one has to share any information they do not wish to share.
- Before presenting their partner to the group each participant should check that their partner is comfortable for any information to be shared with the whole group. The interviewee has freedom to respond in any way they wish to the prompts.

Introducing a partner rather than your self can be easier in a group; it takes the focus away from the individual and towards their relationships. When presenting, participants are often very positive about the achievements and interests of others. This is encouraging for participants and brings things out that individuals may not feel able to speak up about themselves.

The debrief: maximising the benefits

Ask each participant to introduce their partner to the group. If the group is fairly small (say up to eight) the educator can also invite the other participants to ask any questions to clarify or expand. Often this will happen anyway.

In larger groups the educator will have to control the time budget for each participant to make sure all are represented fairly. The educator can wrap up with a general comment about how diverse or interesting the group, thanking participants for their interesting interviews, as a prelude to continuing with the next element of the session.

Equipment/resources needed

Prompt sheets can be prepared in advance for each participant. An alternative is to give everyone a blank sheet of paper and write the headings for the prompts on a flip chart/PowerPoint slide and let each participant write their own headings. The pre-prepared sheet saves time and has the advantage of providing guidance on the task.

Skills to make this work even better

In the debrief the educator can be positive about the interesting things being presented and identify the value of having a diverse group to work with.

In an established group who are getting together for a training session (e.g. a practice team) the questions could be altered to focus on aspects of the team, for example, "*where* is your favourite place to be at work" or "*what* was the most important thing you did at work this week".

Or it can be focused to the tasks that follow, e.g. if the session is to be about developing resilience the prompts could be "*how* do you help yourself get over a stressful day at work" and "*why* is that activity important to you."

Pitfalls/when NOT to use this method

This method while very useful to get a group working well together, is time consuming. So, best avoided if the group will only be together for a short period (e.g. one session or one part of a larger group session).

Participants who are not used to group work may find the level of disclosure a bit threatening, so it is important to stress that this is about sharing things they feel OK to discuss with others in the group setting.

Applications in other areas of the session

Different prompts, but using the same structured approach could be used as reflection stops during a session (WHERE has this session got you to now?) or during a training programme (WHAT have you done in this training that has been most useful, HOW … what skills have you developed during this training course?), and so on.

How does this help to build relationships?

A 20 minute, one-to-one conversation builds a relationship rapidly and this helps the whole group to be more connected, more open and more able to have in depth discussions in which real learning can take place.

For participants used to hurrying through their work as fast as possible (which is how it feels in many situations), having allocated time for a more leisurely conversation can change the pace, and allow participants to relax. Having the focused attention of a partner helps people to feel valued as part of the group, which is empowering.

How does this help to structure the education?

This approach emphasises that learning is about relationships as well as content, that the participants are worthy of time and attention in their own right. By providing a firm basis for relationships within the group the scene is set securely for work that follows.

PAIRS INTRODUCTION SHEET

In pairs – 10 minutes each way.

This introduction task helps people feel at ease in the group and helps to create an atmosphere for free discussion and exploration of issues.

The prompts are to help you to encourage your partner to talk about themselves, in different ways and at different levels.

Feel free to use the prompts in a way that seems best for you and your partner. The interviewee has complete freedom to decide how to respond. Before you introduce them to the whole group later, check that your interviewee is happy for any information to be shared. Do not share information they would prefer to keep private between you and them.

Give me a **where** – tell me about a place that has a special significance to you.

....

....

....

Give me a **what** – tell me about something unusual interesting or important that you have done.

....

....

....

Give me a **how** – tell me about a skill or ability that you are proud to possess.

....

....

....

Give me a **why** – tell me why you do a particular activity that is important to you.

....

....

....

Give me a **who** – tell me something central about yourself that makes you who you are.

....

....

....

NB: Both partners might like to clarify any disclosures they would be happy to go into, and any that they would prefer to left out of the feedback to the whole group.

Back in the group – Introduce your partner to the whole group.

5// SHIELD INTRODUCTION EXERCISE

This is an introduction exercise to help all members of a new group get to know each other better, so that they develop trust and a sense of belonging, which will facilitate learning together.

When to use it

This method takes time, around 10 to 12 minutes per participant at least. Therefore, it is best used for those occasions where you want participants to really get to know each other, to remove barriers to communication and to create trust in the group. These effects come from having talked to other people about yourself in a friendly environment. Thus, it is especially useful when forming a new group that is going to work together for a long time, or study for a period of time, for example, a term long module or a full year Study Release Course.

Although this method takes time initially, it saves time in the longer term as groups form quickly, and begin the processes of "Forming and Norming" (see References and Resources below) straight away. This gets participants "over the hump" of joining a group of colleagues they may not know very well.

By adapting the questions this is also a suitable method for re-engaging with a team (for example on a team away day) and for building team relationships over time. Because the method begins with people working in pairs it is less intimidating than whole group introduction methods. Quieter, less assertive participants get equal attention to noisier more confident ones. See also ENGAGE Pairs introduction, for another method to do this.

The set up: how to use this method

Each person is allocated or chooses a partner. Each person has a sheet of A3 (e.g. flip chart paper). On it they draw a shield shape divided into four with a central section for their name in the centre they should write the name they like to be called by and perhaps draw a little symbol or cartoon that says something about themselves (e.g. a paintbrush if they like DIY).

Shield diagram

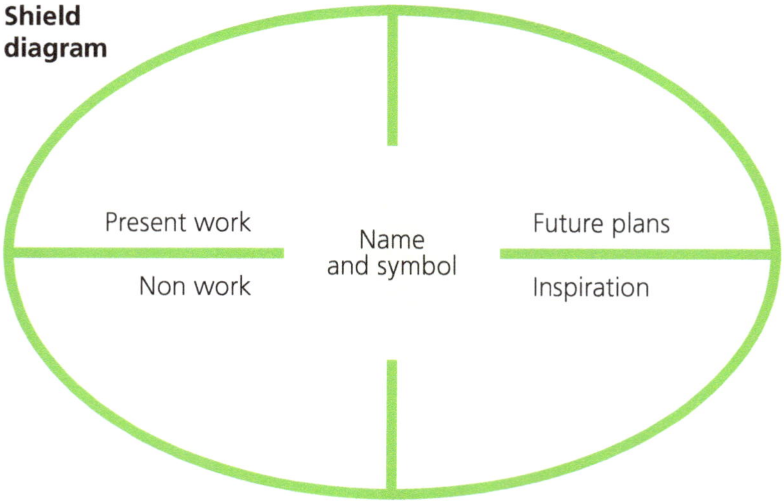

Each participant is interviewed by their partner who gets to know them in more detail by asking questions pertaining to each quadrant and filling in the answers. Allow five minutes for each interview, to allow some depth without resorting to psychoanalysis! The questions work best if they include something about their current work, something about their professional future, something about non-work life and something that explores their values (for example, what inspires you? What is the most important thing about work for you?)

You can make this more fun by also asking "tell me something about yourself that most people don't generally know about (but which you are happy to share with the group).

Below are some examples. These can be altered to suit the requirements of different groups. For example, if a practice team who know each other are on an away day, the questions might be framed to explore their situation within the practice, or their hopes for the future of the organisation.

Examples

- Where are you working now? What are your career plans? Tell me something about your non-work life? What inspires you the most about your work?
- Where are you working now? What is the main aim of your participation in this course? What are your favourite activities outside work? Where do you hope to be in five years?
- What is your role in the team? What inspires you most about your work? What would you like to see developing in the future in the team? What is your favourite activity outside work?

Avoid tricky or difficult questions like "what is the most embarrassing that has ever happened to you?" This will make participants more anxious, rather than developing a comfortable rapport with each other.

Explanations/timings

This works best if the educator explains that investing time in getting to know each other is worthwhile, so that it helps the group to work together more effectively and so that everyone feels more comfortable and involved. The five-minute timing for the interview should be rigorously observed, with the pairs swapping over for another five minutes; the first interviewer becomes the interviewee.

During the debrief timing needs to be watched carefully; if the first participant is very brief, the others will be brief too; if the first person talks for 15 minutes about their partner and every one copies, then the exercise can take a long time and energy will flag (the opposite of what is needed for engaging people!)

If the educator goes first, they can introduce their partner and model how much detail to give and how much time to spend. The other participants will usually follow suit. The educator needs a partner too if the numbers don't allow for that then the educator can introduce themselves using the same shield drawing and answers and model the approximate length.

The debrief: maximising the benefits

After interviewing each other and writing the responses on the shield in pairs the group reconvenes. Then each participant is asked to introduce their partner. If you go round the group in a circle, the people waiting to speak mentally rehearse what they are going to say (which reduces their attention for listening) and the people who have had their turn relax (and may switch off). Instead, ask the participants to introduce their partner and then randomly choose the next person in the group to be introduced; their partner then introduces them and does the same. This keeps people alert as they do not know who is going to be asked to speak next.

The educator can also write down the answers to the question "A thing that people don't generally know about me is ..." At the end of the shield introduction, the educator can use these facts to help the group to remember each other's names. The educator reads out the little known facts, again in random order, using the form ... "which participant has two pedigree Siamese cats at home?"

Equipment/resources needed;

- Flip chart paper, and pens.
- BluTack to pin up the shields when participants are presented by their partners.
- Some space for people to work in when they are being interviewed

Skills to make this work even better

The educator can model good listening skills, reflecting back a clear summary of the individual describes, preferably with positive or interesting features highlighted. If there is time, each pair can use the spaces on the chart to also draw the "arms and equipment" of the individual, e.g. many pairs of hands for a busy working parent, musical notes for someone who plays the guitar …

Pitfalls/when NOT to use this method

While the interviews will be restricted to 10 minutes, debriefing is less predictable, and will take time. So this is less suitable for very large groups (more than 12–14 people). In that case it is best to split the exercise and the debrief into two smaller groups, otherwise energy will flag and it can become boring.

This method is too time consuming and too personally revealing for very short educational activities (less than half a day) or where people will not meet and work together again. As it is time consuming its best used in:

- day long or residential courses
- at the start of a course or programme
- for a new team where people will be working together for a long time
- as part of a team away day to refresh everyone's knowledge of each other and their team roles or aspirations.

Adapt the questions to the specific purpose and group.

Applications in other areas of the session

It can be helpful to refer back to issues that arise in debriefing, as long as this is in a relevant positive and tactful way. For example, if participants mention wanting to develop "educational skills" in the future, the educator can refer to the part of the programme when these skills will be learned. This can be a good demonstration of active listening skills and further build the relationship with the educator.

How does this help to build relationships?

Talking to one person at the beginning starts to build intra group relationships in an unthreatening way. As the group get to know each individual, intra group relationships are also reinforced.

The educator observes carefully and starts to understand the group and its participants; do they engage with this task? Did they listen to the instructions or zone out and have to ask for them to be repeated? Do they need more experience of non-standard group methods to feel comfortable working together? How interested are they in their fellow participants? Do they ask superficial questions or are they really interested in their colleagues as people? This sometimes mirrors their attitudes towards patients; the educator may then decide to ensure training addresses the skills of developing rapport and interest in patients as individuals, which are learnable skills.

How does this help to structure the education?

By being explicit about the purpose and timings of this exercise, educators can help participants begin to understand and value the group process. Modelling accurate timing of the report back and then finishing the exercise on time, because the right amount of time has been planned for, helps participants new to group work to feel "held" and safe in unfamiliar educational settings.

References and resources

Tuckman described the stages of team or group work as being "Forming, Storming, Norming and Performing". There is a quick summary of this here:

https://www.mindtools.com/pages/article/newLDR_86.htm

and a useful Wikipedia section here:

https://en.wikipedia.org/wiki/Tuckman%27s_stages_of_group_development

Tuckman later added "adjourning/mourning " as the stage when a team or group break up having completed their task. (See ENRICH Endings.)

Although the term "team" is used by Tuckman, the same processes occur in educational groups that meet over time. Successfully "Performing" educational groups pay greater attention to the relevant tasks and provide effective support to the learning of all participants, with the potential for greatly improved outcomes. Methods to improve group work in education can be very profitably used in practice and other teams too.

6// WALK ROUND INTRODUCTION

If you want to create the benevolent energy of a pleasant party, try this method for introducing participants for the first time, or for a new purpose.

What it is for?

To enable participants to become engaged in the group and ready to participate in the learning, without doing a long tedious introduction round.

When to use it

This can be a helpful method if a new group is a bit too large for a simple introductions round, which can become slow and tedious if there are more than 10 to 15 participants. It can also be used if participants do not know each other, as the interactions are one to one, and so less threatening than speaking in front of a larger group.

This method can also be used during the life of an enduring group (for example a study release course group that meet every week for a longer period) to refresh the engagement by asking people to talk about something of relevance to the days topic, or to talk about a topic will help to deepen their knowledge of each other (for example, their attitudes to an issue, or how they personally cope with a particular type of difficulty).

The set up; how to use this method

Explain that everyone will stand up and walk around the room, when they catch someone's eye they will introduce themselves to each other (and shake hands for even greater engagement) and discuss an additional question to develop some intra group relationships (suggestions below). Explain that after a minute or two the educator will clap their hands (or ring a bell or whatever will be a loud enough signal) to indicate that it is time to walk around and catch the eye of another participant. Repeat a few times, depending on the time available.

Planning ahead

If you are confident you can make up appropriate questions on the day, then wait and see what the room "feels like". If you are new to this approach or less confident plan ahead and identify a follow up question that will be relevant to the topic of the session.

Here are a selection of some potentially suitable questions; educators can feel free to choose other questions, being mindful of how that will relate to the rest of the session. Questions should be open (not closed) and of a form that will trigger relevant discussion.

- How did you come to be at this event?
- What is the best/worst thing about your current work situation?
- Who have you had to leave behind in order to come and work here today?
- What are the two main things you want to get out of this event?
- What are two things you find most professionally satisfying about today's subject?

Explanations/timings

Explain that though they probably won't meet everyone, they will speak to a few people and feel welcomed. Explain that no one has to speak in front of everyone, acknowledging that some people find that difficult. Acknowledge that it feels a bit weird wandering round the room to say hello to people they don't know and point out the advantages.

It usually takes a minute to explain the process; educators can decide how long to let the group part run. Observe the process and ensure that participants speak to several people and do not just get into a conversation. The time allocated depends on the educator's view of how many people need to talk to each other. Perhaps allow about a minute for each introduction, hence five to 10 minutes for the whole exercise. People do not need to introduce themselves to everyone. The ice will be broken and they can introduce themselves to anyone else during breaks. The educator should encourage participants to do this if they are not already known to each other.

The debrief: maximising the benefits

At the end of the exercise the educator can thank everyone for introducing themselves and encourage participants to use breaks to introduce themselves to anyone they did not get to meet initially. This helps to develop intra-group relationships.

If a specific topic has been discussed the educator can debrief by asking an open question such as "What kinds of issues came up when you discussed ...?"

Equipment/resources needed

Space to move around and meet other people. If in a confined space and participants do not know each other (for example, at a first meeting, or at a session at a conference or meeting) simply ask participants to say hello and introduce themselves to the people on either side and in front or behind them. Even a few people getting to know each other increases the engagement in the room.

Skills to make this work even better

The educator needs to be sensitive to how the introductions are going and whether to allow the participants to continue and when to draw the process to a close. Leaving it too long can create feelings of awkwardness, as people are looking to find anyone they have not already met. If it is too short, people will feel rushed or that the exercise was pointless. If using this with an established group to trigger discussion about the days topic, encourage participants to seek out others that they know less well, or have not got to know so well.

Pitfalls/when NOT to use this method

Occasionally participants may feel awkward doing this

- if they are not used to small group methods
- if there is furniture in the way
- if they are used to courses when they sit behind a desk take notes and say nothing. If you suspect that the latter is the case then introduce your rationale for this method carefully and make sure that your set up is simple and very unambiguous.

If in doubt model the process yourself to the group – "I am Anne and I have left behind my new car to come today (I came on the train!)"

As this is an introduction aimed at facilitating small group working, make sure you plan in advance and move the chairs around to the arrangement that suits the task before participants arrive.

Problems could also occur, if, during the debriefing, it becomes apparent that participants have very different expectations of the session. However, while this may initially identify conflicts, it is much easier to deal with them if they are out in the open and up for discussion. Buried in silence, such disagreements can cause the group to disengage and the learning opportunity can be compromised.

If any participants have mobility issues be mindful of this and place them somewhere in the centre so that other participants can come to them.

Applications in other areas of the session

A variant of this would be to use it later in the session as an energiser. For example, after introducing new material one way to maintain engagement during the session could be to ask participants to go round and speak to others about how they might apply the new learning in their own workplace, or to identify new questions raised by what they have been learning.

How does this help to build relationships?

When participants have opportunities to talk about themselves and their interests to other members of the group relationships start to form and trust is enhanced. Encouraging talk between people who do not know each other well develops a greater sense of belonging and "esprit de corps" which is a strong motivator for learning together.

How does this help to structure the education?

Having brief exercises such this at suitable points in the session can provide a sort of "punctuation mark" offering opportunities to get participants to get involved at the start, to summarise the impact of the learning so far, to stretch their legs. This method helps to avoid boredom and gives opportunities for the educator to signal what is coming next.

For example:

"Now we have seen how this subject relates to your work in the area of … we will consolidate this by talking with each other about how to apply this in our own workplace; after that we will move on to …"

Having an overt structure helps to keep the pace moving effectively and reduces the risk of getting too bogged down in one area. It helps participants to continue to feel invested in the session if they know where it is going and how it will relate to them. Participants who are not used to smaller group methods will find this element of structure reassuring. Breaking up the session in this way also keeps the educator awake.

7// BROKEN CARDS INTRODUCTION

This gets participants off their chairs and was described to me by one participant as "the only ice breaker I have ever done that actually broke the ice".

What it is for?

This is a quick icebreaker (although it requires preparation beforehand) and can be used as part of an introductions process or to get people moving around and talking to each during a session (when it might also belong in the ENERGISE section).

When to use it

When you want to get people moving around and talking to people they are not used to sitting next to, especially as part of an introductions process or to liven things up. It is especially useful if participants always tend to sit with people they already know.

The set up: how to use this method

Beforehand get some postcards/old used Christmas cards/greetings cards which have a picture on one side and are blank on the other side.

For an introductions exercise write a "get to know each other" question on the reverse (for example, "What is your favourite film/book/meal/holiday, and why"). If used as an energiser during a session use educational questions such as "How could you fit this learning into your daily work? or, "How does this change your thinking?" or, "What three things will you take away from what we have done so far?"

Then cut each card into four sections (or two if they are not too big). Ensure you have enough cards so that participants can all get a section of card.

Mix up the sections of card randomly and distribute to the group asking them to keep the cards face up. Ask them to walk around the room and find who has the other sections of their card. Then ask them to turn the cards over, match them up to read the question, and spend a few minutes discussing that question.

This approach mid-session can help if participants get into a bit of a rut of always talking to the same "buddies".

Explanations/timings

Explanations need to be concise and in order; explain everyone is going to get a section of the card face up, that they then have to stand up and find who has the rest of the picture on the card then discuss the question on the reverse.

The benefit increases if you explain why you chose this particular method and why it is important to break the ice anyway. This is done so that everyone gets to know each other, to speak to people they may not know very well, so that they might hear different ideas, or so that the group can discuss the learning they have done so far. (See ENGAGE Everything with a purpose.)

It usually takes a minute or two for everyone to get sorted with their fellow card holders. Allow a few minutes discussion, stopping when the room starts to get a little quieter, before everyone runs out of things to say. Leaving them with more to say keeps energy levels and engagement up.

The debrief: maximising the benefits

The benefits of this ice breaker occur if the ice is broken! This will be judged by how much chatter and good humour there is in the room.

In an introductions exercise a brief debrief question like "Did anything interesting come up?" may suffice, before going on to further activities which could use the new groups of four that have been formed.

If educational questions are used debriefing can be initiated with a general question like "What issues came up when you were talking?" Facilitation can then relate this to the content already introduced, or if used near the start of the session this can provide the focus for a ENGAGE Hopes and fears or ENGAGE Establishing educational needs at the outset exercise to help focus the agenda for the session.

Equipment/resources needed

The educator needs to get cards ready ahead of time, divide them into suitable pieces and shuffle the well so that so that there will be a good mixing of the group members. Make sure the sections to be matched are the same as the number of group members so that no one is left out or made to feel like a spare part.

Skills to make this work even better

This method can be extended. In a new group of any size greater than, say, eight participants prepare cards in sets with the same image or the same type of image, each card cut in half; initially participants find the partner who has the other half of their card and discuss the question on the back. The participants are asked to find everyone who has the rest of their "set", for example, local beauty spots, cards with flowers on, arty cards… Let them work out what connects the parts of the set as this will promote further mixing and discussion amongst participants.

The question to discuss in a group of four or six could be the same, or a different question … the educator can say "all people with flower images discuss this … people with steam trains discuss this …, etc). The questions need to be purposeful, lead into the next section of the session and the debrief needs to bring out any important issues.

This method can be done simply with different coloured index cards, or even with a deck of playing cards with selected cards chosen, a question written on the back and then cut up so that participants have to find a match.

Pitfalls/when NOT to use this method

The questions need to be appropriate to the purpose of the exercise (introduction or energiser?) and of interest to the participants. There has to be space to move around. It works best if the group size is relatively large say 10 to 12 or above. Not suitable for very large audiences or lecture halls. The educator must pay attention to numbers and ensure that the number of cards/sections/card sets matches the number of participants and is appropriately divisible. If this does not happen properly someone could end up feeling very left out which is extremely counterproductive and distracting.

Applications in other areas of the session

Can be used as an **energiser** as described above, perhaps with questions suitable to the stage of the session. With adapted questions/ card sets could be used to make an evaluation process more interesting, see EVALUATION Snow ball evaluation methods.

How does this help to build relationships?

The more members of a learning group get to know each other and understand each others' points of view, the more they will feel that they "belong" in the group, which can then develop into a community of practice. This deepens learning and models important parts of the informal and hidden curricula. This includes **knowledge** (what have other people learned? How did they prioritise that?), **skills** (we can learn effectively when working with others) and **attitudes** (others may have different yet very valuable viewpoints, feedback from more advanced participants can help others, sharing learning can reinforce it, everyone is important here).

How does this help to structure the education?

Exercises like this, while enjoyable, are very serious in their intent. They can provide punctuation points within sessions so that new sections of the learning session are signalled and prepared for. Questions can be structured appropriately so that learning is reinforced or deepened. Planning such moments within sessions help educators to think through the structure and process of the session, so that effectiveness is increased within the same time budget.

8// USING PICTURES AS A STARTING ACTIVITY

A picture is said to be worth a thousand words and certainly gets the creative right side of the brain involved, as well as the analytical left side.

What it is for?

This is a method for engaging participants attention at the start of a session and setting the "tone" of what is to come in an interesting way.

When to use it

At the beginning of a session or at the start of a new part of the session or activity.

The set up: how to use this method

Have a table or tables set up at the side of the room. Small groups may only need one table, larger groups may need several. Get a lot of pictures (no words), with as much variety as possible; place them on the table. This could be postcards, photographs, pictures of art works, pictures from magazine, old greetings cards with the pictures cut off … anything and everything.

Explanations/timings

Ask everyone to choose a picture that they personally feel expresses their feelings about the question you offer them, so that everyone gets a chance to talk about their own personal take on things, so that everyone's position can be taken into account at the start of the session or at the beginning of a new phase of the session.

Examples could be:

- "How are you feeling right now?"
- "How are you feeling about your training so far?"
- "What is your current placement like?"
- "What would you like your future to look like?"

The debrief: maximising the benefits

In a small group, ask everyone to explain how they came to choose that particular image and what it means to them. In a large group ask people to explain their choice in groups of four, then in the larger group invite anyone who wishes to share their choice and reasons.

Encourage participants to elaborate with phrases like "go on" or "anything else", although these may only be needed if participants are very brief. Usually participants are happy to explain their choice. Those that go first encourage quieter ones to elaborate. Offer no judgments, rather model acceptance and interest; no choice is better or more worthy or more useful than any other. They all give useful sharing and a way for the educator to increase their awareness of the "tone" of the group for that day: is the group comfortable and ready to work, or are there stresses that need to be acknowledged, and possibly, addressed.

Equipment/resources needed

Make sure there are at least triple the number of images compared to the number of participants so that there is plenty of choice for everyone.

Skills to make this work even better

This engagement method can be used at the start of any session. It can also be a useful one to use prior to doing an evaluation with the group; using an image orientates participants to feelings and holistic assessments (right brain) and can lead to more fruitful evaluations. (See also the EVALUATE sections).

Pitfalls/when NOT to use this method

If you are with an unfamiliar group, or if it is a brief or one-off session, this may be a relatively time consuming energiser/introduction. Choose another one instead if needed.

Applications in other areas of the session

Images can be used later in the session to sum things up, or to signal the group's response to information that has been part of the session.

How does this help to build relationships?

Participants share very personal things in an exercise like this (hence the need for non-judgemental, encouraging, debriefing) and this can help groups develop richer relationships with each other and help people to understand that other people may have quite different points of view or preferences.

How does this help to structure the education?

Short engagement exercises help to provide punctuation, help to pace learning and give variety.

9// ICE BREAKERS

Ice breakers are techniques to get everyone engaged, talking to each other in a way that helps participants get over the threshold of starting a session.

What it is for?

They are particularly useful if participants are working with people they do not know well, or have not met before. The number and intensity of the ice breakers chosen will depend on the purpose; spend more time (and possibly use more than one method) if the purpose is to start "forming" and "norming" (see General introduction) a group that will exist for a period of time, (more than one day), for example a Study Release Course group. If the ice breaker is for one day, or one session, one will suffice.

When to use it

Use Ice breakers at the beginning of a session, to get things off to a good start, usually after initial introductions, especially if participants come from different backgrounds and need to bond quickly so as to start working on the topic at hand. Also useful if your group is newly formed, or if the topics you are discussing are new or unfamiliar to many people involved.
Ice breakers are also helpful when the educator needs to get to know participants better, for example at the start of a course or when running educational events for a team.
The process of getting to know each other increases trust

The set up: how to use this method

Choose a suitable ice breaker and explain its purpose, which is to "break the ice" so that everyone interacts together and gets to know each other, so that working together will be more effective. Be very clear about the task (what is to be done) and also the process (how is this task going to move people around and get them to talk to more than one person).

When designing your ice breaker, think about the "ice" that needs to be broken. If you are bringing together like-minded people, the "ice" may simply reflect the fact that people have not yet met. If using an ice breaker in a practice team meeting or training day, the "ice" may come from the difference in status between participants, and there may also be different backgrounds, cultures and attitudes to work: thus the "ice" may come from people's perceptions of each other. Focus on what important ice may need to be broken for your training session or course; it is not necessary to deal with the whole iceberg or get a Nobel Peace Prize afterwards. Focusing on similarities, or things that everyone can talk about (for example, their favourite food or what kind of professional problems or successes they have) is usually enough.

Explanations/timings

The specifics of this will depend on the ice breaker chosen (some examples are given below). Allow enough time for interaction but stop before everyone goes quiet which can feel awkward. Less than 10–15 minutes is usually needed for a group up to about 25 to 30.

The debrief: maximising the benefits

Not much debrief is usually necessary, but a synthesising comment about how everyone mixed a lot, or made a lot of noise, or that participants have certainly been able to share some important things, will provide both a summary and a structuring comment to lead into the next part of the session.

Equipment/resources needed

This depends on the ice breaker chosen. Below are some examples with comments about possible benefits. There are many more on the internet and it is easy to make up new ones inspired by these ideas.

1. Allocate groups randomly on arrival/ registration, for example, by giving each participant a different coloured sticker/ picture/number which is matched to a group area or table. This means participants are less likely to stick to talking to people they know already and gets better cross fertilisation of ideas. You can ask them to do one of the ice breaker tasks below to get the group talking.
2. Ask people to move around the room talking to as many people as possible with the following being possible tasks:
   - share your biggest current challenge at work
   - share two things about yourself that you think no one at your table knows about you
   - share what you appreciate most about your colleagues or participants they may have met before
   - share what you like about your current job
   - share the most fun situation you have experienced at work
   - are you a cat person, dog person, bird person, or gerbil person
   - what is your favourite pet and why?
   - what is your favourite type of holiday and why?
   - what is your favourite Sunday dinner?
   - Tell your table mates or colleagues three things about yourself. Two of them are true and one of them is a lie. Ask people to guess which the lie is.
3. Word association. This helps people explore the breadth of the area under discussion. In pairs ask them to generate a list of words related to the topic; for example, in a safeguarding training session ask participants what words come to mind relating to child abuse, (be precise with language here; decide whether you want to ask what feelings come up, what thoughts come up, what words pop into their minds, what pictures the subject conjures up for them). Give them one minute, and then ask pairs to team up with another pair and share their lists. The debrief could take the form of writing all the findings on the board (perhaps by theme e.g. angry feelings, sad feelings, guilty feelings and so on). Summarising thoughts or words that come up may lead to a summary of the form "this is a difficult and sensitive topic that will bring up some difficult thoughts and feelings for us. This is natural and important; if you feel overwhelmed or troubled by things we are discussing please feel free to take a short time out of the discussion and come back in when you are ready". The debrief and summary will clearly vary according to the topic.

Other examples can easily be found at:

https://insight.typepad.co.uk/40_icebreakers_for_small_groups.pdf

https://www.icebreakers.ws/small-group

http://www.socialworkerstoolbox.com/40-icebreakers-for-small-groups/

http://www.dvrcv.org.au/sites/thelookout.sites.go1.com.au/files/Games%20manual%20FINAL.pdf

https://www.mindtools.com/pages/article/newLDR_76.htm

Skills to make this work even better

There are many ice breakers possible and even a quick Google search will yield numerous possibilities. Choose carefully; if too frivolous some groups may lose interest or feel patronised. If too serious, or too focused on the medical tasks at hand, the opportunities for group formation and bonding will be more limited, because people will not have the chance to be themselves and share aspects of their lives with each other. Be wary of ice breakers like "what is the most embarrassing that has ever happened to you?" as they risk raising anxiety and tension, especially in cautious or inexperienced participants. What you are aiming for is something that reduces anxiety, that everyone has an equal way of participating in and that gives them an opportunity to share their best side.

Pitfalls/when NOT to use this method

Avoid if time is very short, if participants already know each other well and are likely to be ready to get on with working together (use other engaging techniques such as ENGAGE Hopes and Fears).

Applications in other areas of the session

Ideally ice breakers are not needed later on because the ice is broken. However, some ice breakers can also be used as ENERGISERS to re kindle or maintain energy and focus over the course of longer sessions, or to explore new areas of the topic. For example, if the topic has been developing a new consultation skill, an ice breaker like "what is likely to be the biggest challenge you have practising this skill in the future?" or "what feelings or thoughts come up now?" can re energise the group and also help the educator to identify any residual difficulties to be addressed in the session. Often attitudinal issues come out in this way ("This is all very well in theory but …") and this enables the educator to explore/challenge such issues while they are fresh in everyone's minds.

How does this help to build relationships?

Participants get to meet and talk to several or even many members of the group informally, often sharing personal ideas or information. This helps to build good relationships so that the importance of the group being a social, collaborative way of learning is emphasised. Learning together is more effective, if the methods and techniques used are different to those that individuals might use when learning alone. Ice breakers can be one component that fosters a sense of "belongingness" which is important in maximising engagement and success in learning. Using ice breakers that allow feelings and thoughts about the topic to be expressed early on, helps participants to feel that their concerns are recognised and valued; they become active collaborators in the session. This has the potential to strengthen learning relationships.

How does this help to structure the education?

Ice breakers provide punctuation points and when the purpose is explicit helps participants to understand how the educational session is going to be paced, how they may be expected to relate to others in the room and also helps to set the emotional "tone" of cooperation, collaboration and conversation that make groups work well. The "hidden agenda" is that we will be learning together and that individuality is to be accepted and celebrated.

10// GEOGRAPHICAL INTRODUCTION

This is a good introduction method and can be used when people are meeting for the first time.

What it is for?

It would also make a good team building exercise to do at the start of a team training day. In teams or units staff may change, they often do not get a chance to know each other as people very well and this exercise would be a good way to overcome that.

When to use it

This introduction method is most useful at the start of a session, for the start of a programme or when beginning a study module that continues over a couple of days, for example a residential.

The set up: how to use this method.

Begin by acknowledging that the people in the room are not all from the street that your building is in! Tell the group that you are going to ask them to arrange themselves as if the room is a map, and they will go and stand in the part of the map that corresponds to the city where they did their initial training (such as Medical school or nurse training). Then ask people to move all the chairs out of the way (or use an adjacent empty part of the room if the room is large enough) and spread themselves out to put themselves in the right position. Encourage people to talk to each other to get themselves orientated. Ask the group to agree where North and South are.

Explanations/timings

The explanation should be brief but include the points that people can help each other find where they should be placed, be ready to help the group decide where North should be. Depending on the size of the group, getting everyone into position may take about five minutes. Explain clearly that seeing where people have journeyed from helps us to get to know them, so that we can work together more effectively and cordially.

The debrief: maximising the benefits

Ask the group what they notice, who is close together, who is far away, and who has travelled furthest from their educational starting point. What does it feel like if you are huddled near to others? What do they think it might feel like to be furthest away? What does the furthest away person have to say about their journey?

Equipment/resources needed. Only a suitably large space is needed. If the room is small, and if available this exercise could be done in nearby hall or outside in a garden or (safe) car park.

Skills to make this work even better

The educator can anticipate that there may be a lot or a little variety in the positions taken by the participants. Think ahead about any participants who may be anxious about "belonging" in the group or who have come from a very different environment to others. Ask them about their position first and thank them for coming all the way to work with the other participants.

Pitfalls/when NOT to use this method

If the only room available is very small this might be difficult; people need room to move around. It will work better if an initial simple introduction has been done (if people do not know each other). In an established team, if you are sure that everyone knows each other's names, explaining the purpose of the exercise may be enough. If participants are very wary of group methods or getting outside their comfort zone, it may be better to choose an alternative introductions method.

Applications in other areas of the session

This method could be used to get people off their chairs when the group is flagging and needs energising. See ENERGISE Using line ups.

How does this help to build relationships?

As participants and educator get to know each other as individuals they start to form relationships. Developing relationships between group members and between group members and the educator deepens commitment to the learning process and deepens learning.

How does this help to structure the education?

Explaining the purpose of this clearly, enables educators to use this exercise to lead into the next part of the session (which will often be ENGAGE Hopes and Fears and ENGAGE Establishing learning needs at the outset). Explaining that first we get to know each other, so that we can work together better so that we can establish what the needs of the group are for this subject, clarifies the structure and process and helps participants to relax and participate fully, knowing that the educator has a clear plan. (See also ENGAGE Everything with a purpose.)

11// LARGE GROUP INTRODUCTIONS FOR FORMAL PRESENTATIONS

Even in very large groups, attention to interactions between participants can increase attention and engagement with your important subject matter.

What it is for?

This is an approach to increase engagement in the subject matter when teaching/lecturing very large groups (realistically over about 30 people).

When to use it

If talking to a very large group (in a large lecture theatre) or a formal presentation in a fixed slot, maybe at a conference, you may feel that all the introductions necessary will be done by the chair of the session. Indeed that may be the case.

Occasionally though, your task may also include helping participants to think differently, to see how something might apply to their specific situation. Encouraging participants to have some opportunity to interact and engage directly, however brief, can change the atmosphere in the room and increase the impact of your presentation

The set up: how to use this method

Explain why you want to do more than just introduce yourself; maybe to increase friendly interactions with people who you have not met before (for example, participants in a large conference) or as a prelude to getting them to discuss something in your paper or presentation (such as the relevance of your presentation to their specific workplace). Be clear in your own mind what your purpose is and introduce this very succinctly.

Simply ask people to introduce themselves to the person next to them and to the person in the row immediately behind them.

There will be some nervous laughter when people turn round to find a head turned round introducing themselves to the row behind them, but your participants are intelligent people and they will get the hang of saying hello to two people.

A variant can be to ask about groups, for example, "How many people here are from such and such a speciality/ location/ special interest group? Or use information gleaned from the conference programme "I see many people here are interested in ....", or "This session is about….. tell the person next to you why you chose this session". Use the introduction to make contact and engage with the audience, they will then be more likely to listen and engage with your subject matter.

Explanations/timings

The explanation should be very brief, under a minute. Allow a minute for people to say hello.

The debrief: maximising the benefits

This need only be brief, acknowledging that it is always good to meet new people and that now there will be more people to say hello to in the dinner/tea/coffee queue.

Equipment/resources needed;

None.

Skills to make this work even better

To increase engagement further, consider asking people to say hello and answer a question such as "Why did you decide to attend this particular presentation", or, "what is the key issue for you in this area", or "what attracted your attention in the title of this presentation?"

This will help focus attention further and may stimulate conversation afterwards too.

Pitfalls/when NOT to use this method

Do not waste time on this if the speaker before you has just done this or something similar, if time is very short, or if the setting is ultra-formal and unfamiliar. This method could be tricky when speaking to audiences outside General Practice. GPs are quite at home with this sort of thing, however, a judgement should be made with other audiences such as a group of surgeons or histopathologists!

Applications in other areas of the session.

This introduction is a variant of the ENERGISE Buzz group approach, and can be used during a session to get further discussion and thinking. When people interact, they learn and retain more.

How does this help to build relationships?

This method can help to build rapport between speaker and audience even in a very large group setting, and can definitely help to loosen up the atmosphere and encourage people to talk to each other outside the meeting.

How does this help to structure the education?

Having a clear start and purpose to discussions: focused question help to give shape to your presentation, which makes it more intelligible to listeners.

12// BUZZ GROUPS

Using buzz groups is a way to ensure that everyone in the room gets to participate, even quieter members or those who are not particularly interested in the subject matter.

What it is for?

Buzz groups provide opportunities for those who are not engaged to interact with someone who is more engaged, which can have a modelling and peer group norming effect. Buzz groups "wake the group up" and they provide a good way to get those with "activist learning styles" involved. Activists sometimes get restless if not given something to do, or may dominate the group if there are quieter reflectors and theorists around, who may take longer to get their thoughts out. It can also be a good "way in" for quieter people or those participants who protest that, even though they are not saying anything, they are "listening and taking it all in". Even for good listeners, participation in discussion is important: it provides an opportunity to have their ideas tested and weighed by others. It also means that the ideas of quieter members are heard by participants with a different approach. That can have many benefits; those who speak loudest and more often are not the only ones with good ideas worth hearing.

When to use it

Buzz groups are a useful way to engage participants at the start of a session and can be used at intervals during a session to discuss further iterations of a subject or different aspects. This one is a good way to maintain interest and energy and keep participants engaged.

The set up: how to use this method

Ask participants to form pairs. This can be with people next to them. This risks them only talking to people they already know or see as their buddies. One alternative is to allocate pairs, to ask people to stand up and walk round to find a person to talk to (the educator could also even ask them to specifically talk to people they do not know so well). If they sit in rows ask them to talk to the person behind them. This mixes up the discussion.

Then tell them exactly what you want them to talk about; the nature of the task needs to be clear, specific to the moment and any question used need to be open ones to promote discussion.

Decide if you want them to share information or decision making ("what approach do you take to someone with asthma who is not using their inhalers regularly?), or issues connecting with emotions and relationships ("Which members of the administration team do you have the best/ worst relationships with?"), or attitudes and values ("Should you ever give a patient your personal mobile number?").

Explanations/timings

Make sure the question is succinct and the task very clear. Try go ask ONE question rather than several. You can be strict about timings (Take two minutes to list the tasks of the practice manager) or you can see how the room sounds (see pitfalls) and stop the discussion BEFORE everyone stops talking or goes on to another topic. It can be useful to be more open ended if you are not quite sure how engaged they are with the question: for example asking what happens about "extra" patients in their practice may trigger quite a lot of discussion, which it may be worth allowing to run on a little). Judgement is required.

The debrief: maximising the benefits

Do not simply repeat the question or task that the buzz groups have been asked to do. Ask an open but related question like "What issues came up?" or "What did you spend most time talking about?" "What other issues came into the conversation?" and take it from there. You can then use this method to widen the discussion, or deepen it. If the educator asks "what if "questions. For example, if the session is about managing practice teams and how to manage disciplinary issues a question such as "what if one member of the administration team is always a bit off hand or rude?" can widen the discussion or signal the subject matter to come. A debriefing summary such as "it seems a lot of us have difficulties helping patients to change their behaviour towards more healthy approaches; this session will focus on strategies that can help this" can signal the focus of what is to come next and link it to the expressed concerns of the participants.

Equipment/resources needed

This is a very low-tech approach! The educator can write the question on a flip chart and record answers there, but this is not always necessary and may interrupt the flow of the discussion.

Skills to make this work even better

Develop specific, provocative questions relevant to the groups concerns will make this an effective technique. Using recent news events/ knowledge of specific problems participants are likely to encounter or provocative questions, can help participants dive in quickly and start working.

Another strategy is to start the discussion in pairs and then ask pairs to join together to form groups of four to share their ideas further. This increases the exposure of the ideas of otherwise quiet members and enables participants to hear a wider range of ideas.

Pitfalls/when NOT to use this method

Do not use this method if the question is too specific and the group members may not all have relevant experience of it. For example, asking buzz groups "how do you fill in the e portfolio covering fitness to practice", in a group where not all members use a portfolio, will frustrate the participants.

If the group is, on the whole, not engaged with the subject matter, then in buzz groups the discussion may fall into the "what has this got to do with me" approach, or may rapidly drift off into something more interesting. If this is relevant to the task in hand then the buzz group output can give the organiser the opportunity to reframe the session to make it more relevant to what the group needs. However, sometimes the buzz groups just gossip, go off on tangents or in some other way fail to engage with the task. This particularly happens if the task is too small and the time allowed too long. The group leader needs to listen unobtrusively to the progress of the conversations to gauge whether the buzz group task is appropriate, being carried out, or whether the groups are drifting.

If drifting away does occur this is important information for the educator, and may help them to re frame what is happening or to pay attention to other psychological processes. For example, the group may not wish to engage in the task because some other issue is more pressing for them (sometimes recent examination experiences or a something relevant in the national news). Recognising and accepting the importance of such concerns and debriefing that concern properly first, enables the group to process the other items and then move on to the material planned for the session.

This uses similar skills to the listening skills needed to establish the agenda with a patient; use those skills in educational contexts too.

Applications in other areas of the session

Repeating buzz groups at different stages of the session can help to encourage engagement and energise the group, especially if they change partners for subsequent questions.

How does this help to build relationships?

Participants feel more engaged in the session, and they get to know their fellow participants better which improves relationships. Closer relationships facilitate deeper learning and discussion of more sensitive and difficult areas.

How does this help to structure the education?

The careful wording of the questions, of the debriefing questions and of any further questions to the group, mean that the educator can structure the learning in an effective yet unobtrusive way. This might mean starting with factual and practical stuff and then leading participants into applying knowledge. This helps them to analyse usefulness, and evaluate the significance and meaning of the material within their own work (see ENRICH Using taxonomies of learning).

13// HOPES, FEARS AND DREADS

This method explicitly addresses the question of what the participants are bringing to the session.

What it is for?

It aims to bring out into the open any concerns, desires, pre conceptions or worries that participants have about the training they are about to receive.

While it takes a few minutes, the pay back is potentially huge. The educator demonstrates interest in the participants and their view of the issues/concerns/worries arising from the topic at hand. These concerns are seen as being inevitable, and useful to discuss. Participants are immediately involved in the planning of the session and will be more engaged in it.

The educator also demonstrates engagement with participants hopes for the session, which helps to orientate the educator to where the participants are "coming from" and this also helps to link the content to their educational needs, which increases their engagement. This approach can be combined with or followed by the engagement technique of ENGAGE Establishing learning needs at the outset.

When to use it

I have heard it said that **every** group session should begin with a "hopes and fears" exercise. That is an extreme position. However, effective training must begin with knowing where the learners are at in their thinking and feelings about the subject matter.

A skilled educator takes the information from this exercise into account during the session, which:

- increases the engagement of the audience
- links material closely into their *learning needs at that time*
- increases effectiveness of the education.

If you have been given a brief to talk about one particular subject area, or to teach one particular skill, it might seem that this exercise is redundant. Consider this; if participants are not interested in or resistant to learning about that issue, or have attitudes towards the topic that may impede learning, it is even more important to do this exercise and arrive at a shared view of what the session can reasonably be used for and what is beyond its scope.

If this doesn't happen the hopes, fears and dreads will still be there. If their hopes for the session are dashed and the fears/dreads realised, participants can become demotivated, which is very counterproductive.

This approach can be especially effective if the educator is introducing an outside speaker (check if they plan to use this approach themselves first to avoid duplication). The speaker is rapidly orientated to the group and can link what they say to the participants' needs. See also ENGAGE Preparing an educational brief.

The set up: how to use this method.

Ask participants to consider on their own, inside their own heads for (say) 15 to 30 seconds, the question What are your hopes for today's session? What are your fears? Or what do you dread will happen? Use your observation skills discretely as participants wrestle with this question. Who immediately starts scribbling notes? Looks puzzled? Shrugs? These non-verbal clues can help you assess your audience.

Then, ask people in pairs (a neighbour or the person behind them), to discuss the same questions for a few minutes, before starting the group debrief, described overleaf.

Explanations/timings

It is useful to allow people time to collect their own thoughts before they start to discuss things in pairs. The time allocated to the **paired** discussion can be varied; if the material is complex, or challenging, if there is like to be a great variability in the concerns within the group, or if the group do not know each other well, **allow longer** … up to five minutes.

If the subject is well defined, the group more homogeneous and already know each other well, allow a shorter discussion. Listen to the overall sound the group makes, when the sound begins to diminish but before everyone has stopped talking, interrupt for debriefing.

The debrief: maximising the benefits

Do not ask each pair to report back unless the group is small enough to make that approach feasible. Going round everyone in turn can be boring and the group can lose energy.

Ask a large group to report back as follows:

Draw a line down the centre of a flip chart and label one **hopes** and the other **fears/dreads**. Ask the group "What issues came up in your discussions?"

This allows speakers to generalise, rather than being very specific about their own worries or concerns, if they are not keen to share them with the whole group.

Write the **hopes** and **fears/dreads** in the appropriate column. When things die down, ask if anyone has anything not yet recorded. You can comment as you go along about hopes, e.g. by saying "we will be covering that…"

Then, challenge the group to say how they would like a "fear/dread" to be turned into a "hope" for the session.

For example, if a dread is "a long PowerPoint lecture with no time for discussion", that could be turned into a hope of "enough time for discussion" (a heads up for the educator).

Or, if the dread is "it will be boring", then the hope will be that people join in and offer contributions that will make it more interesting.

Specific dreads may need careful handling. In GP training people often "dread" role play. If your session has role-play at its heart this could be off putting. Instead, ask the group to use this concern to create appropriate hopes. For example, that everyone will behave respectfully towards each other, or that no one will have to role play in front of everyone, etc.

At times issues will come up that seem unrealistic or beyond the scope of the planned session.

Educators who work regularly with a group will often know the likely issues that will arise. Have material ready that refers to how that learning could happen (for example, a web resource, book, e-learning or signpost another session later in the course). That way participants' needs are heard and acknowledged as important. Guidance is offered about how those learning needs can be met – even if not during the current session.

Equipment/resources needed

A flip chart and pens should be available for debriefing, and any other reasonable method to capture and display the findings can be used. For example there are hand held epidiascope type devices that one can handwrite on, while simultaneously projecting. Just choose the tech level that works for you!

Skills to make this work even better

Making eye contact, using people names wherever possible, thanking people for their contribution, acknowledging and accepting dreads without belittling them and cross referencing comments to what other participants have said have said, can all help to maximise the benefit of this exercise.

Moving straight into an exercise of ENGAGE Establishing learning needs at the outset allows aims and objectives for the session or course to be quickly agreed, and the group is then focused for learning.

Preparation with your specific audience in mind should mean that the hopes and fears/dreads match up to (at least some of) the material you have prepared. Preparation before a session is about understanding what participants are likely to be concerned about as much as preparing what you are going to "teach". When asking a speaker to come make sure they get a good educational brief. (See ENGAGE Preparing an educational brief.)

Pitfalls/when NOT to use this method

Does not work for very large groups/auditoria or where there is a formal agenda and a formal presentation is expected, for example, if delivering research findings at a large conference, or if you have been asked to deliver a lecture style presentation on a very specific topic, to a specific audience as part of a greater whole. In that situation ensure that you understand your educational brief very clearly before preparing your talk.

Applications in other areas of the session

Referring back to hopes and fears, when relevant, will help to demonstrate that you have been listening. At times a new and important issue may arise unexpectedly; quickly establishing what participants' hopes and fears are, around the new topic, can help to keep things on track or evolve into relevant but previously unexpressed areas. This is a bit like the patients "hidden agenda". If something comes up later on, it is often something so difficult or concerning that participants only bring it up when trust is established.

How does this help to build relationships?

Mutual and respectful listening helps to build rapport and trust between participants and educator. This makes for effective learning.

Getting bad feelings or concerns out into the open is a valuable way of engaging with the audience, demonstrating that you are interested in and listening to them. This usually enables dreads/ fears to be dealt with. Care with language will help this along. Saying things like "yes I know you are interested in case x but today I am only going to deal with this" can put people off. Try "case x is really important and interesting and will be dealt with best in …. setting (make some sensible suggestions), today we will be focusing on ….which most participants seem most concerned about".

How does this help to structure the education?

All education needs preparation and should be guided by the curriculum. Exercises like this can help to focus participants' attention, while also signalling that other material will be covered in future sessions, or in their work place learning or via their private study.

14// ESTABLISHING LEARNING NEEDS AT THE OUTSET

This method enables educators to establish what the priorities for learning are for the specific group of participants present.

What it is for?

The aims and objectives for sessions will of course be considered by educators as they plan, influenced by the curriculum relevant to the whole course of study that participants are engaged with. In planning, educators can also use a Taxonomy (see ENRICH Using taxonomies of learning). Therefore, it might seem a waste of time to negotiate the aims and objectives with participants in each session. However, the stage that participants are currently at in their learning/thinking has a huge effect on what will be achieved in the session and whether participants move forwards in their learning. Participants get bored if the level is pitched too low and frustrated if pitched too high to address their specific needs.

In an ideal world the educational brief that educators prepare beforehand (or that a visiting speaker has been given in advance) will include an assessment of the nature of the material, and the level of complexity, that the participants are likely to be interested in.

However, that is just a start. Participants will bring their own individual hopes and fears, (see ENGAGE; Hopes/fears) and have their own ideas about is most important to get from a session. Finding this out will enable the educator to pitch the session at the right level; enough to challenge some of the most able and yet clear enough to enable the less developed participants to get something useful.

Furthermore, really teasing out what participants are actually struggling with, rather than what the book says they need to know, can help to focus the session round the important subject matter. This can also can save time if certain areas can be treated more lightly because everyone is already happy with them.

This discussion also helps to introduce and engage participants in thinking about different levels and types of learning; is the session to address knowledge gaps? Skills deficits? Explore attitudinal and professional issues? Skilfully done, engaging participants in exploring their learning needs can move them away from expecting simple "knowledge transfer", perhaps better done by private study, and into more challenging areas, which may be actually more useful to them.

When to use it.

Use this approach at the start of a session to ensure that the planned material is adapted to the specific learning needs of the group, and to ensure that the group consider skills, attitudes, values and professional issues when learning. This method can be used before or after ENGAGE Hopes and fears assessment. Because these methods ensure that everyone is asked to consider their needs and discuss them with at least one other person, everyone's participation is ensured at the start. This increases engagement with the whole session.

A similar approach can be taken at the start of a whole programme of learning, for example at the start of a Study Release Course. This will again help to orientate educator and group to each other's thinking and assist planning; however, correctly, some participants will insist that their issue is their "unknown unknowns" and they do not yet know what they want to learn. Educators can write this up as "wanting to explore the subject matter in depth" and "identifying unknown unknowns" as legitimate learning objectives.

The set up: how to use this method

Choose the initial question carefully, depending on how the session fits into a programme of learning, and to the stage of training or skill that participants are at. For example, in a session about the consultation skill of (say)"Breaking Bad News" the question for inexperienced doctors might be "How skilled are you at Breaking Bad news and what would you like to get out of this session today?"

For more experienced doctors the question might be "What experiences have given you the greatest difficulty in Breaking Bad News and what do you want to get out of today"

For very experienced doctors or trainers "What issues come up when you are trying to teach Breaking Bad news" to your trainees?

It is worth revisiting an ENGAGE Buzz group approach here. Ask participants to consider the questions alone first for maybe 30 seconds and then ask people to discuss the question in twos or threes.

Explanations/timings

Ensure a clear (and open, not closed) question; allow 30 seconds for participants to think first, three minutes for discussion in pairs. Debrief timing will depend on the size of the group (see below).

The debrief: maximising the benefits

Each group can be asked to report back, or in a larger group, address the whole group with a general question like "What are the issues that come up?"

Record their questions/aspirations/learning needs for reference later on in the session. This will provide a useful way to reinforce learning at the end. Any issues that could not be dealt with can be identified with signposting to how learners can make progress in those areas.

A skilled educator can also classify learning needs during this discussion into knowledge, skills, attitudes, values, (for example), or into diagnosis, management, teamwork. Teasing this out from participants is akin to taking an "educational history" (similar to taking a history from a patient), which will lead to a more effective educational intervention.

The listening skills are those also used in the consultation; picking up clues and non-verbal information, reflecting back and opening things up, may take a few moments. The payback will be a better structured session that participants really want to participate in.

Equipment/resources needed

A flip chart and pens.

At the start of a whole programme, participants can be given sticky notes or cards to record learning needs on .These can be mapped to large sheets on the wall headed "knowledge skills or attitudes and values" to help reinforce that training sessions are sometimes not the best place for "knowledge transfer". Training for skills or competencies can be ultimately of more long term use. Knowledge gets out of date, but skills can be continuously developed through practice.

When planning ahead, focus on the likely needs of the group in question; get information yourself in advance, or discuss with the person who has asked you to come if you are an outside speaker. The more you know in advance the better tailored your session will be.

Skills to make this work even better

Link what you are going to do today with what is done on other parts of the course if possible, and clarify what your brief/planning has been. This will enable a realistic set of aspirations to be negotiated. Write down what you hear; going back to the issues at the end reinforces the learning points and clarifies what still remains to be learned. It shows that you took the setting of the agenda seriously and adult learners benefit from shaping the learning process themselves.

Pitfalls/when NOT to use this method

This will not work in very large groups or if your contribution has already been tightly defined by your educational brief and your session or contribution is very short. In that case saying "this is what I intend to cover … and we will be learning it by doing ..." is a good start, followed by "Is that what you are expecting? Is that what will work for you at this point?" Really listen to the answers, including the hesitations, the groans that may mean "not another boring presentation on …"

Occasionally, even if you have been drafted in to give a 20-minute presentation on managing a specific issue, the audience may not engage if they remain unsure that these actions are in their remit, or if they are unsure that the issue is relevant to them, etc.

Sometimes, participants can be over general (teach us everything about heart disease!) or wildly unrealistic (a participant once asked that in a one-hour session on nurse prescribing, I tell them all about "diagnosis, examination and management of all the common conditions and the consultation skills that you need to talk to patients about them". In one hour, yes – it took me years to learn all that! Negotiating what was reasonable to cover took a few minutes and was crucial to making the session appropriately limited and reasonably effective).

Teasing out where your session fits in with participants' general training, or what exactly they mean by "everything about heart disease" may take a short time but will be infinitely more rewarding for the group and for you as a speaker if you get to the nub of what needs to be addressed.

The parallels with setting an agenda in a consultation are relevant; unless the agenda is agreed things tend to go awry.

Applications in other areas of the session;

As a session unfolds, educators may notice a falling off of energy, or lack of participation. Checking the focus of the learning as you go along, and that it is still where it needs to be, will help to maintain interest. Also referring back to the recorded aims of the session as you go along will help to keep things moving forward so that the group does not get bogged down on a particular issue (sometimes lead by the needs of one insistent participant). This signposting function (as in the consultation) makes for more effective use of time.

How does this help to build relationships?

This approach creates dialogue, a prerequisite for effective participant/educator and participant/participant relationships. When participants appreciate that the educator is interested specifically in them, and not delivering something generic, there is likely to be deeper engagement, which improves relationships all round.

How does this help to structure the education?

As above, checking on learning needs can help structure the session and by linking learning to a wider programme of study participants can "see the bigger picture" This helps them engage with the learning on offer.

15// EVERYTHING WITH A PURPOSE (EWAP)

This is not so much a method of delivery, but more a way of talking about learning and what is going to happen in the session.

What it is for?

In advance, educators will naturally have prepared; the aims and objectives, the intermediate learning outcomes, the methods, the pace and rhythm of the session will be anticipated. Indeed, everything will have a purpose. EWAP is shorthand to remind us to express this purpose to the participants, succinctly and overtly, at the start and in a purposeful way.

When to use it

At the start of a session, or at the start of a new part or element of a session, when theory gives way to practical examples, or when there is a change of subject.

The set up: how to use this method

Introduce the next phase or the session as a whole using the EWAP approach; this means linking what is to be addressed, to why it is important.

This works best if the sentence takes the form "What … so that …"

Just as "go on" are the two most powerful, yet low effort words in a consultation, "so that" are very powerful words to speak to participants.

Examples

- Today we are going to work on Breaking Bad News ("what") … so that … you will understand what breaking bad news is all about. We will also do some practice (what) … so that you will be better at breaking bad news in future … so that you will have these skills honed ready for the CSA exam.
- Today we are going to hear the presentations you have prepared ("what")...so that you can get some practice in delivering education...so that you will have the opportunity to receive some feedback on your educational skills...so that you will acquire evidence for your ePortfolio for this important competency (Maintaining performance, learning and teaching).
- Today we are going to be working with a poet to explore how we deal with emotions ("what") ...so that you can experience how processing emotions differently can help us develop increased professional resilience.

Explanations/timings

This initial explanation of what is going to happen should be very succinct – basically one sentence. By introducing the purpose of the session, participants are orientated to what they are going to be learning about and the purpose of such learning. Identifying what the EWAP sentence is going to be is also a crucial factor when planning. The purpose of the session needs to be crystal clear in the educator's mind if it is really going to land successfully in the minds of the participants.

Prepare your EWAP statement in advance (what) so that your preparation is focused and your choice of methods appropriate – ensuring that participants are engaged, understand what they are doing and why, and will be learning all the time. (I am sure you have got the idea!). EWAP does not necessarily mean that the session is rigid, prescriptive or teacher centred.

An EWAP sentence could just as well be "Today we are going to do some problem case discussion … so that you will get a chance to explore sharing cases, so that you will understand what other people find difficult and so that you can reflect on the usefulness of problem case discussions as part of your CPD. Such a sentence prescribes no specific outcome (for example "you will learn how to do an audit") yet expresses the purpose of the session clearly.

The debrief: maximising the benefits

The EWAP statement can lead into other engaging strategies, especially ENGAGE Hopes and fears and ENGAGE assessing learning needs at the outset. Knowing what the overall purpose of the session is means participants will be able to engage in reflection on what their learning needs are. In a well prepared session most of those needs will have been anticipated by the skilled educator, who will be prepared with suitable strategies for engaging with those needs. Debriefing the EWAP sentence really occurs in the review part of the session towards the end; referring back to the aims of the session and the learning needs expressed is a good way to encourage reflection and evaluation of the session and what was learned. See the EVALUATION section for strategies to achieve this successfully. Reviewing the learning also reinforces it.

Equipment/resources needed

Plan ahead, put the EWAP sentence on the board or a slide to reinforce it.

Skills to make this work even better

The skills for EWAP are really in planning and anticipation; clarifying the educational aims, objectives and intermediate learning outcomes leads to better training. Time spent thinking through what needs to be achieved and why, will pay dividends. Most of this handbook is really concerned with the "how" of education rather than the "what" (which will be inspired by the curriculum") or the "why" (which will be inspired by the outcomes…doctors who are knowledgeable, skilful, continuously developing, who pass their exams and become independent practitioners in their own right).

Pitfalls/when NOT to use this method

EWAP is always needed. Pitfalls could arise if the EWAP is poorly thought through, or, does not take account of the anticipated or assessed learning needs of the participants. This is why it is also important to assess those needs at the start of the session.

Applications in other areas of the session

EWAP statements can be used at any point when there is a change of emphasis or subject ("we are now going to do some skills rehearsal of the things we have been learning about … so that you can get some feedback, so that your skills will improve so that you will be able to use these skills in consultations and in your examinations).

How does this help to build relationships?

When participants know that their education is in the hands of someone who has prepared, who knows what they are doing and why, trust in the educational process increases. This increased trust in the educator means that participants are typically more engaged and more willing to work on difficult or challenging areas. This benefits everyone.

How does this help to structure the education?

Clarity about the "what and … so that" clarify the purpose of different activities, where the education fits in with wider agendas and makes the choice of activities and methods more purposeful. EWAP statements are useful as "transitional statements" or "signposts" at the start or within sessions, indicating clearly where the session is going.

This approach is sometimes called a "Transparent Method" because the educator's purpose and method is openly shared with the group. Explaining why you have chosen particular approaches ("what is going to happen…so that…") also helps participants to learn these educational approaches for themselves, so that they can use them other settings, for example when delivering training to others, in practice or multidisciplinary team meetings and so on.

16// TALKING STICKS

Time is what stops everything happening simultaneously; talking sticks can help stop all your participants talking (or snoozing) simultaneously.

What it is for?

This is a method to encourage all participants to talk and also to stop "cross talk" where more than one person is speaking at one, which reduces listening and fragments the group.

When to use it

Talking sticks can be used if discussing a tricky topic, or one where everyone wants to speak at once, to enable all to participate. Can be used to break up "rounds" in groups for example, where everyone is introducing themselves because the talking stick does not have to be passed directly to the person sitting next door, (See also ENRICH Making rounds effective).

The set up: how to use this method

Explain the purpose of the "talking stick"; whoever is holding the stick is the person talking and other participants should listen to that person speaking "so that" only one person talks at a time and to encourage everyone to have an opportunity to speak. When the speaker has finished they can choose who to pass the stick to (works well in introduction rounds), or participants can bid for the stick by raising a hand or similar, if they wish to follow on from what the current holder is saying. The "talking stick" does not have to be a stick, it can be any agreed token that indicates that the holder is the person speaking and being listened to. Traditionally I believe it was a conch shell, however, it can be any suitably sized object, i.e. clearly visible to all, easy and light to transfer between parties.

A variant is to give everyone some kind of token; if someone speaks they have to put their token on the floor and cannot speak until everyone else has had a chance to speak.

Explanations/timings

Only a brief introduction/explanation is usually required. Participants get the hang of it quickly if any issues are explained as soon as they arise. If the discussion is about something difficult, the educator may need to be sensitive as to whether some people are talking for too long, and find a tactful way to move to another contributor.

The debrief: maximising the benefits

The educator can summarise the discussion, emphasising the benefits of having heard contributions from all participants, and that people are heard better when there is no "cross talk", (several people talking at once).

Equipment/resources needed

A token of some sort to act as the signal for the speaker to have the floor.

Skills to make this work even better

The educator can demonstrate passing the token to another person – showing that it does not have to be the person next to them. In introduction rounds it can make people switch off if they are "waiting their turn to speak". It keeps groups alert if they do not know whose turn it will be next. The educator can invite reflection on what it feels like to have talk structured in this way and what effect it has on the group process. If everyone has a token in the variant described, the educator may like to summarise discussions and also invite reflection on what happens when everyone gets to speak including quieter members. Does the discussion take a different turn? Does it help people to feel they belong more in a group if they get a chance to speak?

Pitfalls/when NOT to use this method

Not all groups need this, many small groups will naturally allow all members to speak when they want to especially with alert educator looking for clues that someone wants to speak. Probably not needed in very formal situations, but useful as a backup if there is a lot of cross talking, confusion or non-listening in the group. Group exercises when well done can increase the sense of cohesion within a group. This method is not really applicable with very large groups, although the roaming microphone at large conferences is in effect, a variant of the talking stick.

Applications in other areas of the session

As with any "round" asking people to contribute, this can be used to punctuate a session if needed, to invite reflection on what has been learned so far and so on.

How does this help to build relationships?

Sometimes quieter members can find it harder to get a chance to speak and this method emphasises that all can contribute.

How does this help to structure the education?

Formal group methods like this can be used to break up a session, to enable discussion at relevant points and to help ensure all participate. Having a structure to the talk can feel containing and reduce anxiety, and can also enable to group to move on (after a summary) when everyone has contributed, which can help maintain pace and interest in the session.

17// PREPARING AN EDUCATIONAL BRIEF

When organising educational events, an educator often decides to invite a speaker from outside to give a session.

What it is for?

Inviting an outside speaker may be useful because they may have special expertise, they may be particularly effective at transmitting learning, or because the educator cannot deliver all the education personally. This technique gives some pointers about how to prepare a good brief for an outside speaker , so that they deliver what is needed, an appropriate amount of what is needed, and so that they allow space for the participants to ask relevant questions or get elaboration on points they find difficult.

When to use it

This is a preparation method. Use when planning the role of an outside speaker within a programme, conference or event, and for them to use as a trigger to their thinking and planning. If such interventions are well planned in advance they are more likely to meet participants' expectations and needs, so that they are more engaged and learn more from the session.

The set up: how to use this method

Before contacting the speaker to come and talk to your participants, the educator must carefully consider the PURPOSE of their talk; this means achieving clarity in the educators mind about the aims and objectives of the event or session, clarity about what the learning outcomes are being aimed for, and clarity about which methods of delivery are likely to be most effective. Assess the time available and how much material, and what kind of material, can usefully be covered. Will the session be about "knowledge transfer" (suitable drugs for hypertension), developing skills, "Working effectively with your team", or exploring attitudes and values ("How should you respond if a colleague is making a lot of mistakes?").

Explanations/timings

Consider using a template to clarity your own thoughts about what the purpose of an outside speaker is and what you would like them to cover. This should include the exact subject matter expressed as a succinct but clear title, a description of the content and a summary of the time constraints and allocation of time for discussion. There is an example, with a worked example, below (see References and resources)

The debrief: maximising the benefits

Debriefing in this situation is with the outside speaker; the educator should seek feedback on the proposed brief and agree the final form of the session with the speaker. Was the prior information helpful and can the speaker deliver on it? If not, what changes should be made?"

Equipment/resources needed;

Can be done in conversation, by letter or email, ensuring that the loop is closed by the speaker responding and commenting on what is proposed, to allow any further changes.

Skills to make this work even better

Use an explicit division into Knowledge, Skills and Attitudes with stated Intended Learning Outcomes, which are statements of things that participants should be able to do at the end of the session/training that they could not do before (see Reference 1).

Pitfalls/when NOT to use this method

Some speakers may have very fixed views about what their audience should be told and how they should learn. Tactful discussions may be necessary to tailor the expertise of the visitor to the actual learning needs of participants, which may be unclear to "experts". For example, a GP may be more interested in knowing when to refer, than in the pathophysiology of the disease, whereas, an ENT specialist trainee may be more keen to know how to perform a procedure or when to avoid doing certain procedures.

Applications in other areas of the session

This is a preparation method. However, referring back to the brief, especially if negotiated and modified by a "Hopes and Fears" and "Assessing learning needs at the outset" process, can be very helpful in retaining engagement of the participants throughout.

How does this help to build relationships?

If the speaker is well orientated to the learning aspirations of their audience, rapport will develop more rapidly. A good brief helps the participants to trust that the speaker will deliver what they need, so that they develop a positive relationship with the speaker and are more engaged.

How does this help to structure the education?

Good planning helps to ensure a good structure of a course over several sessions, and also means that the structure within the session is explicit and suitable for the learning.

References and resources

1. More information about intended learning outcomes and how to develop them is in *The Essential Handbook for GP Training and Education* by Ramesh Mehay.
2. Below is a potential form for an educational brief, with two worked examples. The first (page 49) shows a brief for a group of experienced General Practitioners coming to learn about the long term effects of a stay on ICU on patients. The second (page 50) is a similar brief but addressed to intensivists in training.

A simple template

Proposed Date and time
Speaker's name
Length of session
Title
Purpose and intended Learning outcomes
Structure of session
Educator/Chair present as well as speaker?
A/V and other equipment available
Size of audience

A brief for a group of experienced GPs; the comments in **bold** explain why the content is there.

Proposed Date and time: 1/10/2018

Speaker's name:
Dr JS Expert Intensivist (who works in ICU and runs clinics following up patients after an ICU stay)

Length of session: 1 hour

Title:
Coming home after critical illness; life after intensive care; what GPs need to understand to help patients recover

Purpose and intended learning outcomes:
Time in ICU or experiencing severe critical illness can have many long term consequences for patients and GPs are often left to "pick up the pieces", to try and help patients rehabilitate on their return home. Sometimes relatives come to the patients GP for information about ICU care , while the patient is still in ICU; it can be hard to know who to approach for information. **(i.e. the background and why this speaker has been invited.)**

The key issues to cover would be

- PHYSICAL IMPACTS – what is expected recovery like and should GPs anticipate any particular physical problems? What mitigates these?
- PSYCHOLOGICAL/SOCIAL IMPACTS – how are patients affected in ICU and what steps are taken to manage this for patients/their carers/loved ones? What steps mitigate these impacts?
- ORGANISATIONAL ISSUES – how are ICU services organised e.g. do patients have a named consultant? Is there any after-care?

(These elements start to focus the speaker around the issues important for this particular audience, and classifying them in this way also orientates the speaker about the ways in which GPs think.)

- PRACTICAL APPLICATIONS; what should GPS anticipate? How can they help patients? What help is available to support GPs/Their patients after ICU?

(These are effectively the intended learning outcomes.)

Structure of session:
The chair will introduce the speaker and ask the participants to reflect on any patients they have had who have recovered from ICU care, and what issues cropped up for the GP and patient once they were at home (i.e. the chair will do a basic ENGAGE Assessing learning needs at the outset).

In the light of the questions raised by the audience, a short presentation (20 minutes) is invited leaving around 35 minutes for discussion and questions. The participants are experienced GPs who will be keen to interact and discuss issues arising. The expected style is an interactive one and participants may ask frequent questions and initiate debate.

(This orientates the speaker to the preferred interests and style of the participants.)

Educator/Chair present as well as speaker?
This note is here so that the speaker knows whether they have to do all the work themselves or whether there will be a educator to assist the process. Its much easier to deliver a talk in a strange place if there is someone there to introduce you, get A/V working, etc.

A/V and other equipment available:
Laptop, projector sound, microphone available. Please email presentations in advance (to someone@preparation.ac.uk) as the IT security system will not permit download from data sticks, etc.

(Letting speakers know this info in advance means no wasted time when they turn up with an incompatible device, etc.)

Size of audience:
Variable usually – 15 to 30. Room seats maximum of 35.

Useful information for a speaker who will naturally approach an audience of 200 slightly differently.

A similar brief intended for a group of Anaesthetic trainees.

Proposed date and time: 1/10/2018

Speaker's name:
Dr JS Expert Intensivist (who works in ICU and runs clinics following up patients after an ICU stay)

Length of session: 2 hours

Title:
Managing the long term sequelae of a stay on intensive care and preventing long term morbidity.

Purpose and intended learning outcomes:
Time in ICU has many long term consequences for patients; there are techniques to minimise these and many ICU departments organise follow up clinics for their patients. This session is to cover the key issues in long term morbidity after ICU care and what can be done to mitigate the problems. Effective discharge processes also need to be covered.

The key issues to cover would be

- PHYSICAL IMPACTS – what are the potential problems/what is the evidence base for this, what evidence/guidelines inform the approach in ICU?
- PSYCHOLOGICAL/SOCIAL IMPACTS – how are patients affected in ICU and what steps can be taken to reduce these impacts? What about the impact on relatives?
- ORGANISATIONAL/QUALITY ISSUES – what should be done to improve outcomes? What care takes place post ICU? What quality criteria should be applied? What standards should discharge information meet?

See https://www.rcoa.ac.uk/system/files/TRG-CCT-ANNEXF.pdf

DOMAIN7 Domain 7: Comfort and recovery 7.1 Identifies and attempts to minimise the physical and psychosocial consequences of critical illness for patients and families 1 M, C 7.2 Manages the assessment, prevention and treatment of pain and delirium 2 D, I, C, M, T 7.4 Communicates the continuing care requirements, including rehabilitation, of patients at ICU discharge to health care professionals, patients and relatives 1 M, T, S 7.5 Manages the safe and timely discharge of patients from the ICU.

(These elements start to focus the speaker around the issues important for this particular audience, allows for the fact this is a 2-hour session and links it formally to the syllabus.)

Structure of session:
Total 2 hours, normally with break of 15 minutes for tea about midway. Aim to have some practical examples and discussions, not just PowerPoint slides.

Educator/Chair present as well as speaker?
No

A/V and other equipment available:
Laptop, projector sound, microphone available. Please email presentations in advance (to someone@preparation.ac.uk) as the IT security system will not permit download from data sticks, etc.

This information will also be posted on the Virtual Learning Centre after the session.

(Letting speakers know this info in advance means no wasted time when they turn up with an incompatible device, etc.)

Size of audience:
40 to 50

ENERGISE

INTRODUCTION

This section is about methods that help to **energise** participants in educational environments. The introduction considers the "What, why and when" issues and then the sections that follow are detailed descriptions of different **methods** ("how" issues).

What does "energise" actually mean? Here are some definitions:

1. To give vitality and enthusiasm, to make someone feel excited, enthusiastic or impressed. "People were energised by her ideas", also having connections to ideas of being enlivened, animated, invigorated, perked up, stimulated, fired up, roused, motivated, moved to action, spurred on, encouraged or galvanised.
2. To supply energy to something, (typically kinetic or electrical energy) and set going. "Floor sensors are energised by standing passengers", also having implications of getting things working, actuated, switched on, started off, triggered off or activated.

All educators would like their participants to be excited, enthusiastic and working hard during educational sessions. This needs energy. Having engaged their interest using relevant techniques from the ENGAGE section, educators can select techniques from the ENERGISE section to ensure that the participants remain full of energy and enthusiasm as the session continues. Good energisers can further develop the benefits of the general principles identified in the introduction to the ENGAGE section as follows:

- **Learners feel that they belong**. Educators choose effective energisers to increase the range and nature of interactions between participants so that everyone is fully involved, so that relationships are strengthened, so that a sense of belonging and learning together is developed.
- **Learners know each other and the educator and have a good rapport**. Energising activities are useful so that participants/educators get to know each other better, so that they are able to share something of themselves, so that rapport increases. Rapport creates many educational opportunities that will be missed if participants are unenthusiastic and de-motivated.
- **Learners' agendas and needs are taken into account**. Suitably chosen energising activities help to further identify and refine the specific learning needs of participants in the group, so that time is used more effectively, being focussed around the needs of the group at the time.
- **Learners participate in a community of practice**. Energisers encourage participation, so that learning is not a passive, but rather, an active process. Actively working together creates a greater sense of a community, so that learning is shared and participants learn from each other, as well as from the educator. This is not to say that the educator does not have special expertise, in many situations they do. However, some lessons are learned more quickly and effectively from peers. Role modelling and peer group modelling are influential, however, the learning outcomes can sometimes be poorly articulated. Educators need to ensure that what is learned is appropriate. Educational activities that encourage participation can help to ensure that learning related to the formal curriculum is also consistently reflected in the informal curriculum and the hidden curriculum.

If the methods in the ENGAGE section help to **unite** the group together, ready for further learning, then the techniques in the ENERGISE section serve to **focus** the groups attention towards the Intended Learning Outcomes and **mobilise** them to active learning. These principles also underpin the skills of effective chairmanship of any meeting, (see also ENERGISE Creating action learning sets). This is another example of the crossover of skills from clinical work to education. Many clinicians will participate in meetings or take the Chairmanship of meetings: the skills used in meetings are transferable to education (and vice versa, educational skills can help make meetings run more smoothly).

Why are the techniques in the ENERGISE section useful for educators? Most simply, straightforward energisers can be use on an "as required" basis to encourage a group whose energy is flagging to regroup and be stimulated to carry on working. This can happen if the session is long, starts after lunch when participants may be sleepy or when they are tired after long shifts. It can occasionally happen that somehow participants are bored by the material: this should be rare if the processes of ENGAGE Hopes and fears and ENGAGE Assessing learning needs at the outset have been carefully carried out. Sometimes outside speakers may not fully engage with the group: energy can flag if there is a mismatch of learning agendas between group and speaker (see ENGAGE preparing and educational brief for ways to minimise this risk).

Even when the material to be covered has been clearly aligned with the group's needs, energisers can be useful as a way in, to start things off and get the group working. In any group there will be differences in the way that participants work and learn best. There are several ways of looking at this, one of the best known being the Honey and Mumford Learning Styles questionnaire. This examines the extent to which learners are Activists, Reflectors, Pragmatists or Theorists (see Reference 1). Activist learners can easily get distracted at the start of sessions, so providing energising activities at the beginning, can keep them on board. Suitably paced and chosen activities will also enable more reflective or theoretical participants to get involved using the "pause, pair, square, share method" (see ENERGISE Using QUESTIONS effectively). After activists have had their say in a "pause, pounce, bounce" approach, (see ENERGISE Using QUESTIONS effectively) reflectors, pragmatists and theorists can be directly encouraged to add their (important but more slowly emerging) insights.

The methods in the ENERGISE section can also be used to convey significant educational content even to a group that starts off suitably engaged. Using short themed energising sections at the start of longer sessions can enable more material to be covered, using methods that stimulate active thinking and reflection. These methods are covered in the ENERGISE Warm Up chapters, which include energising warm ups to stimulate and develop critical thinking, professional virtues and examination of the underlying assumptions of modern medical practice. Educators can use these warm-up energisers as a preliminary to sessions including other topics, so that these difficult subjects are covered in more easily digestible "bite sized" chunks, and so that these areas are embedded within the overall curriculum. This indirectly emphasises the importance of critical thinking, because participants are invited to do this at every session. Moreover, having started in a mind-set of active exploration and critical appraisal, participants are more likely to carry over those approaches to later parts of the session, enriching their learning. In the ENERGISE section there are also exercises that can be used to "warm up" groups when group work and team work skills are the subject matter. Such methods offer real time experiences of teamwork that can go well or badly. The key to success is in the debriefing process.

Some simple energisers, such as line-ups can be adapted to convey educational concepts and ideas in a powerful way (see ENERGISERS Quick energisers and ENRGISERS Using line-ups to explore ideas). Such approaches can be enjoyable ways to demonstrate participants' attitudes and values, so that differences can be examined without the process being too exposing or challenging. For example, doing a line-up to see how participants align along a continuum of "After work I can play….versus I can play anytime" can lead to productive discussions about whether work and play are different, or overlapping spheres. Combining movement, with thinking about the material, keeps energy levels high, and can create memorable experiences for participants, especially when they see that others may or may not share their own assumptions or ideas. These methods have the potential to take education to another level, beyond that of "knowledge transfer", developing the participants' skills in analysing, evaluating, organising and applying their understanding. The next section, ENRICH, deals with this in more detail, offering methods to deepen and enrich the educational experience of engaged, energised participants.

Finally, when educators are teaching on Consultation and Communication skills, there are methods in this section that help to energise participants, so that they are motivated to improve their understanding and performance in these crucial skills. These methods can be used as warm-up activities for sessions on Consultation Skills, or as part of Consultation Skills modules.

The ENERGISE methods are summarised under these headings.

Energisers to maintain energy

1. Quick energisers
2. Eyes closed draw face
3. Tidy up Tunes
4. Group sorting methods
5. Reflecting on something good
6. Buzz Groups

Energisers which help deliver specific educational content

7. Making a learning summary for sharing with the group
8. Using line ups to explore ideas
9. Creating action learning sets
10. Using questions effectively
11. Identifying team and group skills using a survival exercise
12. Teamwork skills using construction exercises

Energisers as warm up activities

13. Warm up theme – critical thinking
14. Warm up theme – the assumptions of modern medicine
15. Warm up theme – examining professional virtues

Energisers for Consultation skills education.

16. Consultation skills – initial listening exercises
17. Consultation skills – intensify understanding of listening by deconstruction
18. Consultation skills – what do you say after you say hello

References/resources

Honey and Mumford *Learning styles and impact on training sessions*, see:

https://www.bradfordvts.co.uk/wp-content/onlineresources/0307teachinglearning/learningpersonalitystyles/honey%20and%20mumford%20with%20slide%20notes.ppt

1// QUICK ENERGISERS

These very quick exercises are designed to use as rapid energisers when the group seems to be flagging or running out of steam in some way.

What it is for?

There can be a variety of reasons for a group to lose energy; after lunch energy often sags, if participants have been sitting down too much, energy can wane. Too much formal didactic input (lecture, death by PowerPoint etc) can lead to boredom or overload.

When to use it

Energising exercises can be planned in advance (for example after lunch) or can be used spontaneously if the facilitator notes that energy is flagging. This is another area where the skills of consulting overlap with those of educating. The educator notices cues and clues that an energiser is needed by picking up on the verbal and nonverbal cues from the participants, (yawning, lack of participation, fiddling with phones, lacklustre verbal contributions, lack of debate or disagreement) and "reading" the general atmosphere. These energisers are useful tools to have in your educators "back pocket". If a session is properly planned, an educator may never need an energiser because the session's activities are structured and paced well.

The set up: how to use this method

Be open about your reasons for deciding to do an energiser; explain that energy seems to be flagging a bit, (seek agreement from the group that they have noticed this too), that this will give everyone a burst of energy, and as most of them are done standing up, the extra physical activity will make them live longer. (The public health argument for increased movement is strong; I have heard that public health meetings are held standing up now!)

Explanations/timings

Once you have everyone's attention the explanation will be brief. The whole thing need only take a couple of minutes. The effect is refreshing. Here are some examples of quick energisers, you will be able to make up your own once you have got the hang of it.

1. **Heads, shoulders knees and toes**. Sing if you want, I do not advise it with adults! Get everyone to stand up in front of their chair and then put their hands up in the air and give them a good shake. Then ask them to touch their heads before shaking hands again, then touch their shoulders and shake the hands, then touch their knees and shake the hands around again. Finally shake the hands downwards on one side of the body and then on the other side.
2. **Stand ups**. Get everyone to stand in front of their chair. Then ask them to sit down and stand up as many times as they possibly can, in one minute, calling out their score at the end of the minute. Time it ruthlessly, calling out when there are 30 seconds, 10 seconds, and 2 seconds to go. Some groups get very competitive about this and want another go…great, the benefit will be increased!

3. **Tai Chi arms**. Ask everyone to stand up, preferably forming a circle if space permits. Ask participants to stand with feet shoulder width apart, arms by their sides palm facing in towards the body (model the activity for clarity). Then ask them to swing their arms up in front of themselves until their hand reach shoulder height with palms facing but not touching each other. Model doing this and ask the group to watch each other until all their arms are moving in synch. Repeat the swinging until everyone's arms are rising and falling together. This simple action makes everyone focus in each other, taking attention outwards, and bond in a common activity. Tai Chi instructors say this helps to move "CHI" i.e. energy around the whole body. After a suitable time ask participants to hold their hands at chest height with arms out straight and slightly cupped hands. Allegedly you can then feel a "ball" of warm energy between the palms. Not sure if that is true, however, it provides a distracting thought.
4. **North, South, East and West**. Ask everyone to stand up. Then ask them to move around the room touching each wall of the room, before sitting down again. Participants often see this as a race and the extra energy from speeding helps.
5. **Muscle relaxer**. Ask participants to stand in a circle if feasible otherwise in a couple of long lines. Get them to stand sideways as if they were forming an orderly queue for something.i.e. everyone should be looking at someone's back. Explain the activity and check that participants are OK for the person behind them to gently touch them. Usually this is ok in groups that are working together regularly. Get them to gently pat the back of the person in front of them using the palm of the hands in a clapping motion, starting on the shoulders and then patting down the arms and upper back. This is a gentle action that relaxes the neck and shoulder muscles.
6. **Energiser line up**. There are other uses for line ups, using questions triggered by the content of the session, see ENERGISE Line ups. When used as an energiser use a neutral subject matter. Ask everyone to stand up, then ask them to line up across the front of the room in order of height. Other neutral alternatives could be in order of birthdate starting at January first, in alphabetical order using the initial of their first name, etc.
7. **A comic energiser.** Ask everyone to move around the room and tell a joke to two other people. Alternatively, have prepared a set of cartoons (*The New Yorker book of cartoons about doctors* can provide useful material, see below); give everyone a cartoon and ask them to share it with two other people in the room and discuss what they think it says about doctors.

The debrief: maximising the benefits

Little debrief is needed; simply acknowledge that now everyone feels a bit more lively the session can proceed to its next activity.

Equipment/resources needed

Space to move around in. If space is extremely tight, with very fixed chair ordering, use one of the first few examples which can be done with participants at their own chairs.

Skills to make this work even better

Acknowledging that the group is flagging often brings sighs of agreement; reflect on how that happened and whether it could have been prevented. Was the room too hot, the sessions too boring, or the activity unengaging?

Ask the group if they know any good energising activities; I learned from participants in this way and asking them for help is in itself an energising method. This engages the resources of the group itself, meaning that the educator does not need to provide all the answers. This will help participants to be less passive and they can use similar approaches when organising educational events themselves e.g. for staff.

Pitfalls/when NOT to use this method

Be aware of any mobility issues that may limit some people's activities; choose/adapt a method that can be done seated. Participants may feel an energiser is a bit silly; the facilitator must explain clearly why they are doing this (perhaps the epidemic of sitting down disease is better known than it used to be!) and model the activity themselves too. Apart from a bit of stand up and shake your hands around, these activities are not really suitable for highly formal or large group occasions such as big conferences/lectures.

Applications in other areas of the session

Generally one only needs to do this once. If the group are really flagging so much that the educator feels the need to do this more than once, then there needs to be an investigation about why participants are so demotivated. Ask them. Discussion of the problem will often reveal some other pressing issue distracting them that needs attention and time. Although that may feel like a digression it will pay dividends in the longer run if problems are dealt with.

How does this help to build relationships?

If it works as planned and everyone livens up, the group will feel more trusting of the educator; they have demonstrated attentiveness to the group and to participants' needs. Doing something slightly silly together helps to bond the group and shared laughter is also very energising.

How does this help to structure the education?

An energiser provides punctuation and a springboard into the next planned activity, a kind of signpost.

Resources

The New Yorker Book of Doctor Cartoons
ISBN: 9780679765738

2// EYES CLOSED DRAW FACE

This is a short energiser which can be helpful at the start of a session.

When to use it

This is a good, brief, wake up if everyone is a bit sleepy after lunch. It can also be used as an orientation to subject matter such as feedback (how good is my drawing?) or even issues connected with loss of the senses or disability.

The set up: how to use this method

Every participant is given a piece of paper and something to draw with. Crayons or thick felt pens work best. Explain to participants that you are using these materials because they key into a playful, childlike part of ourselves which makes us more fluid. Also, this engages the more creative right brain, rather than the analytic left brain. Make it clear that it is not a competition.

Explanations/timings

Explain that the task is to draw a portrait of themselves, while having their eyes closed. Ask everyone to put their pen/crayon on the paper near the middle, and about a third of the way down. Demonstrate this with your own paper.

First ask them to draw a loop to represent their face. Then remove the pen/crayon from the paper (eyes still closed) and then replace it to draw two eyes, then the nose and then the mouth. Finally ask them to draw on some hair. Then ask everyone to lift up their portraits so everyone can see them and open their eyes.

The debrief: maximising the benefits

There is usually initial laughter, which is helpful and also tends to wake people up and re-engage them with the group. No extensive debrief is required, mainly an acknowledgement that we can do much better than we think even with our eyes closed, and that having a bit of fun is a good way to start the next session.

If using this as a way into a session on feedback, coping with sensory loss (or whatever is coming next) then this needs to be followed with an explanation of the purpose of the sessions so that the link is explicitly made.

Equipment/resources needed

Paper for each participant and crayons or pens. Works best with thick bright colours so that others can see the outcome. Biro or pencils make lines that are too thin. Charcoal sticks could work but can be messy.

Skills to make this work even better

Best not to over-egg this one, keep it simple and playful and be transparent about the purpose; there should be no sense of any psychological trickery. Explain that salesman call the after lunch moment the "graveyard slot" sometimes, because everyone is a bit unresponsive after lunch. Explain that this task is a short fun way to wake up our creative side, so that the session will go well.

Pitfalls/when NOT to use this method

Not needed routinely or in every afternoon session. Use if there is likely to be exhaustion (for example, a very dense morning session beforehand) or if it is hot, or lunch has been large etc. Do not use more than once with any given group of participants. Groups who are ill at ease with each other, or wary of the educational process may not like the playful aspect and may feel it is demeaning in some way. The set up and explanation is very important with exercises like this, so that the purpose and meaning are transparent.

Applications in other areas of the session

N/A

How does this help to build relationships?

Laughter and a bit of shared silliness increase connections. Education can be serious and fun at the same time.

How does this help to structure the education?

Provides punctuation and acknowledgement that training is sometimes energy consuming and that it is normal to feel a bit tired at times.

3// TIDY UP TUNES

Everyone likes music; sharing favourite songs can bring people together.

What it is for?

This energiser harnesses the power of participants to contribute something of themselves to group sessions, by asking a different member each week to nominate the piece of music they feel passionate about, and would like to share with the group: while the group sets up, or at the end when everyone is getting ready to go.

When to use it

This is an energiser to use at the start of a session, when everyone is coming in and sitting down, or at the end when participants are putting the room back to how they found it and getting ready to leave.

The set up: how to use this method.

At the start of a programme the educator can choose a piece of music to play as participants come in and when they are tidying up at the end (hence the term "Tidy up Tunes" Reference 1). The educator should explain why they feel passionate about this particular music. THEN, nominate a member of the group to choose the music for next week. When they play the music ask them to explain why they are passionate about their choice, and ask them to nominate the next person.

Explanations/timings

How much music gets to be played will depend on how long it takes the group to assemble/ tidy up, normally only a few minutes. Once the initial explanation is done it should take no time at all for the playing and handover to happen each week.

The debrief: maximising the benefits

The educator will maximise the benefits of this by modelling acceptance and enthusiasm about the passions that participants are sharing. Being able to contribute, (not just be passive recipients), creates more energy for learning, and also increases participants' sense that they belong, that they are individuals, with important contributions to make.

Equipment/resources needed

Some kind of AV system able to play CDs, DVDs or music videos, or a laptop with a speaker. Most Postgraduate centres have suitable kit installed.

Skills to make this work even better

Thank participants for their contribution, especially if introducing something new or unexpected, and if possible, refer back to it during the session, reinforcing the value placed in their contribution.

Pitfalls/when NOT to use this method

This is generally for use with a group of participants that is basically stable over a period of time and who have got comfortable enough with each other to consider stepping slightly outside the box.

Applications in other areas of the session.

Educators could use their imagination here, I guess, and use music in innovative ways.

How does this help to build relationships?

The relationships between participant and educator will be nurtured when the participant's contribution is recognised and valued. Peer to peer relationships will be enriched when participants can be themselves and share their interests. Participants will start to appreciate and share the contributions of their peers, which reinforces good relationships.

How does this help to structure the education?

Having a short musical interlude is a non-verbal signal of the start and finish of the formal parts of the session, helping to contain and structure the education process. This is also a signal as to when personal conversations and chat are welcome (when the music is on) and when attention needs to be paid to the session (when the music stops).

References

1. I am indebted to Matthew Creighton (my son) for the term "tidy up tunes", which he invented as a way to get the washing up/ clearing up done. After dinner, someone present nominates a tidy up tune, which plays while everyone gets on with tidying up together. It is interesting to hear what people choose and makes the chore more fun. With modern phone and internet technology there is no limit to the choices that can be made!

4// GROUP SORTING METHODS

Sometimes a big group is just too large to work well; splitting groups up can be very productive.

What it is for?

When working with a whole group, of any size above about six to eight (in which case the educator can keep tabs on everyone's participation and make sure to encourage and include everyone) there is a risk that some members will "switch off "and stop engaging with the group or the subject matter.

While the techniques described in the ENGAGE section will often be enough to overcome this, in large groups it is inevitable that some participants will be listening but not contributing. Does this matter? Quieter participants often say it doesn't matter because they are "listening". Clearly forcing quieter participants to contribute against their will in a large group is counterproductive. However, "just listening", does not give the **participant** the full benefit of working in a group: the full benefit is only obtained when they start contributing their own thoughts too.

Firstly, these thoughts are likely to be valued by other members; it is a condition of collaborative working that everyone contributes, just as everyone benefits. Secondly, one of the key benefits of working collaboratively, is the opportunity to test your own ideas out amongst friendly, supportive colleagues. Ideas can be compared, put in context, challenged and developed. This is only possible if everyone gets a chance to get their ideas discussed.

The methods described here are ways to divide the whole group, during a session, into smaller units. This makes participation easier and if the size of the smaller unit is a pair, then participation is virtually guaranteed. This enlivens the group up, widens participation and enables quieter members to develop their confidence in speaking over time. It also prevents discussion being dominated by a few (louder) people. Participants who perceive themselves to less "mainstream" are often less able to get their voices heard in the larger group (this may include those of different sexuality, race, gender, social origin) and methods to encourage their participation can be helpful too.

Thus, group sorting methods are an essential tool for any facilitator. Explain that the aim is to mix people up, so that the pairs and subgroups bring everyone's skills and talents on board, so that learning will be more effective for everyone.

When to use it

Educators can use these methods to ensure everyone participates at certain crucial junctures: when developing a common agenda for the group, when there is a controversial topic, when a variety of views is likely and all need to be heard, when the group as a whole becomes quieter or less engaged, or, when a majority of participants have not contributed to any whole group discussion.

These methods to "mix up" the group, allowing discussions with different people. Participants naturally sit next to their friends in groups. This can mean they do not hear views that are very different to their own. This is why it is better to allocate groups rather than asking people to "get into groups of four". Allocating saves time too, as asking people to put themselves into groups always takes far longer than expected

The set up: how to use this method

Before dividing the group, explain what the task for the smaller units will be. If you delay doing this until you have allocated the groups people stop listening and the details are lost as everyone wanders round the room. Make sure the question or task is brief, clear, and unambiguous and takes the topic at hand into deeper territory or into opportunities to practice or develop the ideas.

Usually use OPEN questions ("what is your response to the idea that …") or ask the group to apply learning ("we have done the theory of sick notes, here are some tricky examples to discuss"), or divide the subject matter between the groups to synthesise at the end (" this case brings up ethical issues…group A will discuss how Beneficence applies in this case, Group B how Maleficence might apply, Group C will discuss the role of Autonomy and group D will discuss how Justice might apply in this case). Or the different parts of a SWOT analysis (Strengths, Weaknesses, Opportunities, Threats) could be allocated to different units – there are lots of different ways to divide up learning tasks.

To ensure everyone engages, use units of two. Either ask people to work with the person next to them, better still ask them to work with the person in the row immediately behind them. If energy levels are low, get everyone to stand up and walk around the room for 15 seconds and then find a partner different to the person they were initially sitting next to.

This can be built on using the **"Pause, Pair, Square, Share"**approach. Ask participants to reflect alone on the subject and then discuss in pairs, then get pairs to team up into groups of four to share and discuss their ideas further. The time in a four can be used even more effectively if they use that time to decide to decide which ideas they want to feedback to the whole group, or which ideas they give most priority to, which factors they have found most useful to consider, and so on.

To get a range of views/contributions to a topic, use units of four. Work out how many smaller units would be formed if the whole group was working in fours, for example, a group of 20 would be five groups of four, a group of 28 would be seven groups of four. Walk along the row giving everyone a number up to the number of smaller units you are aiming for (1, 2 , 3, 4, 5 for a group of 20, up to seven for a group of 28). Ensure everyone knows which number they are. Ask them to go and join everyone with the same number, indicating clearly which part of the room they are to stand in (e.g. numbers 1 by the door, numbers 2 by this window and so on). Then they can get on with the task allocated.

To facilitate a longer group discussion, or exploration of a topic that has already been introduced to the larger group, use units of six to eight. Using a similar method as above, walking along a row and either giving the smaller units letters (you will be in group A, B, C, D) or a unit name (apples, bananas, cherries, olives), again ensuring that participants do not just sit next to the person they started with. Such groups are useful for exploring implications, and applying new learning in practical ways. For example, after a whole group session considering the principles of an effective screening programme using the Wilson Jugner Criteria, the smaller groups could be asked to apply those principles to a series of actual or proposed screening programmes to evaluate them. This simultaneously reinforces the initial learning and expands it to deeper levels.

Explanations/timings

Explain the task clearly first; this should be clear and precise so should only take about one to two minutes.

Dividing groups always takes longer than expected, in planning allow up to five minutes for everyone to get settled. As groups get used to this way of working, they getter better at moving to where they need to be to start the next task.

The debrief: maximising the benefits

The energising effects of dividing up the big group are lost if the debrief consists of everyone repeating their discussion all over again. So generalise away from the specific content and ask a general question like:

"What issues came up in your discussions". Keep saying "Did anything else come up?" until no more new ideas arise. Observe where the contributions are coming from, and ensure that people from different subunits get a chance to contribute. It may occasionally be necessary to say "thanks to that group for such a useful contribution, can we hear what another group made of things?" Before finishing create an opportunity for anyone to contribute a burning idea by saying "before we move on to....did anyone talk about something that we have not yet mentioned?"

Equipment/resources needed

Moveable chairs help a lot. Otherwise the main resources are in the preparation – having suitable questions or exercises ready in advance. In addition, group sorting methods can be used to energise a group where an important discussion point develops, but which the educator has not anticipated. For example, in a discussion about screening, the group might start to consider ethical issues, or cost effectiveness or failures of screening, in an unanticipated way. Picking such questions up and running with them keeps energy flowing and links the education to what participants are currently ready to learn.

Skills to make this work even better

Having good questions or exercises for the group tasks is key. Plan beforehand (See ENERGISE Using questions effectively) and reflect afterwards on how well the trigger question or task worked. It has worked well if there is a good buzz of discussion, when the debrief raises lots of issues, or if the topic chosen is ignored because the units say something like "we actually found that the key question for us was....instead". That outcome is very helpful; groups often become disengaged (necessitating the use of smaller buzz groups!) when the content is drifting too far away from what they themselves are principally concerned about.

When a new issue of concern is identified (usually during ENGAGE Assessing learning needs at the outset, but sometimes only arising during the session), the educator has choices about what to do with the digression.

The educator can:

- pick up the issue (and redirect part of the session)
- park the issue in their minds, coming back to it later in the session where it will more naturally be covered
- put the issue in context, and signal another part of the session or programme when that issue will be covered.

Keen consultation skills buffs will note that these are the exact same skills that are needed when picking up cues during consultations; cues can be picked up immediately, or, parked and returned to later in the consultation, or used by the consulter to create part of a whole context or picture that helps the understand the patient more fully. Consultation skills and education skills have a lot of common ground.

If there is more than one educator available, rotating between the groups can be helpful. Involving an outside speaker in small group discussions can be very fruitful – ensure that they rotate to all the groups if possible so that everyone gets to discuss things with the visitor.

Pitfalls/when NOT to use this method

It is relatively difficult to form small groups of six to eight if there is fixed lecture theatre style seating, if the room is very crowded or cramped, if the group is not working together over a period of time or if time is very short. In those situations smaller buzz groups of two to four members are feasible to organise and may generate better discussion.

If you really want to get smaller units working in a difficult room then plan the seating arrangements you are going to use in advance (which saves time in the session) as it may be possible still to use the room in a different way.

Be careful to set a realistic and clear task. It is easy to end up being vague or asking several questions (better to say "What options can you come up with for working with the family in this case" than "this is a difficult one, what shall we do? Who might get involved? Anyone had any experience or got any ideas"). Multiple tasks or questions lead to confusion.

Timings need attention; plan in advance how much time a task is likely to need. Pairs will usually finish in under 10 minutes, fours up to 15 minutes if the task is complex. Listen to the sound of the whole room; if it goes quieter it is probably time to debrief. If there is a lot of laughter/cross talk/people all talking at once, it may mean the group has gone way off task and needs debrief time.

Small groups of six to eight can work well for anything between 15 to 30 minutes as part of a session (although small groups of six to eight participants can work well for up to 90 minutes if they have a skilful facilitation, usually from an educator).

Applications in other areas of the session

Breaking into smaller units can be done more than once during a single session to explore different aspects of the topic. If there is more than one educator, then groups of six to eight can be formally facilitated. If not, ask the sub group to designate a chair/rapporteur if needed.

How does this help to build relationships?

By mixing up the participants into different subgroups, they get opportunities to work, and build relationships, with a larger number of participants/colleagues. Anyone who dominates the group or is difficult to work with is also "diluted "by this approach, which makes others less likely to become irritated. Quieter members value the opportunity to contribute, feel more valued and become more likely to contribute to whole group discussion.

How does this help to structure the education?

This approach provides excellent "punctuation" through a session, keeps it moving, ensures that all participants get a chance to positively contribute and makes for lively sessions that are more memorable.

5// REFLECTING ON SOMETHING GOOD

Sometimes, groups benefit from time to cherish what is going well for them

What it is for?

This method is useful to re energise a group who may know each other to some extent, or who work together, in times of stress, or at the start of a new section of training. The aim is to express positive appreciation for what each person brings to the group. This can be used in a similar way to energise an MDT or practice team too and can have very positive effects on general morale.

When to use it

At the start of the session or day programme, to create "positive energy" in the group.

The set up: how to use this method

Give everyone a piece of paper and ask them to write their name on it. Put all the papers into a bowl or hat. Explain that people will be chosen at random, taking turns. The educator/facilitator should demonstrate what to do by picking one paper at random and saying: "I have got Jane; Jane I notice that you bring these three things to the team (for example, always on time, enthusiasm, friendly to those who join.)"

Finish by saying: "Thanks for bringing those things to the team Jane, I appreciate that."

Then Jane picks a name out of the hat and does the same until everyone has had a one minute praising (as the One Minute Manager calls it! See Reference 1).

Explanations/timings

Take one to two minutes per person

The debrief: maximising the benefits

This may not need much of a debrief except to say it is good to be appreciated, or what a lot of strengths we have in this team, how did it feel to realise that you were appreciated? and so on.

Equipment/resources needed

Paper and a "hat"

Skills to make this work even better

Model the appreciation at the start carefully. Include three things, be specific (you are so helpful whenever I need to get a room set up for a meeting rather than "you are nice") and ask participants to follow the same pattern.

An alternative approach is to ask people individually to spend a few moments reflecting on something that went well at work in the last few weeks. Then ask them to stand up, walk around the room and find a partner to share the thing that was good at work. Ask them to talk to two or three people depending on the time available. When stress levels high or morale low it can be amazingly fruitful to focus on a few things that actually were rewarding, effective or enjoyable.

Pitfalls/when NOT to use this method

Participants probably need to know each other a bit before doing this so that they can contribute in a way that has meaning and is not superficial. If the group are very unfamiliar with each other the alternative version may work better.

Applications in other areas of the session

A similar approach can be used in a team building session: What has been good so far today? What have you appreciated about what your colleagues brought to the discussions. Use as an alternative to this method at the start, not as a repetition.

How does this help to build relationships?

Everyone loves to feel appreciated; discovering what people recognise and appreciate about each other can do wonders for building relationships. Actually taking time to praise someone can help to reframe a negative view, and put a relationship on a better footing, with negative feelings becoming less prioritised. Within a team, knowing that people appreciate and value each other's contributions, is a very powerful motivator.

How does this help to structure the education?

Having a good starting exercise helps to give the session structure and kicks it off to an energised start.

References

1. *The One Minute Manager Builds High Performing Teams,* Ken Blanchard, ISBN 978-0007105809. The *One Minute Manager* Series are very useful brief books covering many aspects of management and teamwork. Well worth a look.

6// BUZZ GROUPS

Getting a good "buzz" in the room can raise energy levels quickly.

What it is for?

This method enables every person in the room to participate and contribute, even if they are not comfortable speaking in front of a large group or if they usually prefer to listen. The method has been described in ENGAGE Buzz groups. However, buzz group can be excellent energisers within sessions and that is what is described here.

When to use it

Plan ahead and decide at which point in the session to use buzz groups. This can be at the start as part of a general orientation, or at points in the session when new material is introduced or the focus changes to a different aspect of the session.

The set up: how to use this method

Use a suitable group sorting method (see ENERGISE Group sorting methods). Ask the participants to divide into pairs or groups of three to discuss a specific issue or question. The key to successful participation in a buzz group is to ensure that the issue the group is asked to consider is posed in a way that will always generate more than a simple answer. Questions are better if both open (i.e. that cannot be answered with a simple yes or no) and also clear and specific. Question that begin with How? How many? What difficulties come up when …? What approaches …? are all useful. Statements can also be used. For example, "tell your partner about how a problem is managed in your department."

Explanations/timings

As the question is to be succinct and short, the set up takes a very short time. Work out how long the Buzz groups will need to discuss the issue. Buzz groups are usually best if kept short say three to ten minutes depending on the topic) as otherwise they tend to drift off topic.

The debrief: maximising the benefits

Observe the group and stop the discussion when the room starts to go quiet or if there is a lot of laughter (usually a sign of going off topic) or if its clear participants are changing the subject.

It is usually best not ask groups to simply describe/feedback their answers to the initial question. It is helpful to "generalise away" from individuals specific experiences and so the debrief question should be of the form "what themes are emerging?" or "what issues are coming up". It can be useful to have a second person (another educator or a group member) to record the themes on a flip chart or similar. It is likely that many groups will come up with similar ideas, so before debriefing, use a question such as "have people come up with some ideas that are not yet recorded?"

Be alert to any non-verbal signs that quieter people have something to contribute and encourage them to speak. Continue until no new themes emerge. If it seems that there is more to come but people are wary, ask "did anyone's **partner** have an especially interesting idea that has not been mentioned yet?"

Sometimes people are more willing to speak about ideas they have heard (not their own) or if they know the person they were working with is quiet. This method still highlights the owner of the idea without exposing them too much.

The length and detail of the debrief needed will depend on the complexity or sensitivity of the issues and whether the group is being used to work on specific material or more as an energiser/warm up. Educators need to make a judgement about what is right for the particular circumstances.

Use phrases like "anything else, what else came up, what did other people talk about?" to ensure that as many buzz groups as possible feed into the general discussion. If there are very dominating members who talk all the time consider using a "talking stick" methods, (see ENGAGE Talking sticks) or invite contributions saying "There was a lot of discussion, so I will ask you once you have contributed to stay quiet until other people have made their contributions".

Equipment/resources needed

None

Skills to make this work even better

Thank each contributor, be accepting of what they say and be encouraging about what participants are talking about. Questions like "did anything unexpected come up?" or "before we move on are there any final thoughts that came up" can often pave the way for interesting and useful contributions to emerge.

Pitfalls/when NOT to use this method

In very large groups or conferences it can be used to engage people, but it is not really possible to have a group debrief if numbers are very large. Sometimes if there are odd numbers of people someone ends up alone; the educator should be alert to this and find them a partner or create a group of three as soon as possible, to ensure all can participate. If used at the start of a session, people coming in late may also find themselves confused about what to do and the educator will need to act quickly to get them incorporated into a small group to start work immediately.

This method is not helpful if there is likely to be complete consensus or agreement about the subject matter (e.g. is it wrong to shout at colleagues?) because this will not generate any discussion or new ideas. Hence, closed questions should be avoided. Leading questions are best avoided too, as it can make participants feel manipulated. If the issue is workplace behaviour a better question would be "how do some colleagues end up feeling so angry they get aggressive? Or "Could we propose some expectations about how colleagues speak to each other, even if they are upset?"

Applications in other areas of the session

This is a very useful technique to "wake up" a group that is getting bored, disengaged or where there has been too much contribution from one or two speakers. It ensures that everyone gets to participate. Sometimes the buzz groups resist the question posed and say something like "we felt X was more important". This is a valuable contribution to assessing where the group are at in terms of their current learning needs; see this kind of thing as a further opportunity to explore or to link concerns to the topic appropriately.

How does this help to build relationships?

Having a one to one discussion of an important questions opens up areas for discussion, may allow difficulties to be aired safely and encourages the participants to see each other as collaborators in learning. Mixing the group up helps to establish a sense that everyone can talk to everyone, that everyone has a contribution to make and that everyone "belongs". This can have good effects on adherence to learning and possibly to differential attainment.

How does this help to structure the education?

Buzz groups are a useful way to punctuate a session with active participation. Planning the buzz group questions ahead of time (even if some are also spontaneously generated on the day by the content or discussions) can help educators plan and focus the rhythm and structure of the session, so that is lively and moving onwards. A buzz group can be used as useful signposting of the need to summarise the impact of what has been discussed so far, to signal a change of emphasis or change of topic, or to lead into a new contribution from an invited speaker or a new group exercise.

7// MAKING A LEARNING SUMMARY FOR SHARING WITH THE GROUP

Recording a summary of the learning from a session can help to energise participants.

What it is for?

This is a method to help energise one or two members of the group by asking them to make a summary of the session's learning to share with the whole group afterwards (either by email, WhatsApp or by placing it on a shared drive, Virtual Leaning Centre or similar arrangement). If one person is designated to do this, a summary of the days learning suffices. If two people are involved ask the second participant to identify how the learning relates to the curriculum, to defined competencies and record that too.

This helps to familiarise participants with the curriculum and also reinforces learning; the person doing the summary pays extra attention and the group receiving the follow up email get a succinct summary of learning. Sometimes, the scribe "learns" different things from a session compared to their peers; this is also a useful outcome because on receiving the summary a participant can then reflect in their portfolio entry about what they thought the crucial learning was for themselves. This deepens reflection for all participants.

When to use it

It is particularly helpful to use this method in the initial phases of a Study Release Course because it helps to reinforce participation and active learning when participants know they may be asked to summarise at the end. By providing a summary that can be readily imported into the ePortfolio for reflection, it both reinforces the role of the ePortfolio as a record of learning, and creates easy opportunities for reflection. Having a second person linking learning to the competencies helps the participants to be familiar with what the competencies entail and will help them identify relevant learning in other situations.

This is also a useful technique for encouraging reporting back of useful learning when participants have attended conferences, meetings or have used other learning methods.

The set up: how to use this method

Explain to the whole group that one person will be asked to summarise the session's learning points to be circulated afterwards, and optionally, that a second person will be linking this learning to a Competency framework as defined by the relevant Royal College. Emphasise that the summary needs only to be one or two paragraphs long – a summary not a repetition. You can designate the rapporteur at the end of the session (which may increase the energy levels of all concerned if they know anyone may be called upon to do this) or choose someone at the start.

This is not a task for volunteers; everyone in the group should systematically take turns to do this for the benefit of themselves and others. It is probably worth designating a stronger learner to do the first few of these as this "sets the tone and standard". Keep a register of who has been doing this to ensure everyone gets a chance. Sell it to the group for the benefits to the rapporteur (they will pay more attention, learn more and automatically have a good ePortfolio entry), and the benefits to the group (they do not need to make notes, they will have something easily imported into their own ePortfolio for reflecting on). Furthermore, this will be linked to the relevant competency, so it will make gathering evidence for their ARPC panel very much easier.

Explanations/timings

A few minutes is needed at the start of the term to explain this process. Thereafter, it is merely a matter of agreeing who is to produce the summary for that session.

The debrief: maximising the benefits

If someone is designated to linking learning to the competency framework, ask them to summarise which competencies they think were involved at the end of the session and suggest participants note those to inform their reflections in their portfolio entries.

At the end of the session reinforce to the rapporteur that they should send the summary to the administrator for dissemination by the end of the same working day. This reinforces that this is a quick summary not a huge essay. It also offers opportunities to practice good time management by "doing todays work today".

Equipment/resources needed

Paper, pens and access to group email, which is readily dealt with by the course administrator. It can be useful to give the person identifying competencies a copy of the relevant competency framework.

If the session is very clearly about one particular competency (for example, a session mainly developing competency in ethics) then give the competence rapporteur a page with the word picture descriptors on. Then ask them to highlight which areas have been covered (almost like a bingo card). This can also be photographed and sent with the summary email or shared on a group such as WhatsApp, or similar.

Skills to make this work even better

The benefits of the summary process will be greater if the educator is included in the email and gives feedback on the summary, adding any competency links that may not have been identified. The feedback should be SMART*, of course, and could relate to accuracy/succinctness/brevity and to any important learning points included or left out.

*Specific, Measurable, Achievable, Realistic, Timely

Pitfalls/when NOT to use this method

This method is less helpful for participants who do not work together regularly, who are not connected by some kind of group email or chat, or who are not needing to provide evidence of learning in an ePortfolio (for example a training session for a practice team). In that latter case, summarising learning at the end of the session with the whole group, or reviewing expressed learning needs at the end, will also be good ways to reinforce learning. Participants, who wish to, can then use that summary for their appraisal evidence.

Applications in other areas of the session

If an unexpected learning point arises, or if the group respond strongly in some way to particular experience in the group, it may be worth specifically asking the rapporteur to note that for people to reflect on afterwards.

How does this help to build relationships?

Being the rapporteur for the group emphasises that membership of the group brings responsibilities to other participants. Effective learning is not an individual isolated process; it also requires debate, sharing and the active collaboration of others. Receiving the summary is a kind of "gift" from the session that helps people to remain connected with each other afterwards. This is supportive in its own right: involvement in quality CPD is one of the crucial ways to avoid burnout.

Anyone absent from a session for any reason automatically gets included in the follow up summary, which keeps them connected to their group, and to the learning they may have missed.

Providing even brief feedback connects the educator to the individuals of the group, which reinforces their sense that their learning is of direct concern to that educator. The experience of being personally noticed and valued, builds a strong relationship and increases engagement with the learning.

How does this help to structure the education?

Learning summaries demonstrate how learning builds over time. Identifying the competency that has been covered links education to the curriculum and assessment processes. This should help participants to understand the links between formal learning, the membership examinations of their Royal College, and the application of learning to daily practice.

Appendix

One example of a learning summary from a session. What feedback would you give as an educator to the writer?

Sandra Johnson

From: Scott Ellis
To: Consultation skills learning group
Subject: Learning summary – 16/11/18

SUBJECTS

1) Upcoming events
2) Time management; introduction
3) Triadic Consultation skills

1) LOOKING FORWARD

CSA mock. Everyone needs a trainer, actor and a case (dates 11, 12th January). We have all been allocated case topics and have to create our own cases with our trainer to bring to the mock for others to act out.

2) INTRODUCTION TO TIME MANAGEMENT

Medical leadership – we are all leaders – self-awareness, self-management, self-development, acting with integrity. We talked about time bandits – what some of these were in our lives and the work life balance – should be more like a dove tail than an unbalanced seesaw. Made a chart to show work day – most of this taken up by sleep and work. Talked a lot about time management and wrote down what we need to do to pass the year. Discussed difference between importance and urgency. Talked about importance in terms of how importance is related to having a policy, strategy and operations/tasks. Talked about multi-tasking – is it possible?

New concept: the concept of bang a nasty job off at once, in a bid to reduce stress levels – acronym BANJO!

3) TRIADIC CONSULTATIONS

Talked about triadic consultations, the difficulties - focused on triadic consultations particularly focused on children presenting with their parents at any age ('children' from the age of 16 up to 25 for example) ; importance of setting up the room, having a structure, how to involve both people . More about triadic consultations - both parties perspectives need to be explored and accepted. Consider seeing the parties separately - talked about techniques of how to speak to one party, e.g. adolescent on their own to see if they want further follow up by themselves (if appropriate).Need to be mindful when discussing examination options in a triadic consultation; is the patient happy for their relative/friend/cater to be in the room? Advantages of the third person is that they can act as a 'chaperone'.

Talked about triadic consults with regards to Interpreters and how to transfer interaction between the interpreter and patient (explored difficulty in having non-professional interpreter e.g. relative). W/r to CSA – aim for "toward child behaviours", i.e. involving the child explicitly. Often child not in room in examination scenario, could be spouses come together – may be talking about drinking, still need the triadic skills for effectiveness.

8// USING LINE UPS TO EXPLORE IDEAS

Line-ups are a good way to engage activist learners (See ENRICH Using learning styles) near the start of the session, while also allowing learners with other styles to participate.

What it is for?

Line-ups can be used as simple energisers (see ENERGISE Quick energisers). However, the line-up technique can be used in much more nuanced ways, to support the delivery of the formal content of the session, and to explore the ways in which participants understanding of ideas changes over time.

For example, participants could be asked to line-up with one side of the room being designated as "I have never given any personal information about myself to a patient, in any circumstances whatsoever, except for my name and GMC number"; the opposite side being "I have shared personal information with patients, would give selected patients my personal mobile number and would happily share my own experiences of illness or mental health issues if it was relevant to that patient." The middle might be "I have shared occasional experiences with patients and the practice website includes information about my non-work life".

Participants line up on a continuum, discussing with people on either side of them whether there are some personal things they would share (which? And in what circumstances?).

When to use it

This method is useful at the start of sessions exploring subjects that require critical appraisal of ideas from participants,(see the section on critical appraisal of tests and investigations in RESOURCES, below) and at intervals during that session. The method can also be used when exploring responses to potentially controversial material, where the range of opinions is wide and where learning may be expected to develop participants' attitudes and values over time. The method can also be used to trigger debate amongst participants when they realise that other people do not have the same approach as they do themselves. While at one level it may seem very obvious that people hold different opinions: in practice, many participants are surprised to find that other members of the group have different beliefs and behaviours to themselves, even in common clinical situations. Further examples are given below in Resources, which will make this clearer.

The set up: how to use this method

As in most situations, the initial set up, and the subject for the line-up need to be carefully chosen by the educator, so that the maximum rage of responses is elicited, so that the potential for discussion, debate and attitudinal change is maximised.

Explanations/timings

Explaining the line-up subject should take less than a minute if the issue has been prepared by the educator in advance, with two opposing statements, represented by the extreme ends of the line-up. Explain the issue and that you are asking them to line up so that the range of views in the room will be seen, so that participants can learn about different views and ideas.

Allow a few minutes for participants to discuss their positions and to change their positions as they realise that they may need to be towards one end or another.

The debrief: maximising the benefits

When the talking has died down and the line-up appears relatively stable, stop the talk and make a general summarising comment about how participants have distributed themselves.

Invite participants to comment on how they came to choose their position. ("How" questions are often more comfortable and easier to answer than "why" questions). Educators can either wait for volunteers or use the "pose, pause, pounce, bounce" approach (see ENERGISE Using questions effectively).

Use an accepting approach, thank participants for their contribution and accepting their views in a non-judgemental way. Initially, aim for the widest number of views (using easy access questions).

Then, commenting on the range of views can lead into the specific content of the session. In the case suggested above the introductory line up about how much personal information patients can share about the clinician, could be the introduction to a session on fitness to practice and integrity, or to the subject of how clinicians manage their own personal health issues, or to a session on how clinicians should behave in respect of social media.

Equipment/resources needed

Space to move around in is ideal. Most rooms will allow this as even in a formal layout there will be room in the aisle or across the front or back of the room.

Skills to make this work even better

Debriefing can go beyond a simple exploration of the spread of ideas, although that, in itself, can be extremely revealing and helpful. Educators can increase the challenge of follow up questions by asking participants to pair up with someone whose view seems different/ furthest from their own.

Ask the pairs to discuss their views. A range of possible trigger questions can be used here as long as they are open questions that allow exploration of the issues.

Examples of follow up questions could include:

- **"What if?"** What if you were working in a small town? (to the participants who would never share any information) What if your health problems included drug abuse? (to the participants who would share freely).
- **"How would you justify your position?"** Explain to your partner what justifies your position on this topic. Extend by saying: "How would you justify a more/less flexible approach?"
- **"What implications does your position have for the place you work in?"**
- **"What evidence would make you change to a different position?"**

Pitfalls/when NOT to use this method

This method is not likely to be helpful in a highly formalised educational setting, where participants do not know or trust each other. Exercises like this benefit from the structured introductions and engagement processes outlined in the ENGAGE section. In a large auditorium, participants could be asked to do a thought experiment, where they mentally choose a position for themselves at the start (ask them to write down a number from one to ten to indicate their preference), repeating the exercise at the end, to see whether new information changes positions.

While this is a very useful technique, as with all methods, variety is the key. Be sparing and deliberate about using line-ups and they will maintain their effectiveness and interest.

Applications in other areas of the session

Repeating a line up at the end of the session using the same question could give participants the opportunity to enact any changes in their positions. Using line-up more than once during a session could also be used to illuminate positions on different but related questions. In the example above, a follow up issue might be at one extreme "I never post any photos of myself on social media and I have deleted my Facebook account", with the other extreme being "I maintain lots of social media accounts, and only mention work/patients in disguised ways".

How does this help to build relationships?

Participants learn to appreciate that there are a wide range of approaches to many issues, and that a variety of positions can be justified. In discussing the follow up questions, participants are invited to enter into the thinking of another person, and share their own thinking. This builds relationships between participants. When ideas are shared with the group, the educator, modelling accepting, non-judgemental attitudes, also builds participant educator relationships.

How does this help to structure the education?

Using line-ups as punctuation helps to give the session pace and structure, making it more interesting and helping to maintain engagement throughout.

Resources

Here are some examples of ways that line-ups can be used to deepen engagement with specific subject matter. Educators can easily develop their own examples when familiar with the technique.

In a session on end of life care or assisted dying; the two extremes could be:

- "If there was a legal, properly set up "Dignitas" type service in this area, I would be willing to participate as one of the clinicians"
- "I would never do anything, whatsoever, to hasten a person's death."

In sessions discussing professional development and career aims; the two extremes could be:

- "I am a clinician and I don't want to be burdened with administration and management, I should spend all my time looking after patients".

  "Organisation influences how well the service works for patients; I want to be fully involved in ensuring it works well. I can learn new skills if needed".
- "Care should be provided on the basis of need not ability to pay the costs, so I want no part in private medical care at all".

  "Why shouldn't I gain if people have money to spend on their health? I am happy to seek out lucrative private practice opportunities".

  "A clinician's duty is to do everything possible for patients and I expect to work pretty hard, staying late at times".

  "A clinician's first duty is to themselves and their families and they never work beyond their allotted time."

Another way to use a line-up is to illustrate "Normality" as a concept when the subject is critical appraisal of tests and investigations.

When using a line-up in this way, the aim is to demonstrate how, although participants may all be considered "normal", some of their characteristics will inevitably put them at the extreme of a Bell Curve. Ask participants to line up several times, changing the issue each time in a way that may be expected to differentiate people in different ways. Give the participant at the extreme ends of the range a card, with a red exclamation mark on, to illustrate that they are an "Abnormal outlier".

Here are some examples of issues that will spread the participants out:

- Line up in order of height – tallest this end, shortest that end.
- Line up in order of birth month – January at this end, December at that end.
- Line up in order of the date of your birth in the month (i.e. one for the first, two for the second, etc.)
- Line up with those of you who cannot sing and feel singing solo in public is a form of torture here.
  At the other end those who love singing and actually have a gig coming up soon!
- Line up in order of how many educational establishments you studied at between the ages of three and 23.
- Line up in order of those who like their food as spicy and hot as possible at one end, and those who prefer unspiced, creamy, mild foods at the other.

After a few rounds, it will become apparent that if you go on long enough, everyone will attract a red exclamation card for something. Most test results give a normal range which is defined as two standard deviations from the mean. It will be clear that in some respect or another, everyone who is normal will none the less be at the extreme end of some kind of bell curve. It follows for this that if we do enough blood tests, even a *normal* person will probably have at least one *abnormal* result. Demonstrate this so that participants can develop their understanding of what tests and investigations actually mean. This can illustrate the potential harm of over investigation, finding and chasing irrelevant results that are in fact, arising by chance.

For most tests, about five per cent of people who are normal will lie outside the two standard deviation range, i.e. if there are 20 tests done, one would be abnormal entirely by chance. This also explains "reversion to the mean" if the same test is repeated several times.

9// CREATING ACTION LEARNING SETS

Giving participants the opportunity to work in self-facilitated small groups can galvanise learning and develop useful skills for working together effectively.

What it is for?

Giving participants the opportunity to work in self-facilitated small groups can galvanise learning and develop useful skills for working together effectively.

Dividing groups into smaller Action Learning Sets method can achieve several objectives.

- Participants learn the skills of self-facilitated learning in groups, so that they can continue to educate themselves in the longer term – small group work, often problem-based study, seems to generate Continued Professional Development of the highest quality. Working in such groups is a good protection against burnout.
- It is a way of using educator resources more efficiently.
- It is a way to engage and energise participants to do educational activities at times when formal educational events such as study release courses are not running.

When to use it

Action learning sets are small sub groups of the total participant group, meeting without an educator, facilitating themselves. Such groups work best when they can meet over a period of time, with the same participants. So they need to be set up when there is a realistic possibility of the participants still being in continuing training for the duration of the group. The total duration of the group will depend on its purpose and practical arrangements; it should be at least three or four meetings, but could meet weekly for up to a year, within a training programme. Some groups, which initially start during formal training programmes, develop into long-term CPD groups that may continue to meet after the end of the formal training programme. Such groups, may provide education and developmental support to their members for years after they were initially set up. The educator can approach organising such groups so that they are well prepared for this way of working: as the effects may last for many years on occasions, this is a very effective use of educator time.

Setting up learning sets at the start of ST3 (in General Practice) provides excellent opportunities for self-directed learning skills to develop, for supportive groups to form and for educators to use their time effectively. The same method could be used at other stages of training.

The set up: how to use this method

Before setting up action learning sets, participants need to be aware of and have skills in participating in small groups. Thus, previous training exercises in how to run a group are essential. This will normally be experiential learning (for example a Survival task with focussed debrief about the teamwork skills required) and highlight the need for everyone to take responsibility for chairing functions, timekeeping, scribing, keeping on the task, or for those roles to be specifically rotated around all members of the group.

Allocation of the members of the group should be done by the educators(s) aiming for a mix of strengths, a mix of personalities, a mix of learning styles and a mix of abilities. Try to avoid having people who just "sit with their friends". This makes for a less rich learning experience and is not overall beneficial. Thus, do not encourage groups to self-select.

The **meeting location and time** should be

agreed in advance with the educator if it is to form part of a Study Release Course. Remind members that ST educational time is *paid work* and should be completed with the same punctuality, attendance, diligence and quality as other work they are paid to do.

Explanations/timings

Group work should be prepared, using the EWAP approach (see ENAGAGE Everything with a purpose) having a mixture of methods of working. This could include some quizzes, case discussions, preparation of an audit or protocol, working through partnership issues in a "virtual practice", or ethical discussions. The range is huge. Time should also be allowed for participants to share experiences, work on examination related material and provide support to each other.

If action learning sets are created as part of Study Release Programme, allow about two hours for the action learning set to meet so that there is also time for writing up and ePortfolio entries to be completed.

The debrief: maximising the benefits

A chair and a scribe should be identified each week and the scribe asked to produce a one page summary of learning to be circulated to whole group, not just their smaller unit, so that learning is shared and stronger, more detailed work is highlighted to the whole group. The educator can allocating the chair and scribe, so that that all members get experience of these roles, and the same people do not do everything. Highlight that the purpose of this is so that participants will be well prepared for taking chairing and reporting roles in the professional teams they will be involved with after training. Encourage them to ask for opportunities to practice chairing meetings while they are still in training and get feedback. The chair of the action learning set should be encouraged to seek feedback from the group. A suitable feedback proforma is under Resources (page 30).

Equipment/resources needed

Some "trigger" prepared work should normally be allocated, although as groups become more skilled there is the option to encourage them to devise and deliver their own learning, simply reporting back what they are doing. Adult learners will also naturally use the time to share experiences, talk through difficulties and support each other.

Skills to make this work even better

Link the trigger learning materials (examples given below) to the competency framework. This helps to guide planning, so that the purpose of the work is made explicit to participants and so that participants are assisted to write appropriate portfolio entries. In turn, good portfolio entries are useful, so that trainers to link the competencies to entries, so that preparation for ARPC panels is easier and quicker.

Take feedback on the work set:

- Is it too little or too superficial?
- Too much?
- Does it provoke thought?

(See the EVALUATE section for more details on how to evaluate education).

It can be helpful to set work as an unfolding story, where the group need to respond differently as different information becomes available. Ask the chair to take responsibility for working through this. Start with easy access, low challenge material, so that all can readily engage, and then use Bloom's taxonomy (see ENRICH Using taxonomies of learning) in preparing subsequent work so that the challenge increases and addresses higher order skills such analysis, evaluation or critical appraisal.

Educators may want to consider having some formal facilitation at the initial sessions (perhaps using a trainer or "GP scholar" (see ENRICH GP scholars) so that the group can be guided towards using more effective team/group work methods.

Encourage groups/scholars to report and discuss any group work problems (for example disruptive or non-attending members). Emphasising and giving experience of the need for effective facilitation/chairing, and making the group roles both explicit and allocated, tends to make the work effective. Such roles could be confined to Facilitator/Chair, and Scribe. Ask groups to consider whether they would also benefit from sharing the functions of timekeeper, quality checker (are we getting deep enough here?), group representative (to report concerns or difficulties), someone to manage any resources, task manager (are we on track?) or social secretary.

Pitfalls/when NOT to use this method

This works when groups can reasonably be expected to work together over time, building their relationships and their skills together. It is not really suitable for one off sessions.

Applications in other areas of the session

N/A

How does this help to build relationships?

If sub-groups are well set up in the action learning set activities, learning relationships deepen and develop to a high level. Often such groups will continue doing CPD together after the Course itself has finished, which offers lifelong learning opportunities.

How does this help to structure the education?

The nature, difficulty and content of the work can be varied through the year, starting with clinical issues perhaps, and moving on to more complex areas such as partnership matters, developing resilience, ethics and can include challenges such as preparing an educational session for other people.

RESOURCES

Here are some examples of ways for the chair to get feedback on their skills.

1. Action learning sets /chairperson's feedback

Each week the small group will have some tasks and a designated chair and scribe. This is to help you learn how to work in a group or team and to practice teamwork skills in a supportive environment. Each week one person will give feedback to the chair using this sheet as a guide. The chairs job (supported by everyone in the group who will also need to use some chairing skills) is to:

- **Unite** the group
- **Focus** the group on the task (and helping the whole group to work together effectively)
- **Mobilise** the group to do the things needed (on time, complete the business, make decisions where needed)

UNITING THE GROUP. Did the Chair start the meeting clearly?

Did the chair encourage everyone to introduce themselves and role (if needed) or bring them together in some other way (e.g. " everyone say how their week was, or one good thing at work or one difficult thing") .Did the chair ensure everyone knew what they were there for?

Feedback for this week's chair. What did you notice them doing that helped this process?

FOCUSING THE GROUP. Did the chair focus everyone's attention on the task?

Introducing the agenda, checking for any other agenda items that people wanted to discuss, setting out broad timescales. Did the chair focus everyone's attention on the process? Did the chair ensure that quieter members were also able to contribute and that they were on board? That the process of how to do the task was agreed by everyone, not necessarily decided by the chair but agreed together?

Feedback for this week's chair. What did you notice them doing that helped this process?

MOBILISING THE GROUP. Did the chair help the group to get the task done?

Ensuring everyone contributed, encouraging quieter people to contribute, helping noisier people to listen to what others have to say?

Feedback for this week's chair. What did you notice them doing that helped this process?

Write some suggestions for how they could improve their chairing skills.

2. An Example of work for an Action Learning Set in General Practice training

Here is an unfolding story, starting with some clinical issues around learning disability, and deepening to discuss safeguarding and ethical concerns. As you read it consider how you, as an educator, would explain the purpose of the work and what competencies are being explored. Participants can find that such evolving stories are memorable, and trigger deeper reflections than any web based or textbook learning. The notes in ***italics*** show how the different elements are structured to cover different levels of learning. This covers the GP curriculum statement concerning The Care of Patients with Learning Disabilities and the competencies include Data Gathering and Interpretation, Holistic Care, Working with Colleagues and in Teams, Clinical Management and Maintaining an Ethical Approach.

Learning disabilities Group work

Chair to read out these details of press release.

Carers who worked closely with James Hughes, the disabled man whose decomposing and emaciated body was found crammed into a suitcase in the garden of the family home, today told how they had been taken in by his mother's "lies".

When Hughes, who was 21 but had the mental age of a toddler, stopped attending two care centres, his carers accepted the explanations given by his mother, that he was with other relative Once, she said he could not attend because he had a piece of popcorn stuck in his gums.

On the second day of the inquest into his death, it emerged that James had not attended one centre for six months and a second for five at the time his body, weighing just 28.6kg (4st 2lb) and dressed only in a nappy, was found. It was also revealed that, despite needing constant care, James did not have his own social worker at the time of his death.

Yesterday, a doctor at his local surgery admitted he had "slipped through the net".

James's death came to light only after his mother had gone missing She was found hanged in undergrowth nearby, police then discovered James corpse, wrapped in a sheet and quilt, in a suitcase in the garden.

This morning, his one-to-one carer at the Church View respite centre, which Hughes attended twice a week, said he was "adorable", She said she noticed last autumn that he was losing weight. The centre contacted his mother to express concerns about his health, but his attendance "dwindled". When she went to James's home to give him his Christmas present, Wardle shut the door on her. Wardle continued to make "plausible" excuses as to why Hughes would not be attending the centre.

The inquest has been told that James had a rare genetic condition called ring 22 chromosome. He could not speak and had epilepsy. He wore nappies because he was doubly incontinent, tried to eat almost everything he could grab, and often kept the whole household up all night with extremely disturbed behaviour in his room. Wardle had "doted" on James but, as his main carer, was always tired. She was worried about debts, the threat of losing her home and the possibility of her relationship breaking up.

She was on anti-depressants while drinking heavily and smoking cannabis and had told her son, Daniel: "I've had enough," the inquest heard.

The inquest has been told that James had not seen a doctor for three years before his death. His computer records were almost completely lost during a switch of systems, and he was given repeat prescriptions of a drug for epilepsy without being seen by a doctor. The drug could have been dangerous for a person as slight as James.

His GP's surgery had written to Wardle on a string of occasions asking her to attend reviews of her son's treatment. However, she did not reply and the letters were not followed up.

The inquest continues.

The events described in the press release were tragic for all concerned. James, his mother, the professionals involved. Cases like these form the background to the recommendation for an annual review of those with learning disabilities. This is especially pertinent as many patients in this group are now living much longer, developing co morbidities and complications. They may live in a great variety of circumstances; at home, in assisted living centres, in supported lodgings, group homes, residential homes or flats.

Part one

List the interactions that James and his mother had or could have had with the practice who was looking after them.

What opportunities of improved care do each of these interactions offer? List them and clarify how these opportunities could have been enacted or missed in your own practices. How would James and his mother have been coded to highlight their need for care? How many carers are on a practice list? Where can they turn to for help?

> ***Note for educators:*** *this element roughly corresponds to Blooms level of "Knowledge" or "remembering" using words like describe, or list. These are easy access, low challenge tasks that help to get everyone on board at the start.*

Can you explain what is it like being a Carer? A person with a learning disability?

Use your smart phones or computers to have a look at some first person accounts:

https://www.mencap.org.uk/about-learning-disability/information-parents-carers-and-family/real-life-stories

http://www.healthtalk.org/peoples-experiences/disability-impairment/pam

http://www.healthtalk.org/peoples-experiences/disability-impairment/tracy

https://www.mencap.org.uk/about-learning-disability/information-parents-carers-and-family/real-life-stories/becoming-single-carer

https://www.mencap.org.uk/blog/everyone-should-have-chance-be-relationship

After you have done some browsing (individually or in pairs perhaps), debrief by summarising and sharing what you found.

> ***Note for educators:*** *this roughly corresponds to Blooms level of "Understanding" triggered by words like explain, summarise, paraphrase.*

What did you find most interesting about these accounts/ideas? Most surprising? Any thoughts about professional roles?

Part two

In the following pages you are going to have the opportunity to work through a complex case, looking at different aspects.

The patient; Grace Dowd is a 26 year old woman with Downs syndrome. She has been on your list for some years but you know little about her and she rarely consults. She appears to have been in good health. She is listed for a double appointment with you later during your surgery. The patient before her has just cancelled and the patient after her has sent a message saying she will be a "quite late" so Grace is effectively the last patient on your list today. You take the opportunity to browse her notes and prepare for the consultation.

Her address is 26 Green Street, a pleasant street of small semidetached, housing association houses near the surgery. She is on Phenytoin 100 mg four at night, and has no current or past investigations listed except her weight and height from five years ago (weight 70 kg height 5 feet 1 inch). She has no ongoing active problems apart from the entry for Down's syndrome. Minor issues have been:

- Nits
- Fungal infection of the skin
- Sports medical

What other types of information can you get from your system that may help you to prepare for Graces consultation today? What issues would you like to bring up?

> ***Note for educators:*** *this roughly corresponds to Blooms level of "Knowledge" of what the IT system can convey, with some elements of "Analysing" which uses ideas like categorise, organise outline.*

Part Three

Your records show:

- Aged 10 nits – several consultations.
- Aged 19 skin rash – treated for a fungal infection of the arm.
- Aged 22 thought to have had a fit – she went pale and fell down and was slightly twitchy according to the notes. She was started on Phenytoin in casualty. There are no other letters pertaining to this event and she has been on Phenytoin ever since.
- Aged 23 Attended for medical to ensure she was fit to attend the sports offered at her Community College. At that time she planned to do swimming and this was thought to be OK.
- Her medication is overdue for review and there are two letters to the mother asking her to be brought in for a review one in each of the preceding years.
- She is not on the learning disability register in your practice.
- Her address shows two other people on your list.
  - John Dowd, now deceased. He died suddenly last year from a sub arachnoid haemorrhage. Little other history.
  - Jane Dowd a 65 year old woman who has severe CKD and attends a local dialysis unit three times a week. The CKD is due to polycystic kidney disease.
  - Jane Dowd had an episode of severe depression after her husband's death and took an overdose. She is on Fluoxetine 40mg and Trazodone at night as well as BP drugs, sodium bicarbonate, one alphacalcidol, Diazepam to help her sleep, Vitamin B co, Thiamine, She is under investigation for a high GGT at the renal unit.

Are there any other issues you would now like to pursue?

> ***Note for educators:*** *this roughly corresponds to Blooms level of "Applying" knowledge in practice. Sometimes this takes the form of being able to ask or generate the right questions, than simply to know some answers.*

Part Four

Grace comes in with another adult holding a clipboard – this is "Maria" her carer. Grace has been living in a group home for learning disabled adults it seems, in a distant part of your practice. This happened because her Mother became too ill to care for her. Maria announces that they have come for a "routine annual medical".

- What would constitute a "routine annual medical" here?
- What important conditions may not be spontaneously presented by Grace, but would be important not to miss?

> ***Note for educators:*** *this roughly corresponds to Blooms level of "Applying" knowledge in practice.*

Grace complains of tiredness alot and likes to stay in bed as much as possible. She is settling in well at the home, enjoys attending community college twice a week to do Art and Basic Skills. Maria reports that "Barry, who is Grace's favourite staff member" says she is constipated and her tummy hurts.

On examination you find:

- Grace is a bit pale.
- She has cool extremities and has dry skin. She is rather obese BMI 37
- Her abdomen shows a possible swelling, mildly tender, on the left hand side, but Grace is very ticklish and laughs alot so it's hard to feel much.

Maria gets a call on her mobile phone during the exam and goes out to take a call. While she is out Grace says: "Glad she's gone. She won't let Barry stay in my room. We are going to get married one day and Barry says it's good to practice sex beforehand". When Maria comes in the room Grace immediately clams up and says nothing else.

What are your thoughts now and what would be your next steps?

> ***Note for educators:*** *this roughly corresponds to Blooms level of "Analysing" information and understanding the implications as well as "Evaluating" which includes ideas of interpretation and making appropriate and defensible judgements.*

Part Five

Your nurse got some blood but remarks that Grace found it extremely distressing and yelled and screamed throughout although she did remain still and co-operated. She said after that "Barry will be cross with me if he hears I have been naughty, he says I am dirty girl."

The blood tests come back:

- HB 10 MCV 77 ferritin 3
- TSH 20 T4 18
- Vitamin D level less than 15 (NR 50 to 150)
- Phenytoin level 100 (normal range for the lab is 30 to 70)

How does this link with her history and physical examination?

Outline a clear management plan for Grace.

1. Her immediate treatment.
2. Her follow up; what issues may arise here?
3. What about her psychological situation? Her social care?
4. What services locally should be involved in Grace's care?
5. How have you decided to tackle to issue of her having sex with a staff member at her home? Isn't she entitled to a relationship just like anyone else?

Note for educators: *which elements of Bloom's taxonomy are involved in these tasks?*

How could the practice improve its care for learning disabled patients? What makes these patients difficult for health care professionals to deal with? What developments in our skills or attitudes could help?

See also https://www.mencap.org.uk/PANTSCampaign

Note for educators: *this roughly corresponds to Blooms level of "Creating" which refers to ideas like design, produce, make, invent and improve.*

10// EFFECTIVE QUESTIONS FOR GROUPS

Using effective questions is a way of opening up discussion, directing it productively, focusing attention on relevant issues and can also be used to reinforce learning and aid recall.

When to use it

Effective questioning focusses discussion effectively so that the group is directed appropriately to consider important issues. Good questions are helpful in all aspects of the session; initial set up of the day, in pairs or small group exercises, in plenaries and when revising learning points at the end of the session.

Planning effective questions can happen as part of the educator's preparation. Well developed questioning skills are also valuable for educators to use opportunistically during sessions. For example, interesting issues may arise in an unplanned way, or, participants may voice unexpected concerns or difficulties. Good questions open up debate and permit deeper levels of discussion, critical appraisal and evaluation.

The set up: how to use this method

First decide your question; questions should be open (which means they cannot be answered with a single word), and create an element of uncertainty or debate within them.

Consider starting questions with a word like "Who, Where, What, How and When" so that the field is left open for discussion, yielding richer content.

Aim for "easy access, high challenge" questions, so that the question is readily understandable, so that lots of answers are generated to begin with, so that the educator can get a large **quantity** of ideas first. This makes participation easy and less intimidating to quieter group members.

Then use follow up questions to rank ideas, to prioritise ideas, to extend ideas, to test ideas in practice and even work out when they might not apply, so that the challenge of the questions are increased. This means examining **quality** of ideas after first getting a quantity of suggestions.

Increasing the challenge works well if questions start with:

- What if …? (changing a key variable like age, co-morbidity, geographical area)
- What evidence supports …?
- What are the implications of …?
- How does this link to other things we have learned about?
- How would you justify ...
  - – an opposing point of view?
  - – a more drastic approach?
  - – a more kindly approach?
  - – a more flexible approach?
- How could you use this in practice?

Explanations/timings

Use a **"Pause, Pair, Square, Share"** approach. Always allow some individual reflection time first to allow all participants to collect their thoughts, to think for themselves, ensuring that all have something to contribute.

Then ask them to discuss in pairs, deciding which ideas are then most important. The in groups of four (square) ask each pair to justify to the other pair why their ideas are valuable and important…explaining the reasoning. This exposes participants to different points of view and different thinking processes.

Weaker students learn about how stronger students think and are exposed to a greater range of ideas, while still having to think about ideas for themselves.

When inviting sharing from the smaller units to the whole group accept each contribution and thank the contributor, aiming for the maximum quantity of contributions initially. Then use more challenging questions as above to extend and explore the ideas.

The debrief: maximising the benefits

Try to simply avoiding restating the question, explore the issues that come up and follow up with questions or statements to encourage contributors to share their reasoning. This can be remembered as ABC:

- Accept and thank the contributor,
- Build their response (tell me more, any more details?)
- Challenge them to provide evidence or to summarise their position in one sentence or ten words.

Equipment/resources needed

N/A

Skills to make this work even better

Encourage the participants to write down their thoughts as they have them, even better if they have a dedicated notebook for the training sessions. This encourages commitment, creates a record of learning ideal for e Portfolios.

When debriefing in the whole group, the educator can use a "Pose, Pause, Pounce, Bounce" approach. Pose the question, Pause to allow reflection individually and then in pairs, then squares(fours). Pounce on one person to feedback and then Bounce those ideas between the other contributions. (For example, thanks for the idea that courage is required to go and see a dying patient, anyone got other thoughts?")

Before starting the discussion, explain that you will be stopping from time to time to summarise what has been said and that participants should record key points and who said them as they go along.

Use questions like:

- What made you think the most?
- Who had the best evidence for their point of view?
- What contribution was most similar to your own?
- Who do you agree with most?
- Who would you still like to hear from?

This approach allows quieter and introverted participants to actively participate much more, and reinforces the points raised.

Finish with a statement like: "Write down ten words to sum up what you have learned/taken away from this discussion."

Pitfalls/when NOT to use this method

Probably not for very large groups in lecture type situations – these are rare in ST training but occasionally occur in conferences, etc.

Applications in other areas of the session

The think, pair, square, share approach can be used to trigger discussion or to consider application of learning at different stages of the session and can provide useful recap and reinforcement of learning too (See EVALUATION).

How does this help to build relationships?

This method of learning is collaborative so that participants find themselves learning and sharing their knowledge in the same session. Hearing good ideas from peers is often more powerful than hearing the same ideas seemingly dictated from a senior.

How does this help to structure the education?

This approach provides an excellent way to structure learning into smaller component parts, providing pace and changes of tempo through the session.

Resources

For more details see *The Really Lazy Teachers Handbook* by Jim Smith.

11// IDENTIFYING TEAM AND GROUP SKILLS USING A SURVIVAL EXERCISE

We do not usually face the challenge of a plane crash, shipwreck or being lost in a desert; yet a simulation exercise considering how to survive is a good way to energise a group and orientate them to the skills of effective teamwork.

What it is for?

This method is used as a way of energising groups to really think hard about what is required for effective teamwork, or effective education in smaller groups. Everyone works in teams and recognises the effective and less effective team players. However, it is often assumed that a good team player was "just born that way".

The task of educators is firstly, to demonstrate what skills are required for good teamwork, so that those skills can be identified and understood. Secondly, educators need to offer opportunities for those skills to be developed, with feedback, so that participants understand that these are learnable skills. Methods such as ENERGISE Creating action learning sets and the team skills methods in the ENRICH section, give participants opportunities to practice team skills and get feedback, so that they can develop their team roles, so that they can be more effective in clinical settings.

When to use it

A simulation approach to a team task can be used with any team wishing to develop their skills further. In an educational context, this approach is often best used at the beginning of a programme or module where the development of teamwork is emphasised, so that the skills needed are highlighted, so that the problems arising from failure to use these skills are experienced and so that participants get opportunities to practice new skills in a non-threatening environment. It is very suitable for a residential and can be followed up later with ENERGISE Teamwork skills using constructions.

Asking participants to work individually at first, then in a small group, and then as a large group, highlights the strengths and weaknesses of each approach, so that the educator can help the group identify helpful and non-helpful team work behaviours. The advantages of small group over individual and large group learning are also experienced directly by the participants; learning from experience in this way is a powerful and time efficient way for educators to get their points across.

This is a complex and many faceted exercise, not a quick method; allow plenty of time especially for the debriefing.

The set up: how to use this method

In this exercise, the participants are asked to imagine themselves being a group who have survived a crash, or shipwreck, in a desert or other hostile environment. Individually, then as a small group, and later, as a whole large group, they are invited to consider a list of equipment that is available to them and rank these in order of usefulness. (Examples are given in the Resources section below). The most useful item should be ranked number one, the second most useful number two and so on.

Give every participant a copy of the challenge task to read. Ask them to commit themselves to their *own personal* ranking of the equipment in order of importance. In addition, they should record their decision as to whether they wait to be rescued, or set off in search of help and shelter themselves ("Stay or go").

Divide the group into smaller units of around six (minimum) to eght (maximum) participants. Very small groups will not have enough spread of behaviours and larger groups tend to mean that quieter participants simply do not get a chance to participate comfortably. Then ask the small groups (each having a private room or space to work in) to agree a group version of the final ranking, and a group decision about "stay or go".

Reconvene as a single large group and invite the small groups to share their rankings and their "stay or go" decision". Record these clearly on a flip chart for all to see. Using different colours for different groups will highlight who decided which ranking. Debrief the changes that individuals made and how the small group decided its final ranking, (see the debrief for more details).

Ask the whole, large group, to agree a final ranking, as there will inevitably be differences between the small group rankings. The large group should also make a "stay or go" decision. The final decisions should also be recorded on the flip chart.

Finally, **write the "expert rankings"** on the flip chart and invite reflection on how those rankings differ from individuals' decisions, and how they differ from small and large group rankings.

Explanations/timings

Allow a couple of minutes to explain that they are the survivors of a crash, and that the task is to rank the equipment list they have available, in order of usefulness. They have ended up somewhere with *no mobile service, no internet* and *no battery recharging available.*
(For example, one of the large meeting rooms in a Grange over Sands Hotel – true).

Explain that the purpose of this task is to give them experience of different ways of working, (individual, small group and large group), so that we can explore what happens in different contexts, so that we can learn more about how working together as a group or team enhances learning. This is so that the team and group work they do in education and clinically will be more effective, and almost always, more enjoyable, (See ENGAGE Everything with a purpose).

Then, after giving everyone a sheet with the information on (see Resources below), allow participants at least five minutes to do their individual rankings and possibly a little more. The time it takes participants to read and digest the information given to them varies a lot… observe participants carefully and see when they stop reading and start making lists; allow at least five minutes for the ranking process. Insist that they write down their ranking privately and fully: check they have done this before allocating them to small groups. They can be allocated randomly (see ENERGISE Group sorting methods) or educators may choose to try and balance groups (with quieter and louder participants, for example).

Allow 20 minutes for the small groups to make their own ranking decisions: time this strictly, asking them to complete a ranking which they can report back at 20 minutes.

Allow the large group no more than 10 minutes to decide the final rankings and decision about "stay or go". Be strict about timing.

Writing up their rankings and "stay or go" decisions on the flip chart takes time, allow at least five minutes for this.

The debriefing process can easily require 20 to 25 minutes.

The debrief: maximising the benefits

Although doing the rankings can be quite interesting, and energise groups to start working together, the real benefits of this exercise are only realised during the debriefing, which needs to be meticulous.

When all the rankings are recorded, (individuals will have their own, the small groups' results will be on the flip chart), **invite individuals to compare their own rankings to that of their small groups and the other small groups**.

Then ask open questions like:

- "What changes in ranking were made from individual's ideas, after discussion with their group?"
- "How did you come to change your mind?"
- "How did the small group decide on their final ranking?"
- "Who was most involved/least involved in the ranking in the small group?"
- "What behaviours did you notice that helped the group to decide?"

The educator needs to facilitate this discussion to include team role issues, such as, someone being asked to be the scribe to record decisions, agreements about the process, (all agree or vote or loudest get their way?), some kind of chairing function to ensure everyone's ideas are heard, encouraging behaviours ("that's a good thought"), attention to timekeeping and staying on track with the task (not getting side-tracked).

Then ask the whole large group to make a single large group decision about rankings and "stay or go".

When the large group decisions have been recorded, ask the group to reflect on any changes in ranking or changes to the "stay or go" decision that they may have made. Then invite reflection about the process of the large group compared to the smaller groups.

Refer back to previous issues: did everyone get to participate in the large group? Does anyone feel that a person who contributed well in the small group did not contribute at all in the large group? What might this mean for how the large group" thinks and decides"? How did the "stay or go" decision go?

Finally, put the "expert score rankings on the flip chart and ask the group to identify similarities and differences in the various rankings. Have the "expert" crib sheet to hand to explain the expert reasoning, if you are not a survival expert yourself.

Typically, the shared brain power of the small groups tends to mean that small groups **improve the quality of their rankings over that of individuals.** Use this phenomenon to stress how the group "knows more" than individuals, and that learning together means that everyone benefits from the different things participants bring to the group.

Educators can then emphasise the difference between the **task** and the **process**. Developing understanding of the **process (how we do things)**, means that the skills of teamwork can be deployed more effectively on the **task (what we are going to achieve)**. Groups that have effective processes, (everyone agreeing about how to do the task, paying attention to everyone, encouraging contributions, attending to timekeeping and staying on track) tend to complete their tasks more effectively.

Very often, the large group rankings are in some or several ways worse than individual or small group rankings. Ask the group to identify the behaviours that meant certain rankings or decisions are worsened. Usually, this is because one or two confident participants in the large group sway the rest. Sometimes large groups make more risky decision for example deciding to "go" when staying is more rational, usually because of the strong feelings of a few people.

Finally, the educator should invite the group to **make a list of the most helpful behaviours/skills** used in smaller groups or teams, and record these clearly on a flip chart. End by pointing out that anyone can learn how to do these skills. These skills will be useful in small group work in educational settings, and they are crucial skills for effective teamwork in clinical settings too, (see also ENERGISE Creating action learning sets).

Equipment/resources needed

Each group should ideally have their own room to work in, although in a very large room it might be possible to have two groups working, if they are very well spread out.

In advance, prepare the information sheets, one per participant, and one for each educator.

Before the session, the educator should prepare a large table on a flip chart: the equipment listed at the left and then columns for each small group and the large group to list their ranking decisions, (there is an example below). The educator should have the expert ranking to hand, and the rationale for those rankings as participants will always want to know how expert rankings have been made.

Skills to make this work even better

It can be extremely useful for the educator to observe the small groups in action, just as they will be observing the large group in action at the end. It can be useful to have more than one educator available and for each educator to observe each small group, rotating between them. Educators should note actual examples of helpful or unhelpful behaviours, and refer back to these during the debriefing, as they are valuable ways to reinforce group skills.

Examples could include:

- I saw the whole group listening attentively to the person speaking.
- I heard X say "It would be useful to hear more about Y's thinking"
- I noted P saying "we only have ten minutes left"

Unhelpful behaviours could also be noted:

- I saw a period when there were three conversations going at once, so not all contributions were heard.
- I heard two people say something useful that the group ignored.
- I noted the group starting to talk about irrelevant subjects.

When allocating groups, educators could choose to deliberately "unbalance" groups by having all the confident louder participants on one group and all the quiet ones in another. This could be a risky strategy unless the debrief is very carefully done, as unbalanced groups are more likely to generate at least one group that is dysfunctional. Such a group may fail (sometimes spectacularly) at the task, which is demoralising and can make participants feel upset and disengaged. It is not useful to have a dysfunctional, angry group at the start of a training programme. Unbalanced groups can mean that the potential benefits of learning to work with others of a different style are reduced. To explore team roles and strengths more explicitly, but in a less threatening way see ENRICH Teamwork styles).

Pitfalls/when NOT to use this method

One pitfall is that one or more participants know all the correct answers. This may be because they have done the exercise before, (although many participants will keep quiet about this because they realise the value of the discussion), or because they have genuine expertise. However, having genuine expertise may not be recognised by either the small or large groups. One colleague who used this exercise using a desert situation after a car crash, noted one participant say mildly, "It is much better to stay put and be rescued". He was ignored and subsequently said nothing at all. The group made many errors in their rankings and took the (fatal) decision to set off walking across the desert. In discussion later, it emerged that the participant who was ignored, had extensive desert survival training and experience from his military service. Because he was a quiet, reflective person, the louder members of the group discounted his contribution.

This method, for energising people to understand and develop their group skills, takes considerable time. It is best used when groups will be working together subsequently, so it is not really suitable for one off sessions, unless the learning will be properly followed up with more opportunities to build on the skills explored.

Applications in other areas of the session

It is possible to note helpful and unhelpful behaviours at various points in the session. In subsequent sessions it is useful to refer back to the importance of task and process and the importance of the skills used in the process of achieving tasks.

How does this help to build relationships?

Participants get to know each other better through this kind of intense small group working, especially if the debriefing is thoroughly and sensitively carried out. Having the opportunity to contribute in a smaller less threatening group can be very encouraging for quieter, more reflective participants. This approach can encourage good participation by all participants.

How does this help to structure the education?

The initial explanation of the purpose of this session, (see ENGAGE Everything with a purpose), can be used to introduce the concept of team work skills, and to explain to participants how these skills can be developed during training. This makes the cumulative structure of training explicit, and can be used to link the training to assessment and curriculum requirements, for example, the relevant Royal College curriculum. Some participants are very focussed on specific "knowledge" and may not realise the importance of learning skills and developing helpful attitudes to other team members. Team work training can help them understand how skills development fits into professional training.

RESOURCES

It easy to google survival exercises. Suitable examples are available at

- https://www.mindtools.com/pages/article/team-building-problem-solving.htm which includes some useful information about the "stepladder technique" for gathering ideas and a worksheet for a "lost at sea exercise".
- http://www.wilderdom.com/games/descriptions/SurvivalScenarios.html

In the section below, a plane crash scenario is given in full, with the information for participants and the correct answers for educators! The key point about these scenarios is that all use unfamiliar environments to emphasise the role of group skills in solving problems; thus the discussions and debrief are arguably more important than the team exercise itself. Educators can decide whether to ask groups to name themselves and make the exercise competitive (who lives who dies? Who has the best survival/group skills), or, to play down the competition element and facilitate it as a means to identify, understand and develop group/team skills. This needs a more cooperative approach, which may, ultimately, be more effective educationally.

Survival: a simulation

You and your companions have just survived the crash of a small plane. Both the pilot and co-pilot were killed in the crash. It is mid-January, and you are in Northern Canada. The daily temperature is 25 below zero, and the night time temperature is 40 below zero. There is snow on the ground, and the countryside is wooded with several small rivers criss-crossing the area. The nearest town is 20 miles away. You are all dressed in city clothes appropriate for a business meeting. Your group of survivors managed to salvage the following items:

- A ball of steel wool
- A small axe
- A loaded .45-calibre pistol
- Can of cooking fat
- Newspapers (one per person)
- Cigarette lighter (without fluid)
- Extra shirt and pants for each survivor
- 20 x 20 ft. piece of heavy-duty canvas
- A sectional air map made of plastic
- One 2 litre bottle of 100-proof whiskey
- A compass
- Family-size chocolate bars (one per person)

Before joining your group **rank** the equipment above in order of importance for your survival. The most important item should be ranked 1, the second most important 2 and so on. The least important should be ranked 12.

Your task as a **group** is to list the above 12 items in order of importance for your survival. List the uses for each.

You must also decide whether the **whole** group stays put and waits to be rescued or whether the whole group leaves to seek help. You **must** come to agreement as a group before reporting back

Explanation/educators notes

Mid-January is the coldest time of year in Northern Canada. The first problem the survivors face is the preservation of body heat and the protection against its loss. This problem can be solved by building a fire, minimizing movement and exertion, using as much insulation as possible, and constructing a shelter. The participants have just crash-landed. Many individuals tend to overlook the enormous shock reaction this has on the human body, and the deaths of the pilot and co-pilot increases the shock. Decision-making under such circumstances is extremely difficult.

Such a situation requires a strong emphasis on the use of reasoning for making decisions and for reducing fear and panic. Shock would be shown in the survivors by feelings of helplessness, loneliness, hopelessness, and fear. These feelings have brought about more fatalities than perhaps any other cause in survival situations. Certainly the state of shock means the movement of the survivors should be at a minimum, and that an attempt to calm them should be made.

Before taking off, a pilot has to file a flight plan which contains vital information such as the course, speed, estimated time of arrival, type of aircraft, and number of passengers. Search-and-rescue operations begin shortly after the failure of a plane to appear at its destination at the estimated time of arrival.

The 20 miles to the nearest town is a long walk under even ideal conditions, particularly if one is not used to walking such distances. In this situation, the walk is even more difficult due to shock, snow, dress, and water barriers. It would mean almost certain death from freezing and exhaustion. At temperatures of minus 25 to minus 40, the loss of body heat through exertion is a very serious matter.

Once the survivors have found ways to keep warm, their next task is to attract the attention of search planes. Thus, all the items the group has salvaged must be assessed for their value in signalling the group's whereabouts.

The ranking of the survivors' items was made by a former instructor in survival training for the U.S. Army. This survival simulation game is used in military training classrooms.

Rankings

1. Cigarette lighter (without fluid)

The gravest danger facing the group is exposure to cold. The greatest need is for a source of warmth and the second greatest need is for signalling devices. This makes building a fire the first order of business. Without matches, something is needed to produce sparks, and even without fluid, a cigarette lighter can do that.

2. Ball of steel wool

To make a fire, the survivors need a means of catching he sparks made by the cigarette lighter. This is the best substance for catching a spark and supporting a flame, even if the steel wool is a little wet.

3. Extra shirt and pants for each survivor

Besides adding warmth to the body, clothes can also be used for shelter, signalling, bedding, bandages, string (when unravelled), and fuel for the fire.

4. Can of cooking fat

This has many uses. A mirror-like signalling device can be made from the lid. After shining the lid with steel wool, it will reflect sunlight and generate 5 to 7 million candlepower. This is bright enough to be seen beyond the horizon. While this could be limited somewhat by the trees, a member of the group could climb a tree and use the mirrored lid to signal search planes. If they had no other means of signalling than this, they would have a better than 80% chance of being rescued within the first day.

There are other uses for this item. It can be rubbed on exposed skin for protection against the cold. When melted into an oil, the fat is helpful as fuel. When soaked into a piece of cloth, melted fat will act like a candle. The empty can is useful in melting snow for drinking water. It is much safer to drink warmed water than to eat snow, since warm water will help retain body heat. Water is important because dehydration will affect decision-making. The can is also useful as a cup.

5. 20 x 20 foot piece of canvas

The cold makes shelter necessary, and canvas would protect against wind and snow (canvas is used in making tents). Spread on a frame made of trees, it could be used as a tent or a wind screen. It might also be used as a ground cover to keep the survivors dry. Its shape, when contrasted with the surrounding terrain, makes it a signalling device.

6. Small axe

Survivors need a constant supply of wood in order to maintain the fire. The axe could be used for this as well as for clearing a sheltered campsite, cutting tree branches for ground insulation, and constructing a frame for the canvas tent.

7. Family size chocolate bars (one per person)

Chocolate will provide some food energy. Since it contains mostly carbohydrates, it supplies the energy without making digestive demands on the body.

8. Newspapers (one per person)

These are useful in starting a fire. They can also be used as insulation under clothing when rolled up and placed around a person's arms and legs. A newspaper can also be used as a verbal signalling device when rolled up in a megaphone-shape. It could also provide reading material for recreation.

9. Loaded .45-caliber pistol

The pistol provides a sound-signalling device. (The international distress signal is three shots fired in rapid succession). There have been numerous cases of survivors going undetected because they were too weak to make a loud enough noise to attract attention. The butt of the pistol could be used as a hammer, and the powder from the shells will assist in fire building. By placing a small bit of cloth in a cartridge emptied of its bullet, one can start a fire by firing the gun at dry wood on the ground. The pistol also has some serious disadvantages. Anger, frustration, impatience, irritability, and lapses of rationality may increase as the group awaits rescue. The availability of a lethal weapon is a danger to the group under these conditions. Although a pistol could be used in hunting, it would take an expert marksman to kill an animal with it. Then the animal would have to be transported to the crash site, which could prove difficult to impossible depending on its size.

10. Quart of 100 proof whiskey

The only uses of whiskey are as an aid in fire building and as a fuel for a torch (made by soaking a piece of clothing in the whiskey and attaching it to a tree branch). The empty bottle could be used for storing water. The danger of whiskey is that someone might drink it, thinking it would bring warmth. Alcohol takes on the temperature it is exposed to, and a drink of minus 30 degrees Fahrenheit whiskey would freeze a person's oesophagus and stomach. Alcohol also dilates the blood vessels in the skin, resulting in chilled blood belong carried back to the heart, resulting in a rapid loss of body heat. Thus, a drunk person is more likely to get hypothermia than a sober person is.

11. Compass

Because a compass might encourage someone to try to walk to the nearest town, it is a dangerous item. Its only redeeming feature is that it could be used as a reflector of sunlight (due to its glass top).

12. Sectional air map made of plastic

This is also among the least desirable of the items because it will encourage individuals to try to walk to the nearest town. It's only useful feature is as a ground cover to keep someone dry.

How to score

Each team should list its rankings in order, prior to seeing the answer sheet. To award points, look at the ranking numbers on this answer sheet. Award points to each team's according to the numbers here. For example, the map would earn 12 points, while the steel wool would earn two points. Lowest score wins (and survives).

"Stay or go " – teams that stay are likely to survive. Those that go ARE DOOMED.

12// TEAMWORK SKILLS USING CONSTRUCTION EXERCISES

Can clinicians build actual bridges? Sometimes an unfamiliar task can lead to unexpected learning opportunities.

What it is for?

This method challenges small subgroups of participants to complete a shared, but unfamiliar, task, so that they are energised to work together, particularly if there is a competitive element, where subgroups compete against each other for the best construction.

The educator observes groups working together, so that in the debriefing discussion and feedback participants can reflect on the skills and attitudes needed for effective team work. The educator can then link those skills to the wider professional context, so that participants understand how these skills are also needed in other group/team settings, including Study Release Programmes, multidisciplinary team meetings of all kinds, partnership or clinical team meetings, and even in planning committees and boards.

When to use it

This can be used early in a Study Release Course when group formation is a priority (for example in the later stages of a group residential) or, can be used during the course as a way of deepening reflection on the skills needed for effective team work, or, as a way of demonstrating to the group that their team work skills have improved after training in specific aspects (for example effective chairing, turn taking, ensuring all contributions heard, planning the work and priorities)

The set up; how to use this method

This works best with teams of around six to eight people. If the group is large divide it into smaller units. Explain that the task will be to make a structure that conforms to certain rules/ criteria, using the materials they have been given, so that they get an experience of working as a team. Be very clear what materials are available, (examples are given in RESOURCES below), and where other tools or equipment such as scissors/sellotape are to be found/ shared.

State that the finished piece will be assessed using fixed criteria and explain what these are, so that every group starts with the same information. Compare this to a task that a clinical team might be required to do (for example, create a set of easily accessed instructions and equipment required for Resuscitation), so that participants understand why they need to learn teamwork skills, so that they understand how those skills will be applied in clinical practice, or in learning situations such as Action Learning Sets (see ENERGISE Creating action learning sets).

Explanations/timings

Give each team an information sheet that gives the list of materials, timings and any specific criteria for the build (see examples below in RESOURCES). Explain the task beforehand: this usually takes about 5 minutes, as there will be questions from the participants. Then allocate participants to groups and give them somewhere to work: groups can be in the same room if it is large enough or separate rooms depending on facilities available. It works better if they can have separate break out rooms so that each group works out its own approach. Note, it is not forbidden for group members to wander about and see what others are doing, although this need not be mentioned. Indeed it is a key skill in developing a project to see what other people are doing/have done, even if their approach is not followed. It is efficient to learn from the mistakes of others!

Explain there is a set time for this exercise and stick to that time ruthlessly, stopping the build as soon as time is up, even if it is not complete. The Great British Bake Off approach to timing is the one to follow.

During the build, educators observe the group processes carefully, and note any examples of helpful skills ("Let's hear what E has to say about this…") or dysfunctional behaviours (a quiet person being ignored), so that these behaviours can be quoted and discussed during the debriefing. It is usually useful to have more than one educator available for this method, so that more helpful/unhelpful behaviours can be observed, so that debriefing discussions will be richer. Rotate educators between groups, so that all groups are observed by all educators. Note down specific behaviours or words used, so that group feedback will be SMART (Specific, Measurable, Achievable, Realistic and Timely).

The debrief: maximising the benefits

Debriefing is in three parts.

Firstly, the assessors visit each group in turn to give feedback against the agreed criteria, so that the group's own reflection on the group process happens in private; what went well, what they struggled with, how they found solutions or identified problems. Do not allocate marks at this point.

Secondly, take all the groups in turn to see each other's build. At this point, give the overall mark to the group whose build is being assessed. It is better to give the mark **after** the feedback: evidence shows that if given the mark first, learners tend to ignore the feedback (see EVALUATE giving feedback). Invite comment and discussion from the whole group about each build.

Thirdly, with all participants together, invite reflections on what issues came up for the groups when doing the build, so that the educator can facilitate a discussion that reminds the group of the essential functions that group members need to fulfil for effective teamwork.

These include:

- **chairmanship functions** to ensure that everyone contributes, important contributions are not ignored and that tasks are planned and prioritised (chairmanship may be designated to an individual or distributed amongst team members)
- **timekeeping functions** to manage and monitor the time available (teams often fall down in this one)
- **allocation of work** so that tasks are clearly identified and allocated to participants(s) to complete.

Equipment/resources needed;

The main requirement is for space for teams to work in, preferably one room per group. The exact materials suggested are in RESOURCES below. Educators who become familiar with this technique can easily make up their own exercises or collections of materials. In most training centres or hotels this can even be done using "found materials" i.e. stuff that is there already (like water bottles or paper). Do not rely on this though, it is better to be prepared in advance. Items like scissors, string, or sticky tape should be brought with you, in case they are not available on the day. Bring a model car or person to use when assessing stability.

Bring instruction sheets one for each group (examples below) and also one assessment sheet for each observer.

Skills to make this work even better

This exercise can be used in several ways. The first is to use it at the start of training, which tends to demonstrate the lack of high level team work skills. This can form the basis for an introduction to teamwork roles and skills.

Alternatively, it can used after another team building exercise such as the survival exercise (see ENERGISE Survival exercise) to allow groups to demonstrate skills that they have learned.

Creating the groups can be done randomly, or the group members can be designated by the educator (for example, to obtain balanced groups, ahead of them working together in action learning sets see ENERGISE Creating action learning sets).

Later in training, this approach could be used in the ENRICH Team work styles exercise. In that situation the groups are deliberately skewed to only contain people with a specific teamwork style.

A further refinement of this method is to have a "plant" in the group to take a particular teamwork role or to "act out" in a dysfunctional way. For example, one member of the group could be asked to disagree with all suggestions, or to say absolutely nothing unless directly invited, or to spend as much time as possible looking at their mobile phone during the build. Choose the person and their dysfunction carefully so as not to cause too much upset. During debriefing to the individual groups ask "and what did (the person invited to say nothing whatever) bring to the build? Or what effect did X disagreeing with things have? Or "what effect does using a mobile have on the group process?"

One option is to "change the rules" half way through by giving each group an extra item they must incorporate into their design, so that the group's ability to respond flexibly to changing circumstances is also explored, so that the link to the changing circumstances of the workplace can be emphasised.

The debriefing process can also be used to introduce ideas the teams may not have thought of. For example, it is quite rare for doctors to make a formal drawing or plan at the start. Ask the group what a group of engineers or architects would have done first? Ask them to consider the possible benefits of making a time line or project plan before starting, so that they are introduced to the concept of formal project planning skills such as Gantt charts (Reference 1), or Process Mapping, which could be developed in sessions later in the training programme.

Pitfalls/when NOT to use this method

The full benefit of this exercise is as part of a series of sessions considering teamwork roles and skills. It probably would not work so well in isolation or as a standalone session with a group who do not usually work together. It can be used as a team building task in a practice team though; they work together longer term and can take some of the messages into later work.

One pitfall with this method is that if the group is dysfunctional for any reason, the build may fail. This can cause embarrassment in itself, and dysfunctional teams can be unhappy experiences for participants. Think carefully about the balance of the group members and whether they are likely to be able to work together. If groups are dysfunctional in this exercise, try to "generalise away" from the specific team in the debrief: saying things like "if team members think no one is interested in their contribution they tend to go quiet, even if they have useful expertise" can make the point that it is useful to ensure everyone gets to contribute, without highlighting one team.

Avoid any direct blame or criticism of a dysfunctional build. If possible positively connote what they have contributed by highlighting common problems (" Thanks for behaving out of character and disagreeing with everything Jo, I think you enabled everyone here to reflect on what happens if there is a lot of negativity about").

Note, this is a TEAMWORK exercise NOT a team BUILDING exercise. Team building exercises are for creating intra team relationships and bonding, providing opportunities for fun, enjoyment and bonding. Some of the exercises in the ENAGAGE section are good team building exercises. This team WORKING exercise may help build a team if they are successful, but may not have the same effect on a dysfunctional team; they need some team building before they can perform well.

Applications in other areas of the session

N/A

How does this help to build relationships?

Working together on an unfamiliar and unexpected task helps groups to build relationships and the feedback process which emphasises the team work roles and skills, can help groups to strengthen their ways of working together.

How does this help to structure the education?

This kind of task can be used to introduce topics that many clinicians believe are not "teachable" such as teamwork skills. This can be signalled as a prelude to subsequent sessions that will cover these skills in more detail. If used as a follow on from other teamwork exercises, the development of skills should be identified to demonstrate progress.

References

1. A Gantt chart is a type of bar chart that illustrates a project schedule, more information at: https://en.wikipedia.org/wiki/Gantt_chart
2. A process map is a planning and management tool that visually describes the flow of work, a flowchart, for an example, in this case making breakfast see: https://www.process.st/wp-content/uploads/2016/08/2.gif and for more information see: https://en.wikipedia.org/wiki/Business_process_mapping

RESOURCES

Possible team work construction exercises

Bridge building: team task

TEAM instructions

- Your task is to build a bridge as a team, between two stable supports of your choice, bridging a gap of at least one metre.
- The bridge must have at least 60cm clearance underneath (to allow boat to sail up the putative river underneath the bridge) and must allow the toy car to drive over safely from one side to the other in a stable fashion. There is a time limit of 20 minutes to complete the task. The bridges will be assessed for s**tability, clearance, driveability** and **aesthetics**
- Your envelope contains the materials you can use to make the bridge. Tools such as scissors/ruler/ toy car for testing are with the assessors

ASSESSORS should make notes on team work process and on the above criteria, marking each one out of 10, adding up the scores to get the overall team score. TIME this exercise ruthlessly, stopping teams immediately that time is up.

Materials

Sheets of A4 plain paper, several metres of string, a dozen straws, some Blutack/sticky tape, some felt tip pens or crayons, some tooth picks or BBQ wooden skewers, something potentially to be used for decoration; some sticky notes, paper doilies, a magazine with colourful pictures in.

One set of instructions for each group. Marking sheet for assessors.

Tallest tower building: team task

TEAM instructions

- Your task is to build the tallest possible tower, only using the materials you have been given.
- The tower must stand on the floor in a stable, independent way, without falling over and must be strong enough to take the weight of a small model person at the top. You may only use the materials you have been supplied.
- Your tower will be assessed for **stability, height, abilty to support the model person** and **aesthetics**

ASSESSORS should make notes on team work process and on the above criteria, marking each one out of 10, adding up the scores to get the overall team score. TIME this exercise ruthlessly stopping teams immediately that time is up.

Materials

4 Sheets of A4 plain paper, 4 sheets of newspaper, several metres of string, small roll of sticky tape.

One set of instructions for each group. Marking sheet for assessors.

13// WARM UP THEME – CRITICAL THINKING

Critical thinking skills can be developed with these short, energising exercises.

What it is for?

Having a warm up exercise at the start of the session can help to get everyone engaged and actively involved in learning from the start. It can be useful to have warm up exercises in "themes" that run through several weeks or a whole term. Other examples include professional virtues or the assumptions that underpin medicine (see ENERGISE Warm up theme professional virtues and ENERGISE Assumptions of modern medicine).

When to use it

As a theme at the start of sessions over a term or a few weeks, as a preliminary to any learning involving guidelines, evidence, the use of tests and investigations.

The set up: how to use this method

Using a suitable example (a PowerPoint slide set to go with these exercises is available from HEENW Contact avril.danczak@gmail.com for details), work though the ideas that the participants initially have about the problem (perhaps using the Pose, Pause, Pounce, Bounce method outlined in ENRICH Using questions effectively). Then add extra bits of theory or information for participants to explore and understand.

Explanations/timings

Explaining the original issue or problem should take only a few minutes. Then work through the additional information gradually, step by step over perhaps 15 to 20 minutes, involving participants in discussion of their ideas.

The debrief: maximising the benefits

Ensure that all ideas are captured, not just those that crop up first form noisier members. Using prompts like "any other thoughts?" before moving on should help to capture these.

Equipment/resources needed

A PowerPoint resource with the issue and the critical thinking skills needed to solve it. An example can be found in Resources at the end of this section (page 53). Educators need to thoroughly understand the issues themselves before embarking on this. I have certainly obtained some excellent CPD for myself that way!

Skills to make this work even better

Reinforce the learning afterwards by asking participants to list key points, to identify other areas where the same principles might apply, by asking them to link their thoughts with other things they have learned, or by asking them how they might apply this new learning in practice the next day. This could be in general group discussion or by using the "Ideas bring and buy" outlined in ENRICH Making rounds effective.

Pitfalls/when NOT to use this method

This method probably works best as a "mini series" within a course. However, the exercises could be used together, in sequence, during a day or half day on critical thinking or clinical reasoning skills.

Applications in other areas of the session

The skills of critical thinking should be incorporated and referred back to whatever the subject matter. Learning of critical thinking will be reinforced if the methods and approaches are referred back to and reinforced for example, in thinking about screening tests, long-term conditions, complexity and uncertainty.

How does this help to build relationships?

The immediate responses of activist learners may not always yield the best results; it can benefit relationships when activists come to value the contributions of quieter, more theoretical or more pragmatic members of the group.

How does this help to structure the education?

Having a short warm up theme means that everyone knows what to expect at the start of the session and can be prepared to start working on it. Having short themes that last maybe 15 to 20 minutes helps to maintain pace and variety that keep learners engaged and interested.

Reference

Possible subjects could include:

- Investigating anaemia what is the evidence?
- Interpreting blood tests, especially screening tests
- Thinking about scoring systems; strengths and weaknesses of using scores like CURB in primary care versus secondary care.
- Applying evidence intelligently: the importance of context.
- Explaining CVS risk accurately.
- When is a disease not a disease?
- Screening: assessing interventions

See Resources (page 56) for a full example.

RESOURCES

Example – a new screening test

A new screening test has been devised:

- The Test identifies **correctly everyone who truly has the disease** and has a small **false positive rate** of five per cent
- Your patient Mrs W. Well has tested positive for the disease. She wants to know what she should tell her family. Has she got the disease?

Note for educators: initially ask for a hands up "yes or no" do you think she has the disease?

- What will you say to her? Has she got it?

Note for educators: what are the chances that she has the disease – i.e. what percentage likelihood of her having the disease? 95%? Less?

Note for educators: ask the participants: "what information do you need to know before answering her question?"

- **Prevalence** is one in a 1,000 in the population served by you.
- So out of 1,000 patients, **one has the disease**.

Note for educators: now ask again, How likely is Mrs W Well to have the disease? Then share the following slide, showing what various groups of clinicians thought.

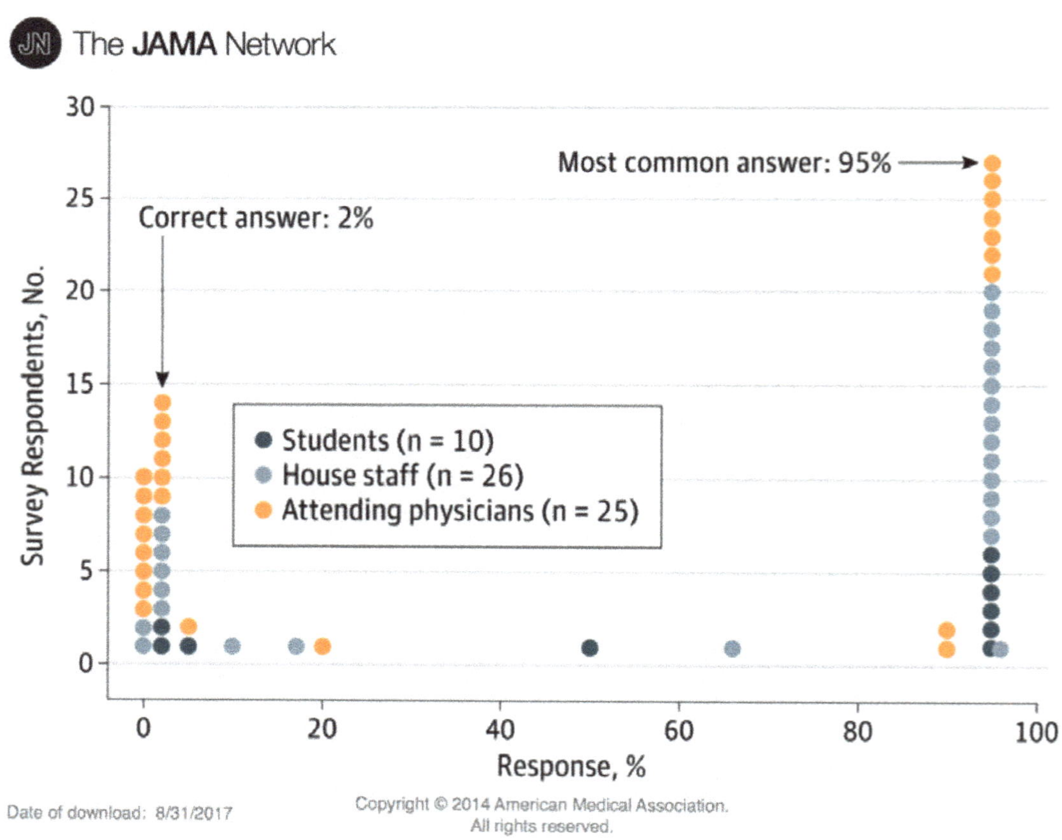

What information do you need to know before answering her question?

- **Prevalence** is one in a 1,000 in the population served by you.
- So out of 1,000 patients, **one has the disease**.
- Five per cent will get a **false positive** = 50/1000
- One **true positive** divided by **50 false positive** = **two per cent**

Therefore, she has a two per cent likelihood of having the disease (put another way, of 100 who test positive, only two will actually have the disease).

Note for educators – debrief: consider discussing

- *Are you surprised by this figure? (Consider going over the reasoning again, many clinicians cant do the maths)*
- *What is the potential for harm with this screening test? (Anxiety, exposure to dangerous confirmatory investigations or invasive biopsy)*
- *What if the potential treatment is toxic? (how many might have an unnecessary treatment or procedure? A harmful treatment or procedure?)*
- *If there is a more accurate confirmatory test (e.g. a biopsy)? How might patient be harmed?*
- *As screening is applied to people who are **well**, what messages about health does screening give?*
  - *you may feel well but be harbouring a disease*
  - *early diagnosis is necessarily better – often little evidence for that*
  - *you cannot trust your health*
  - *only doctors really know how well you are*
  - *we can prevent bad diseases by knowing them early*
- *Or, does this just prolong the time we know about diseases (which is called prolonged lead time)*
  - *does it impact overall mortality, i.e. does it lengthen life to start treatment earlier?*
  - *what is the evidence for that? For example, disease specific mortality for breast cancer has reduced while overall mortality has not – what could be going on there?*

Further examples are gven in the accompanying PowerPoint document – ENERGISE examples of CRITICAL THINKING.pptx which is available by contacting HEENW.

14// WARM UP THEME – THE ASSUMPTIONS OF MODERN MEDICINE

A warmup activity that questions common assumptions is a useful way to wake up critical thinking.

What it is for?

The purpose of this method is twofold. Firstly, having some short discussion exercises at the start of the session is energising. The group gets an immediate task to get on with; choosing something interesting or controversial, while not spending too much time on it, gets things going and also leaves things unfinished. This can trigger reflection later. Educators can invite examination of a series of ideas on a similar theme over a few weeks (see also ENERGISE Warm up Critical Thinking and ENERGISE Warmup Professional Virtues) so that deeper thinking is encouraged. Use smaller bite size stages so that the material is more easily assimilated by participants, so that attitudes and beliefs can be explored and challenged in a relatively gentle way.

When to use it

This method is energising at the start of sessions, so that participants challenge a different Assumption of modern medicine every week, so that they are invited to think critically about aspects of our work that may go unspoken. There are 10 assumptions listed here to explore; obviously educators can select the ones that seem most useful or relevant, or even divide the group into two and have half the group examine one assumption and half the group examine another.

The set up: how to use this method

Explain that modern medicine is built on a number of assumptions that we tend to take for granted. How successful are these assumptions in helping us to look after patients in the "swampy lowlands of Primary Care"?

Point out that not everyone agrees with these assumptions. For example, social scientists would question the assumption that the doctor is a detached, neutral observer.

State the assumption to be discussed (preferably have it displayed clearly – for example, on a PowerPoint slide.)

Possible assumptions to discuss:

1. Patients suffer from diseases that can be characterised in the same way as other natural phenomena.
2. A disease can be viewed independently from the person who is suffering from it and from their social context.
3. Each disease has a cause and finding it is a major objective of research.
4. Given a certain level of host resistance, the occurrence of disease is explained as a result of exposure to a pathological agent.
5. The physician's main task is to diagnose the disease and wherever possible to prescribe a specific remedy aimed at removing the cause or ameliorating the symptoms.

6. The physician uses an intellectual tool, the clinical method known as differential diagnosis.
7. Mental and physical disorders can be considered separately, with provision for a group of psychosomatic diseases in which the mind appears to act on the body.
8. Each disease follows a defined clinical course that can be influenced by medical interventions.
9. The doctors effectiveness is independent of their gender or their beliefs.
10. The doctor is usually a detached, neutral observer.
11. The patient is usually a passive recipient of the prescribed treatment.

(See *Being a Doctor; Understanding medical practice* by Wilson and Cunningham, Chapter 3. Very useful for a background discussion.)

Explanations/timings

After explaining the overall context of the discussion series as above, ask participants to think about the assumption by themselves for a short time ("pause") and then discuss the day's assumption with a partner ("pair") for five minutes, explaining that you would like them to explore the extent to which this assumption is useful in the setting they work in (for example, primary care) and the extent to which it is more or less applicable in that setting.

Then ask pairs to join to form a group of four and to examine their shared ideas or ways in which they thought differently ("square"). (ENERGISE Using QUESTIONS effectively for more details of the "pause, pair, square, share" approach).

Consider using group sorting methods (ENERGISE group sorting methods) to ensure that participants talk to different people each week.

The debrief: maximising the benefits

Ask the group to feedback the issues that came up in their discussion. If they are struggling to see how the assumption may NOT be warranted or useful in a particular setting, have some useful "what if "questions ready to deepen the debate. For example Considering whether a disease can be viewed independently from the person and the social context ask them to choose any disease; then ask how it would affect a young doctor about to do the CSA, a young mother of a 1 week old baby, a famous footballer about to go to the World Cup … would we see the disease process in exactly the same way? Or consider mentioning complex phenomena such as HIV, panic attacks, ADHD…

Equipment/resources needed

PowerPoint slide with the assumption clearly visible.

Skills to make this work even better

The key task for educators is to promote discussion, in a way that sensitively challenges the assumptions participants may bring from hospital medicine, while also being supportive and encouraging. This is not an easy task. Picking up and using their own examples, asking them to identify any exceptions they may have come across, empathising with the complexity and difficulty of modern medical practice, will all help the discussion to go well. The educator can be well prepared by reading Wilson and Cunningham themselves beforehand!

Pitfalls/when NOT to use this method

This is a method that works best when bite-sized chunks form part of a coherent series of discussions that build up on each other. If scattered or not linked together, such a series risks seeming incoherent or disconnected from daily practice.

This method is less useful if the group only meet once, are constantly changing in composition or if they are too concerned with the nuts and bolts of hospital practice to reflect on underlying assumptions and how these may be less helpful in different settings. However, being informed by these discussions can help the educator raise these important issues. Participants may be struggling with practical issues of "How to manage disease X", when some of the difficulties they face may be due to an assumption that does not hold in the case they are discussing.

Applications in other areas of the session.

It is always useful to refer back to discussions if something relevant comes up later.

How does this help to build relationships?

Being able to explore challenging ideas in a safe environment with colleagues builds supportive interpersonal relationships and helps participants to develop confidence in their thinking skills which they will transfer to other environments.

How does this help to structure the education?

Having a short discussion helps to punctuate the session and break it up into more interesting parts. This can help to keep activists on board. Also having a series that goes from week to week gives the SRC a sense of continuity, of structure and of building up expertise. This is itself encouraging and empowering as participants feel their ability to engage with difficult topics increasing over time.

Reference

Being a Doctor: Understanding medical practice by Wilson and Cunningham. RCGP books, ISBN 978 0 85084 365 1

15// WARM UP THEME – EXAMINING PROFESSIONAL VIRTUES

What are characteristics of a "good clinician"? These warm up exercises help participants to reflect on what really matters.

What it is for?

Study Sessions of three hours can be daunting to educators and participants alike. Breaking the time up in a structured way with a variety of activities can maintain energy for learning throughout. Using different methods of learning is one way to achieve this. Another way is to have different strands at different times in the session. Having an "opening strand" can be a good way to energise the group. This means devoting, say, 20 minutes to a theme that runs from week to week, so that the subject is explored in bite sized pieces. Having a strand examining the VIRTUES a professional needs is one described here. See also ENERGISE Assumptions we make about medicine, and ENERGISE Warm up critical thinking.

When to use it

This approach works best as a theme running over several weeks with a group meeting regularly. Start the session with this immediately recognisable and understandable task, so that the reflective process gets going, and so that the whole group engages in discussion). This enables active reflective processes to continue in the rest of the session, so that the discussion gets to deeper levels. This method takes the subject of "Professional Virtues" in small "bite sized" chunks, so that they are more readily digested by participants.

The set up: how to use this method

Start the session with an opportunity to discuss a **professional virtue** (for example, courage, gratitude, humility or compassion – a full list is available at the end of this chapter).

Ask participants to pair up (preferably with someone they know less well, for example, with the person behind them rather than their friend next to them). Ask them to consider what this virtue is about? When have they themselves demonstrated this virtue? How could we do more of this?

Explanations/timings

Explain what a professional virtue is and why such things are important – this may take a few minutes.

Explain the virtue of the week, then get into suitable pairs to discuss it – this should only take a minute or two.

Allow about five to ten minutes for the discussion in pairs and then about ten minutes for debriefing. Educators should judge how long to leave pairs by how vigorous the discussion is.

Stop the pairs discussion for the debrief when it starts to go quieter or if people have evidently gone off topic. Have a wander round and hear what issues are coming up.

The debrief: maximising the benefits

Ask the whole group what issues came up when they talked about what the day's virtue is about; go on to ask for examples of this virtue in practice. Adding anything interesting you heard when wandering around can enable quiet participants to be honoured. Perhaps saying "K said an interesting thing when he mentioned…"). Then invite consideration of how the virtue of the day is important in our professional lives and how could we demonstrate more of it?

Equipment/resources needed

The educator needs some knowledge of the professional virtues and how they may be manifested in good clinical practice.

Skills to make this work even better

One way to develop these ideas further could be to contrast virtues with professional vices, so that participants also develop their understanding of behaviours that are to be avoided: arrogance, timidity, apathy, callousness, indifference, ingratitude, laziness, complacency, overconfidence, self-absorption are all counterproductive in the workplace. Telling participants in advance what next week's virtue will be can give them a chance to think and prepare in advance. Ensuring that this strand is included in the weeks learning summary (See ENERGISE Making a learning summary) reinforces the learning. This strand can be even better if the previous week's virtue is revisited briefly: "did anyone notice some courage happening last week?"…before examining the virtue for the current week.

Pitfalls/when NOT to use this method

This approach needs a group who meet regularly week to week to work properly, so is less useful for a one off session. The facilitator needs to have some knowledge of how the virtues might play out in practice. This is not that difficult, we can usually recognise opportunities to demonstrate a virtue, even if we do not always take those opportunities.

Applications in other areas of the session

Referring back to a virtue when an opportunity arises (for example, it takes courage sometimes to go off protocol even when you know it's the right thing to do) reinforces learning.

How does this help to build relationships?

Virtue is not a usual topic for clinicians. Talking around the subject of our professional practice helps people to open up and share ideas which builds up relationships and awareness of others different points of view.

How does this help to structure the education?

Having a short opening strand helps to break up the session, helps to give pace and direction and contributes to having a good structure for the day.

Reference

The Professional Virtues are summarised in the following broad groupings:

- **Wisdom** – includes judgement, perspective, creativity, love of learning and curiosity.
- **Courage** – includes bravery, honesty, perseverance and zest.
- **Humanity** – includes kindness, love and social intelligence.
- **Justice** – includes fairness, leadership and team work.
- **Temperance** – includes forgiveness, humility, prudence and self-regulation.
- **Transcendance** – includes appreciation of beauty or excellence, hope, gratitude, spirituality and humour.

Educators can be selective about which to cover, perhaps aiming to cover some obvious ones honesty, judgement, humility) with some less obviously applicable ones (appreciation of beauty or excellence, forgiveness, courage) aiming to discuss at least one virtue from each of the broad groupings.

See also:

https://www.viacharacter.org/www/Reports-Courses-Resources/Resources/Character-Strength-Fact-Sheets

https://www.jubileecentre.ac.uk/1585/projects/published-reports/virtue-wisdom-professional-education

https://www.cebm.net/2016/01/5395-2/#.Vq6l1WsGI_s.twitter

16// CONSULTATION SKILLS – INITIAL EXERCISES FOR LISTENING

The phrase "thank you for listening" is a powerful one, recognised by practitioners and patients as signalling that something valuable has occurred. So what is this "listening"?

What it is for?

What happens if we hear but do not listen? These exercises are useful for exploring the meaning of listening and what happens when we are, or when we are not, listened to. By using this experiential method, putting the participants in the shoes of both the listener and the listened to, a deeper understanding of what listening is about can be developed. This exercise focusses initially on the skill of literally "hearing" followed by the deeper skills of passive and active listening.

When to use it

This is useful at the start of a programme or the start of a module about consultation skills, or when working on the development of skills for managing mental health problems in the GP consultation.

The set up: how to use this method

This method is done in pairs and invites reflection on listening by getting pairs to do three exercises. The first is one about NOT listening, the second is about PASSIVE listening and the third is about ACTIVE listening. The latter two are often muddled up in participants' minds and these exercises help to clarify what using different skills can achieve.

Explanations/timings

Part one: not listening

Ask the group to divide into pairs and spread themselves widely around the room, facing each other. This position is important. The exercise will not work so well if people sit next to each other or look over their shoulder at someone behind, etc. Take a minute to get this part of the set up right.

When everyone is in place, explain the task. The task is for one person to be the speaker and one the listener. Ask participants to designate who will be the speaker and ask the designated speaker to raise their hands. Tell the designated speaker the task will be to "explain the repeat prescribing system in their practice and the features about it that improve patient safety". If participants are not working in general practice, another, similar, patient safety-related task can be given.

Before the speakers begin to talk, give every listener a card/piece of paper, explaining that this is the instruction for them alone and must not be shared with their partner. On the piece of paper are the words: "Do not listen to your partner, do not speak, do not move away, do not show them this paper."

Explain that there is five minutes for this task and **use strict timing**. However, it is rare for the speakers to continue for a full five minutes. Stop the exercise before five minutes, if everyone goes quiet, starts laughing or stops talking about the subject (the educator needs to walk round and be aware of what is happening in the group). When that happens, ask participants to swap roles, passing the instructions to their partner before the first time listener changes roles and becomes the speaker.

The debrief: maximising the benefits

Part one: not listening

Begin with asking the speakers to comment on what they experienced. Use a flip chart and note what they say under the headings of what they were **thinking** and what they were **feeling**. Typically, when they are speakers, participants think that what they say is not that good or that their partner is not really interested, or that it's a waste of time. They may feel frustrated, (another word for angry) inadequate, boring, uninteresting, useless or insignificant.

Use facilitation skills, (go on? Anything else? Can you elaborate?), to draw out the widest range of responses, and name the feelings accurately.

Then ask the listeners to describe what they experienced in similar terms. There are often surprising similarities. Explore these.

Make the link that communication involves **thinking** and **feeling**. Point to the list of emotions that were felt; what do patients feel like when they are not listened to? Does some of the anger and frustration we encounter come from this? Explore the experiences of the participants who are listening without really listening; emotions are powerful and when we are not listening the emotions of the speakers transmit themselves to us too. Coping with that and feeling that we are not doing our listening job properly can create feelings of disturbance in the (non) listener. If not recognised and dealt with, such emotional disturbance uses a lot of energy and can contribute to us feeling drained at the end of the day. Effective listening is often less tiring (a bonus!).

Part two: passive listening and Part three: active listening.

The set up and debrief for these is shown in Resources at the end of this section (pages 63 and 64). Always use these three as a sequence, debriefing each one before moving on to the next one.

Equipment/resources needed

Chairs, space to move them into pairs

Prepare the cards in advance with the wording: "Do not listen to your partner, do not speak, do not move away, and do not show them this paper".

Skills to make this work even better

Use the debrief (perhaps on the second time round) to explain the value of experiential learning; one could read about these issues or see a PowerPoint, but learning is much more powerful when derived from actual experiences. This can be a useful cue into the purpose and value of processes which will be used on training courses, such as, role play, skills rehearsal or simulations. These are sometimes viewed as uncomfortable or unnecessary by participants. Use this opportunity to explain that training in the Study Release Courses is like a laboratory; things can be tried out in a safe environment and developed, without risking problems in the patient encounter. Thus, experiential methods create powerful learning opportunities.

Pitfalls/when NOT to use this method

Do not use this method alone. It must always be combined with opportunities to be listened to, otherwise the bruising experience of being not listened too risks overwhelming the learning. The explanation and debrief of passive and active listening are given below in the appendix. ALWAYS combine these three exercises together.

It might seem that this method will not work if people have done it before, or when repeated with the pair swapping roles; in fact, although slightly less intense, the emotions and thoughts are similar even if participants know what is going to happen. This again reinforces the effectiveness of learning by practical experience, with time to reflect and discuss things immediately afterwards

Applications in other areas of the session

N/A

How does this help to build relationships?

This process risks damaging relationships, unless followed up with passive and active listening experiences. If those experiences do occur, however, participants get a chance to be listened to properly (always a good experience) and this helps to build trusting and open relationships within the group. If the exercises are facilitated well and their meaning and purpose drawn out in the discussion, it helps the participants to develop trust in the facilitator and in experiential methods – a good investment for later exercises.

How does this help to structure the education?

This helps to show how a process that we all think we understand, "listening" is quite a complex process and paves the way for consideration of different listening skills that can be used in different way. This signals a methodical approach, and that listening is a set of learnable skills to be developed.

(See also ENERGISE Consultation skills INTENSIFY understanding by deconstructing listening, and ENERGISE Consultation skills – what do you say after you say hello.)

RESOURCES

Passive listening exercise

The set up

In pairs again, timed for five minutes.

- The speaking task – describe all the people that make up the practice or team you are currently working in, and what makes them work well together (or not).
- The listening task – listen to the speaker, but **do not use any words at all**.

Again observe the group for signs that speakers are drying up. See if they can speak for five minutes without the listener saying anything. Stop if everyone stops talking! Swap partners and repeat.

The debrief

Ask the speakers what they noticed about this conversation. Often it is easier to talk at first, but hard to keep going. What did they notice about that? How did it feel? What thoughts did they have? Ask the listeners what it was like for them. Bring out the fact that both parties need to be involved for effective communication; listening intently is a key process. Point out that what has happened is NOT ACTIVE LISTENING, but PASSIVE Listening. Active listening only occurs when what the speaker says is built upon in the rest of the conversation, referred to or represented using active listening skills.

Active listening exercise

The set up

Ask participants to form into pairs again. Participants can change to a different pairing now, if wished, as both parties have listened to each other.

- The speaking task is the same; describe all the people that make up the practice or team you are currently working in, and what makes them work well together (or not).
- The listening task is to listen, use any active listening skills they can but to **ask no questions at all**. Statements can be used – for example, "That sounds interesting …"

Again observe the group for signs that speakers are drying up. Stop if everyone stops talking, although this is extremely unlikely where active listening skills are being used properly. Swap partners and repeat.

The debrief

Ask them what is different between passive and active listening? Speakers; how did you know that the other person was listening? Listeners, what was it like to listen without having to ask any questions? How did your mind feel? One of the key problems for clinicians is that when they listen to patients, they are only using half their mind; the other half is busy trying to decide what question to ask next. This means listening is less effective and content is lost. Paradoxically, simply focusing on listening, and not trying to think too hard, will be easier. Focussed listening will usually yield more information from the speaker.

Finally, ask the group to identify what listening skills were used by the listeners, other than asking questions.

You should be able to come up with a list such as:

- **Encouraging skills** – go on … tell me more … that's interesting … echoing, reflecting back, repetition, the power of the pause.
- **Responding skills** – empathic comments, ("that sounded scary"), reflections of the speakers thoughts "that's puzzling", statements or observations, ("you suddenly stopped when you mentioned person X").
- **Summarising skills** – "so the senior partner is scary but everyone else is really kind … go on", paraphrasing "so overall, you got to know everyone really quickly"

Conclude by reflecting on how important feedback is in communication, so that we know the other person has really heard and understood us. Active listening is a loop; one person speaks, the second responds in a way that makes it clear they **heard and understood** what was said. Encourage participants to reflect on how much information can be gleaned **before asking any questions, open or closed**.

Reference

See *Skills for Communicating with Patients* by Kurtz, Silverman and Draper for a full discussion of listening skills.

17// CONSULTATION SKILLS – INTENSIFY UNDERSTANDING OF LISTENING BY DECONSTRUCTION

How well do we really understand the process of "listening" even though we do it every day?

When to use it

This is a useful approach to helping participants understand the complexity of "listening" by offering them a series of listening experiences to reflect on. This approach can be used at the beginning of a series of sessions on consultation skills, or, as a session during a longer course such as a residential intensive. Taken individually, the elements of good listening could be used as mini "warm up" exercises to be done either at the start of a session or to break up a longer session on consultation skills.

Understanding the complexity of listening helps participants to be more attentive to the process so that they listen better to patients so that more relevant information is communicated. Full and accurate listening is essential so that diagnosis and treatment plans are correct and so that a good therapeutic relationship is built up with the patient, so that clinician and patient can work together effectively.

The set up: how to use this method

This method for teaching "listening" needs a bit of preparation; sequencing and timing are important.

The elements of listening to be considered are:

- rapport
- hearing
- understanding
- remembering
- interpreting
- evaluating
- responding.

Each one of these has a different "set up and debrief". The details for each one are given in Resources at the end of this section (pages 67–71).

Explanations/timings

Explain the elements of listening first, giving examples of each and how they influence the communication between people. Each exercise takes about ten minutes. If run together, this can take about half a session (say two hours).

The debrief: maximising the benefits

Debrief is in two parts. Each exercise needs a debrief about **what** that part is about, **how** it felt to be experiencing that element of listening, and **how** it relates to what happens in the consultation. What will participants try out the next day when they see patients?

At the end, overall, the debrief needs to allow participants some time to reflect on their experience. Allow this alone first, so they get their thoughts in order and then in pairs. Share ideas with the whole group at the end. The final debrief questions can be around issues of learning:

- What learning strategies did you use in this session?
- What will it take for you to succeed in
  - building rapport?
  - remembering what people say?
- How will you reinforce this learning in practice?

Equipment/resources needed

It is useful to have the specific element of listening projected on a screen to aid recall.

The exercises and any equipment needed are listed in Resources at the end of this section (pages 67–71).

Skills to make this work even better

Refer back to these skills in later sessions. Specifically ask participants how it went when they tried to build rapport explicitly in every consultation, or what happened when they named an emotion and so on. This is called "**looping**" and helps to reinforce learning and set it into the wider context of participants work. Be ready to hear about failures and pitfalls too; accept and thank anyone who says "it didn't work". Ask them for more details to clarify the issue. Then "bounce" around the group inviting other contributions; what did other people do when they encountered this? Anyone had the same/different experiences? How did you handle that? What did others do to make this work better?

These exercises are examples of **experiential learning** – participants do something, experience something and learn from their direct experience. Educators can use the opportunity to explain the benefits of this and reinforce the effectiveness of experiential learning.

Pitfalls/when NOT to use this method

This is not suitable for very large groups (over 30) unless there is more than one facilitator to help and debrief. The idea that listening comprises learnable skills is basically accepted in general practice, although not always fully understood by participants. In a different context, you may have to do some work to get "buy in" that this is a worthwhile thing to do. Usually the best way is to start from things that went wrong; that is where people are "hungry" for new learning. See ENGAGE Assessing learning needs at the outset.

Applications in other areas of the session

In a session on consultation skills it may become apparent that there is an issue with one of these basic elements of listening; revising this, using one of these experiential methods can then be used at other stages.

How does this help to build relationships?

Better listening builds relationships amongst participants. They have some fun in many of the exercises, (learning can be enjoyable, who knew?), and this also builds relationships and "esprit de corps" in a healthy way. Participants who are willing to "have a go" often draw others along with them and this builds confidence between people as they develop their "community of practice".

These exercises are a good way to introduce the concepts around experiential learning; that we learning by experiencing things and then reflecting on them together, with the help of a facilitator who can help us explore and understand what we have experienced, put it into the context of our work and add in relevant theory. Reading about listening in a book will not yield the same depth of learning.

How does this help to structure the education?

This sequence of exercises gives structure, pace and varied tasks which makes the time fly by if well organised.

RESOURCES

The specific exercises for each element of listening are described here: in all these there is a brief introduction, what will be done and why; then the task is experienced and the learning summarised afterwards in a short, focused debrief.

Build rapport

Explanation

"Rapport is like money; it increases in importance when you do not have it, and when you do, a lot of opportunities appear." (Laborde)

Ask the group how they know when they have rapport with someone. Rapport has two phases – initiating, then maintaining and deepening.

The task

1. Initiate rapport by smiling (with full face including the eyes), making eye contact and then projecting a silent message of warmth and good will to the other person. Demonstrate this to the group (See also How to communicate basically brilliantly by GP David McConnell). Then ask the group to stand up and move around the room. Choose any partner and practice initiating rapport in turns. Shaking hands can be a way to signal that has happened. Then move onto another member of the group and repeat. Let them do this three or four times.

Then they can sit down; debrief by asking what would you need to do to initiate rapport like that with every patient you see?

2. Matching and mirroring. Rapport is deepened when the parties match their tone, pace of speech and posture. This can work both ways; following the patients tone and mirroring their posture can aid rapport and build the relationship if congruent. If the patent is angry and aggressive this will fuel the fire; in that case the reverse can happen. The doctor can get the patient to mirror them by slowing their speech, being quieter, having a calm and non-aggressive posture. In this way mirroring can help to calm the situation down.

Ask participants to work in pairs, one speaking, the other listening; the listener should unobtrusively match and mirror the speaker. The speaker should have a straightforward task like "Describe what your last clinical day was like".

Debrief

How was that? How could you apply this in a consultation?

Hearing

Explanation

Listening can only occur if you hear what people say to begin with. This exercise is described in detail in ENERGISE Initial exercises for listening.

Debrief

This should emphasise the difference between active and passive listening and all the component skills of active listening including echoing, reflecting back, summarising, etc. See *Skills for Communicating with patients* Kurtz Silverman and Draper for details.

Understanding

Explanation

Understanding can mean something rather global, the result of a series of empathic, effective communications as when a patient says "I am so lucky, I have a very understanding doctor". In the context of these exercises, understanding has a more literal meaning, the question being: do we understand what someone has just said to us?

The task

First, ask the group to consider what the barriers are to this basic kind of understanding; these include language barriers, class barriers, dialect, jargon or slang barriers, lack of shared experience, (someone referring to "my home" might mean anything from a convenient and available doorway to a grand mansion, to a place where they are routinely beaten up).

In pairs, ask participants to spend five minutes listening to their partner and trying to ensure that they understand exactly what was said. The task should be simple; say, "describe the house you grew up in to your partner". The speaker should pause regularly for the listener to clarify anything they did not understand ("What exactly is an outhouse?" or to summarise the key points "so your childhood home had three bedrooms, a big kitchen, a small living room and a small garden of about half an acre in size?"). The speaker can clarify any confusion or omission.

If time is short, this exercise can be omitted and the element of understanding covered briefly in considering the barriers to understanding, as above.

Debrief

Begin by articulating that everyone has been talking about their "home". How do our concepts of "home" differ to that of some of our patients? What listening skills were used in this exercise? Which were most effective from the speaker's point of view? Which were most helpful for the listeners? It is helpful to ask participants to list skills under suitable headings such as supporting skills, encouraging skills or summarising skills.

Remembering

Explanation

For someone to feel really listened to, for a clinician to maximise the use of time in a consultation, and to have the maximum amount of information available to help make medical decisions, it is really important to **remember** what the speaker says to you. It is very common when watching video to hear a doctor ask the same question several times, because they did not really listen to the answer and therefore did not remember it, or to hear a doctor ask for a piece of information a patient has already clearly given. (Patient "I gave up smoking two years ago, I have lived with my daughter since my wife died, and she hates smoking." Clinician "Who do you live with?")

To remember things we need to use our "Working memory". This is a faculty that we can train, like training a muscle, although like muscles, some people have better working memory than others.

The task

Form the group into a circle and have some kind of token (a small object that can be thrown around the group…a pen, small toy, anything). The task is to tell a group story. One person starts saying: "Once up on a time I was …" then they say a sentence. After that they say "and then…" At this point they pass the talking stick/token to someone else in the group randomly (not to the person next to them).

The next person has to repeat exactly what the person before them said and then add a sentence of their own, followed by the words "and then …" to signal it's the next person's turn.

The token is passed round the group and every person has to recount the entire story so far, exactly, before adding in their own sentence.

Using random people means everyone has to listen carefully in case it is their turn next. Ask the people who have already spoken to listen carefully and put their hands up if any detail is missed from their bit of the story; this keeps them listening too. Stop the round when the story becomes inaccurate.

See how many people can speak before the next person finds it too much to remember. It can be worth doing a practice round with just two or three people and then challenging the group to see if they can manage to keep the story going for longer. Generally, experienced practitioners (perhaps demonstrated if you have a co-educator) can do this much better than participants in training, because they have developed their working memory.

Debrief

Asking how people remembered what was said and identify the successful strategies. These might include;

- **paying full attention to the speakers**, rather than thinking about what you are going to say yourself
- **focusing** on the key words (large, barking, dog),
- **making a picture in your mind** of the story that you can go back to (for example, they were in a wood when …). Some theory might include a discussion about how long most patients talk for (it is rarely more than a minute at a time, if you do not interrupt) and also what strategies you can use to develop your working memory. For example, writing down one or two words that sum up what the person has said in each sentence. See References for more information.

Interpreting

Explanation

Really listening to someone means more than just hearing what they say and remembering it. Active listening requires some kind of interpretation; often the full meaning comes from an accumulation of things, or several clues to the overall meaning. This is especially true when people talk about their emotions and feelings. People may not name the feeling outright, "I really resent the way my boss makes me to do overtime", but rather leave you to work it out by saying "Everyday it's the same, I am getting ready to go and she turns up and says oh please will you just do this or just do that before you go, or I am putting you on the overtime shift to cover until M gets here, I was late home every night last month!" Demonstrating empathy and showing that you have really heard, remembered and understood what some has said, is exactly this kind of interpretation. "You sound rather resentful towards your boss".

The task

In this exercise, participants are invited to consider how the same incident might give rise to very different experiences for different people. Explain that the scenario is this;

"A person is standing waiting for a bus. Out of the blue a cyclist veers into them and knocks them over, causing them to get a fractured clavicle, but no other injury. They come to see you with their arm in a sling"

Divide the group into smaller units of three. Give each group some cards, each having the name of a different feeling written on the back. Their task is to work out how to tell the doctor the story of the injury expressing that emotion, but without naming it directly. Suitable feelings to put on the cards could include any of the following:

- Resentful, frustrated, furious, angry, irritated, proud, relieved, submissive, resigned, defeated, exhausted, shocked, vulnerable, exposed, outraged, stoical, motivated, weary, guilty, ashamed, embarrassed, fearful, apprehensive, panicky, envious, foolish, humiliated, overwhelmed, scared, helpless, hopeless, bitter, disgusted, exasperated, satisfied, excited.

When they have worked out how to tell the story (allow about one or two minutes per word, give each unit three or four words to work with) ask each unit to link up with the neighbouring unit.

Then they should take turns telling the story; the participants from the other unit of three have to work out what the emotion/feeling is being described. They should signal this by saying "it sounds like you feel ...". They get one point for each correct answer.

Debrief

- Which feelings are easier to express than others?
- What did you have to do to work out how to make the story express that feeling?
- When listening, what helped you to work out what that person was feeling?
- When the feeling was named, how did the speaker feel then?

Usually having your feeling recognised is a good experience – relate this to patients, who feel better if their thoughts **and** their feelings are understood.

Evaluating

Explanation

Evaluating means being able to consider different elements and weigh them up; which are most or least important? What should we focus on next? This often means summarising a whole section of content in one or two sentences (for example at the end of one section of a consultation), and may also guide the overall direction of the consultation.

There is no specific exercise for this part – perhaps you can make one up.

Responding

Explanation

We can listen to someone at a rate of up to 500 words a minute, but we only speak at about 120 words per minute. Relaxing back, hearing, remembering, interpreting evaluating and thinking before we respond means we are more likely to respond effectively. What is said next, must relate to what the person has just said. If you are thinking about what to say next while someone is talking you are not really listening.

Responding is what we do after we have heard, understood and interpreted what we are listening to. Developing appropriate responses to develop the conversation will be covered in other sessions on consultation skills.

Resources

1. Some basic information about working memory is here: https://www.psychologytoday.com/gb/blog/memory-medic/201203/training-working-memory-why-and-how
2. There is more discussion of how emotions and feelings are expressed in consultations in these useful books – *Consultations Skills That Heal*, Barry Bub, ISBN1 85775664 9, Radcliffe. *Field Guide to the Difficult Patient Interview,* Platt and Gordon ,ISBN 13 978 0 7817 4774 5. *Communication Skills in Mental Health Care*, Coll et al, ISBN 978 184619.

18// CONSULTATION SKILLS – WHAT DO YOU SAY AFTER YOU SAY HELLO?

Not all consultations get off to a good start – sometimes things go wrong right from the beginning.

What it is for?

This method is a way of developing two consultation skills. Firstly an awareness of how a patient's initial presentation can "press our buttons" and create a defensive atmosphere from which the consultation may not recover. Secondly a way to promote discussion and awareness of how we can use our skills to defuse this process.

When to use it

This is useful as part of a consultation skills module, especially when doctors have had some experience of working independently in clinics with patients. May be useful as part of a residential or introductory course as it is quite an energising and interesting exercise. It has the added advantage of introducing experiential methods of working in a way that is not threatening.

The set up: how to use this method

Prepare some cards in advance that have a series of possible "opening gambits" from patients written on. These are the first things that patients say, after initial introductions have been made and before the patient gets down to the business of explaining what exactly they are there for. There are some examples in Resources at the end of this section (page 74).

When the group is comfortable, introduce the session by explaining that the beginning of the consultation is crucial for the rest of the interview – that things can get off to a good or a bad start and that there are skills to deal with this. It is better if they have already got some ideas about how to skilfully do initial introductions and agenda setting.

Use small Buzz groups (See ENERGISE Buzz groups) initially to brainstorm any experiences they may have had where the patient started off in a tricky way (suggest an example like "hello Dr, I didn't realise you would be so young/so old!") and record these difficult comments from patients on a flip chart.

Then distribute cards with possible opening gambits on – a list is available in Resources at the end of this section (page 74).

The educator should initially take the role of the doctor and invite one card holder to sit next to them. The educator starts by saying;

"Hello I am doctor X", then the patient can say "hello"...and read out what it says on their card.

Then discuss with the group what they FEEL about the patient opening gambit and how they think that could influence their response. Then discuss what skilful approach the doctor could use to diffuse the situation and avoid becoming defensive.

Try a few of the openings as a large group, then get the group into threes (doctor, patient, observer) and let them try out more of the opening gambits you have prepared as well as some of the ones they initially generated themselves. Ask the observer to give some feedback about how the interaction went, when observed objectively, asking them to comment on whether the doctor rose to the bait, how well they diffused any aggression, what they said that helped to build a good relationship.

Explanations/timings

Explaining the purpose of the session and the initial brainstorm should only take a few minutes – perhaps ten. It might take 15 to 20 minutes to do the initial opening statements as a whole group. Then allocate ten minutes for practice in smaller groups, with the roles changing round so that everyone gets to try out being the doctor/ patient and receive some feedback.

Allow time for a final de brief to really draw out the learning points.

The debrief: maximising the benefits

Ask the whole group to reflect on what kinds of feelings they experienced as the doctor (e.g. anxiety, anger, detachment, a wish to push the patient away and not get involved) and invite reflections on how we can overcome this – by being aware of the difference between the patients feelings and our own, being aware that all relationships have a feeling component.

Offering some didactic input on identifying the skills needed to build effective relationships could also be appropriate. These skills include expressing empathy, respectful listening, non-judgemental acceptance, expressing concern and willingness to help.

Full details of these skills are found in Skills for Communicating with Patients (Reference 2).

Equipment/resources needed

Some pre-prepared cards will deepen the learning; being prepared means the educator can ensure a wide range of difficult beginnings are available for practice. A list is available in References.

Skills to make this work even better

Link this to further reading about consultation skills, (see References), and to the benefits of discussing these kinds of issues in Balint style groups during training and more importantly as part of Continuing Professional Development. There is further information in the BJGP articles by Eby (Reference 3) and Swinglehurst and Atkins (Reference 4) which emphasise examination and analysis of the specific details of what patients say and how they say it.

Pitfalls/when NOT to use this method

A group needs to be reasonably "formed" and comfortable before doing this, unless they are already accomplished group learners, such as, a group of trainers or experienced GPs.

This exercise needs to be part of a context of learning about specific consultation skills so probably would not work well as an isolated exercise.

Applications in other areas of the session

N/A

How does this help to build relationships?

By experiencing difficult moments and then learning how to overcome them, participants learn to trust each other more and this makes learning more potent as anxiety decreases. It has obvious benefits for building relationships with patients. Having the educator initially taking the role of the discomforted doctor on the receiving end of a difficult comment, normalises the fact that not all consultations start well. Even experienced clinicians have such difficult moments. Participants get to discuss and learn some functional responses before they try things out for themselves and this can increase their confidence. Experiential learning of this nature also improves intra group relationships, as everyone gets to share both difficulties and methods for success.

How does this help to structure the education?

In a series of sessions on consultation skills, exercises like this can reinforce the point that effective consulting can be systematically developed by learning and applying a series of skills, linked together. Effective consulting is not innate, but can be learned, developed and improved through attention to the skills required, as well as the cultivation of attitudes of mind which make for more effective consultations – for example, being non-judgemental.

References

1. See *The Inner Consultation* by Roger Neighbour, ISBN 13 978 1857756791 for more about opening gambits.
2. *Skills for communicating with Patients* by Kurtz Silverman and Draper, ISBN 1 85775 640 1, Radcliffe has more information on how to get consultations off to a good start and how to build effective relationships with patients.
3. *Empathy in general practice: its meaning for patients and doctors,* Don Eby, Br J Gen Pract 2018; 68 (674): 412-DOI: https://doi.org/10.3399/bjgp18X698453
4. *When 'yes' means 'no': why the small details of clinical interactions matter,* Deborah Swinglehurst and Sarah Atkins, Br J Gen Pract 2018; 68 (674): 410-411. DOI: https://doi.org/10.3399/bjgp18X69844

Resources

Some possible opening gambits to prepare in advance and write on cards;

- At Last! I have been ages in that waiting room!
- So, What the dickens is going on here?!"
- Oh… I thought you would be a male/female doctor.
- So, I have come to insist on a referral. I have tried everything, it is not getting any better, I have been putting up with it for ages now and my sister said I MUST definitely get a referral or else I will find a doctor who will!
- I am so glad it is you I am seeing – my cousin says you are a great doctor.
- Thank goodness you are back from your holidays, I have been waiting ages for you to get back
- Well I hope you are going to be better than that stupid doctor I saw last time.
- I always like to see young doctors – you're more up to date aren't you?
- Congratulations! You are that doctor who has just had a baby aren't you? (When the doctor has NOT in fact had a child recently!
- Oh, I thought I was seeing Dr Clever today instead of you.
- I do not really know where to start, everything has gone wrong!
- Oh good, you are the doctor that speaks Polish/Welsh/Punjabi/French aren't you! (To someone who speaks none of these)

ENRICH

INTRODUCTION

This section is about methods that help to **enrich** learning. Formal training has a very limited "time budget", so that making the most of any learning opportunity is crucial.

The considerations described here provide ways to enrich sessions, so that each one offers more "bang" for the educational time "buck".

The ENRICH section is laid out with some preliminary information about what educational enrichment is, and some thoughts on using different planning methods, (the "what and why" issues). Then the following chapters describe some enrichment **methods**, (the "how" issues). I have tried to "enrich" the chapters in this section with some interesting or thought provoking quotations. Some of the chapters are enriched, by being a little longer and more discursive. I hope this will enable educators to explore some of the deeper and more complex ways in which we can use formal training time.

What does enrich actually mean? Here some definitions.

1. To improve or enhance the quality or value of something, including ideas of enhancement, adding to, supplementing, boosting, upgrading or reinforcing. "Her life was enriched by going to the theatre and museums"
2. To make someone better off though the acquisition of cash or other resources.

Enriching may have the connotation of making more money, but this is not the concept being considered here. Enrichment is an idea widely used in education in general, with the expected benefit that it makes learning more substantial, more rewarding and more interesting. It is sometimes considered only for those who have already mastered basic curriculum matters. However, enrichment opportunities can help all participants pursue learning in their own areas of need, interest or strengths. The provision of extended learning opportunities and challenges can deepen engagement with learning and take participants to higher levels of achievement. Even simply exposing weaker participants to more challenging ideas can help them to become more ambitious.

This may be done by adding educational content, by signposting new learning opportunities, or, by identifying learning activities that take participants to areas above and beyond their current achievement level. Several different approaches are described, and educators will surely feel empowered to design methods of their own too.

> "One can choose to go back toward safety or forward toward growth. Growth must be chosen again and again; fear must be overcome again and again."
> **Abraham Maslow**

When training clinicians, we are training for two distinct phases in their careers. Firstly, we are offering education that will help them succeed in their current roles and pass their relevant examinations. However, we must also provide education that enables them to succeed in the future, as their careers continue to develop. This second aim of education can focus on developing self- awareness, reflective capacity and improving learning skills. These elements are especially important in the context of educational enrichment.

When thinking about planning educational events or even whole courses like a Study Release Course, our initial approach is usually a linear one; what will we start with? What will come next and then how will we finish things off? This approach is very important in setting up the bare bones, the structure of the education, and, like bones in the body, provides a firm basis for everything, the means of movement and progress and something reliable to build on.

However, we all know from our own learning, or from listening to our participants, that deep learning and true change, often seem to come from something that happened on the side; a chance remark, an unexpected happening, even from something that went wrong. These "side" events can provide real illumination for participants. Can we build this in? Or do we just rely on happenstance and the "wisdom of the group" to bring these things out? How do enrichment activities "fit in"?

Enrichment activities can help participants **feel that they belong**, because many enrichment activities promote deeper relationships between participants and between participants and their educators. When **learners know each other, and their teacher and have a good rapport**, enrichment activities can really take off so that participants can engage at the level that is right for them and in ways that enable them to deepen and extend the scope of their learning. Enrichment activities allow flexibility in relation to **learners' agendas, so that their needs are taken into account**. This matters because what participants are ready, able and needing learn next, is more important than what the Educator wants to teach next. Enrichment activities also reinforce the value of a **community of practice**. This is a group of people brought together by a learning need, whose collective learning becomes a bond amongst them, and whose interactions affect their clinical practice in ways that vary with individual. Their learning experience helps them in a variety of ways: individuals are able to develop in the direction that is necessary for them.

Educators can enrich learning experiences, and make them deeper and more embedded, if a variety of different methods are used, so that the bones of a linear plan, are fleshed out with interesting and "out of the box" approaches. This involves tolerating a certain kind of uncertainty, because as we provide an enriching variety of experiences, different participants will digest these in different way and with different outcomes at different times. Our educational aims become "offering opportunities, to experience and think about..." rather than "Participants will be trained to..."

If general planning is linear, the enrichment principle is to LAYER the learning horizontally over time, so that different aspects and greater depth, "flesh out" the learning described by the bare bones. The dividends are huge. Creating enriched learning experiences makes them more exciting, more memorable, more influential... and more unpredictable. As with other methods, educators need to plan carefully, so that they think through how, and when, their chosen technique is to be used, and so that they are meticulous in the way that experiences are set up, debriefed and linked to other aspects of education. Language matters, so that educators need to be clear and positive about the expected benefits of enrichment activities, and so that they can also be honest that different participants may see things differently, and gain different value from the education on offer. This open approach makes enrichment more successful. Walk your talk; if preparation is asked for, then make sure it is incorporated into the session. If a non-medic is involved do not be apologetic or undermining, rather be really positive about what they can contribute and how we can learn from them, (see ENRICH Involving patients in education and ENRICH Artist in residence). If you think reading poetry can be a thrilling way to process emotion, be excited when you explain what is on offer (see ENRICH Poems to process suffering).

Educators also need to consider the support offered to participants, especially that which helps with their sense of belongingness and their ability to recognise the flexibility in the educational offering. This is so that increasing the challenge of the educational experiences, does not overwhelm participants, because they feel themselves to be in a supportive and cooperative environment. Many of the methods described in the ENGAGE and ENERGISE sections help to provide this sense of cooperative, supportive learning environment. This is an important precursor to most enrichment activities, so that participants feel confident that they can respond to more challenging, or more complex, material.

Enrichment activities can be explicitly linked to the requirements of participants' future workplaces, so that skills like team work, the development of resilience and professionalism and the value of transcendent experiences in the arts and culture are seen in context. These experiences are valuable in their own right, and also as key ways in which we develop professionally over time. Enrichment means going beyond knowing the right answers, so that participants develop an appreciation of the importance of ***asking the right questions***. True expertise in continued professional development terms rarely involves neat and tidy "right answers". Rather participants need to be exposed to the uncertainties faced by the mature practitioner, so that they are able to develop their skills in a relatively protected professional environment, so that they develop the right skills to manage the challenges of independent practice (see also Reference 2).

Enrichment needs to be contextualised to the type of clinician. For example, a session on screening, with General Practitioners, could include basic information about what screening programmes are, and be extended to cover the criteria that the National Screening Committee use to establish the benefits of proposed screening programmes. Enrichment could go deeper by inviting participants to apply such knowledge to existing screening programmes or proposed ones. This could be extended by considering which stakeholders are involved in screening programmes and whether they have conflicts of interest. Going further could examine the ethical issues (contrasting autonomy with justice and use of resources use for example), and could then extend in a variety of directions: breaking the bad news of a screen detected abnormality accurately, perhaps, or developing explanatory leaflets listing the harms as well as benefits of screening, or perhaps developing the formal shared decision making skills of participants.

> "Error in judgment must occur in the practice of an art which consists largely of balancing probabilities."
> **Sir William Osler**

To a group of cardiologists "screening" may have different connotations and they may consider screening for atrial fibrillation or depression post MI to be unproblematic and sensible. The criteria for effective screening and the national arrangements for assessing proposed screening programmes could be enriched by examining the uncertainties involved, the potential for harms, or the sensitivity and specificity of screening tests when they used outside hospital, in populations where the prevalence may be much lower.

Enrichment may also mean addressing some of the "informal and hidden curriculum" areas that may contribute to the stress of clinical practice, (see General Introduction for a description of what the informal curriculum and hidden curriculum may contribute to educational activities). Addressing the hidden and informal curricula is important, so that participants can recognise some of the "dark sides" of clinical practice, so that they can develop relevant coping skills, professional behaviours and the ability to work with others effectively before they become independent practitioners. Educators can use training time to help participants engage with issues such as failure, things going wrong, knowing what to do "when we do not know what to do", illness, stress, or criticism and complaints. This is so that they get some practice in dealing with these before they happen (which is inevitable), so that they can begin to develop helpful strategies for dealing with the demands of clinical practice.

Furthermore, if educators have offered participants the opportunity to work in a supportive environment, and in action learning sets where they have learned to work together, they are more likely to be able to build and develop supportive communities of practice in their own working life, after becoming fully qualified.

Another aspect of the "dark side" of professional practice, comes from the context we work in. Clinical work inevitably exposes us to the deeper issues that our patients are forced to encounter. These include attachment and loss, fear, the changes wrought in our lives by birth, aging, approaching infirmity and death. Many art forms offer us enjoyable ways to process and understand these challenges through transcendent experiences of all kinds. Using the Arts, offers us tools for reflection, using holistic, right brain approaches that differ from the analytical, cold, left brain thinking that may dominate "scientific" practice. The arts can help clinicians process their own experiences of clinical work, unconsciously, so that they can also understand the experiences of their patients at a deeper level.

Using creative writing, exposure to the visual arts, cinema and even dance and theatre have all been used to enrich the educational offering, so that clinicians are supported to deal with the emotional and relationship aspects of their work, not just the decision making and knowledge based aspects.

Finally, another "dark side" of clinical practice is the bullying atmosphere that sometimes prevails in some of the high stress environments clinicians work in. Prejudice, racism, sexism and failures of teamwork and leadership, all feature here. One step is to equip participants to recognise these issues when they occur. This is only a preliminary. Educators need to offer training in effective teamwork and collaboration, so that teams and organisations move away from blame cultures, towards collaborative, collective solutions. The purpose of training in resilience and teamwork skills is precisely to develop these aspects of professional work (see ENRICH Weaving in resilience techniques and ENRICH Teamwork styles).

> “Success is not permanent; failure is not fatal.” **Sir Winston Churchill**

Complex matters of teamwork, failure and difficulty are ignored at our peril. If we pretend they are not there, they will not disappear: rather, what will happen is they slide into the territory of the hidden curriculum. If a helpful hidden curriculum is not provided, the "dark side" of clinical practice is simply expressed in off message outcomes: do as little as possible, patients are demanding and horrible, we are powerless to change anything. This is a harmful curriculum. Our informal and hidden curricula need to transmit hope, inspiration and educational "nutrition", so that our participants are orientated to a "growth mindset" (Reference 1). Our enrichment activities should make us, as educators, redundant, so that participants take increasing control of what they think, what they do and how they develop. Participants should understand what "good looks like", and have the tools to work with others to achieve positive change in their work and in their own true professional development.

Here are the basic methods, educationalists can develop their own and be really creative in this area.

Enrichment methods to enhance learning

1. The power of preparation
2. Using taxonomies 1 – KSA and Miller's Pyramid
3. Using taxonomies 2 – Bloom's Taxonomy
4. Making rounds effective
5. Making experiential learning of new skills effective
6. Enhanced educational speed dating

Enrichment methods to prepare for professional practice

7. Using a film to teach professionalism
8. Weaving in resilience techniques
9. Teamwork styles – red, green, yellow and blue
10. Using sculpts
11. When a clinician becomes the patient
12. Endings

Enrichment methods that widen the view

13. Conferences and how to make them enjoyable and effective
14. Enrich with a gift
15. Creative writing
16. Artist in residence
17. One-to-one meetings
18. Involving patients in educational sessions
19. Using poems to process suffering

References

1. *Black Box Thinking: Marginal Gains and the Secrets of High Performance: The Surprising Truth About Success*, Matthew Syed. ISBN 978-1473613805
2. John Launer has a useful blog on the importance of the arts here: https://pmj.bmj.com/content/84/995/504

1// THE POWER OF PREPARATION

Preparation methods can enable participants to achieve maximum benefit from an educational session, by directing their attention to key issues before they arrive.

> “He who is best prepared can best serve his moment of inspiration.”
> Samuel Taylor Coleridge

What it is for?

Wise words from a great poet and Lakeland explorer. Sometimes whimsically called the “flipped classroom”, methods that enable participants to prepare beforehand, can really enrich the educational process.

When to use it

Preparation methods work best when the participants are a known group, for example a cohort on a Structured Training Programme, or, attendees at a team training event, and when the topic is planned in advance. This means preparation can be sent to participants ahead of time, or listed in the course programme.

Clearly educators will usually plan ahead. This method is to consider the various ways in which ***participants can plan ahead*** and be better prepared for the content of the session, so that they will understand any basic knowledge required, so that they can brush up on anything they feel uncertain about, (enabling them to contribute more comfortably in the group), so that the session itself can use the power of the group learning to address more complex areas. This could mean going beyond “knowledge transfer” and addressing attitudes and values, or, higher levels of learning, such as analysis, evaluation, critical appraisal or application of learning to the workplace. This offers more interaction and more opportunities for feedback. See also ENRICH Using taxonomies of learning.

This approach is called the “flipped classroom”; study and learning are done beforehand, so that classroom time is used to enrich, reinforce, develop and anchor the learning through discussion, feedback and practice (Reference 1, page 9). In Miller’s Pyramid terms, (Reference 4, page 9), this means that the “knows about” part happens before the session and the “Knows how and Shows how” elements can be the focus of learning during the session.

As we might anticipate, preparation is most often actually done by the stronger participants, and in a virtuous circle, they get more benefit from their educational sessions. However, studies in schools suggest this approach is particularly beneficial for weaker students. When they are orientated to the material they feel less at sea during the session and also benefit more from it. Find ways to encourage the weaker students to do the preparation, perhaps by inviting reflection on it at the start of the session, or asking participants in small buzz groups to use the preparation as a trigger to thinking about what they consider their learning needs for the session are, (see ENGAGE Establishing learning needs at the outset). When Educational Supervisors are included in the loop and receive course programmes in advance, they could also nudge participants to do any preparation by using tutorial time to talk about their preparation on that topic.

The set up: how to use this method

When considering the aims, objectives and intended learning outcomes of any session, educators can also consider what ***advance preparation*** would help participants. Ensure they get adequate notice so that they do have time to prepare. Preparations can be graded in complexity from simple thought experiments to active gathering of information about the topic, or simple audits or diary keeping. Even having a good title for the session, can help participants think ahead and orientate themselves to the possible challenges of the subject matter.

If the session subject matter is "Breaking Bad News", the subject line could be made more intriguing if it is called "When Breaking Bad News is hard to do: challenges, skills and ethical dilemmas", or, "Breaking Bad News; the good skills, the bad feelings and the ugly truth". This paves the way for more formal preparation.

Suitable preparation, can start with simple, low effort exercises, and grade up to more complex, high effort tasks. Bloom's taxonomy can be used as a guide to complexity (Reference 3, page 9).

Some options for preparation are listed here, with the relevant Blooms Taxonomy level in brackets for guidance.

Reflection (Remember)

"Before the session reflect/think about the problems you encounter with Breaking Bad News"

Thought experiment (Understand ... what it is like)

"Before the session, think about a time when you had to break Bad News; how did it go and what would have made things run more effectively. Have you ever received Bad News yourself? What helped you hear it appropriately?"

Hyperlink to suitable background information (Applying Principles)

"Before the session look at this link about how to give Bad News:

https://patient.info/doctor/breaking-bad-news

https://www.medscape.com/viewarticle/856955_3

Hyperlink to the patients' point of view (Analyse, Differentiate)

"Before the session read these accounts by patients of what it was like to receive bad news and reflect on what is was like for them; reflect on your own experiences of receiving bad news".

https://www.researchgate.net/publication/23238740_Receiving_Bad_News_A_Phenomenological_Exploration_of_the_Lived_Experience_of_Receiving_a_Cancer_Diagnosis

https://experiencelife.com/article/when-your-doctor-says-i-have-bad-news/

https://www.kidney.org.uk/perceptions/kidney-failure-a-presonal-account/

Background Reading (Evaluate)

"Before the session read the Chapter about Breaking Bad News in Skills for Communicating with Patients by Kurtz Silverman and Draper; which elements of this chapter have been most helpful to you?"

Deeper Material (Analyse)

"Before the session, read "What doctors Feel" by Danielle Offri (Reference 2, page 9), and consider what effect breaking Bad News might have on the doctor as a person".

Investigate practice (Create)

"In the week before the session keep a diary of the patients you see where you have had to break bad news to them (i.e. any news that "significantly alters their view of the future") with brief notes on what happened".

Obviously these are possibilities; it would be far too much to suggest all of these before one session! In practice, its best to choose between one and three pieces of possible preparatory work, to enable choice, while being realistic about what some participants will manage. It is very unusual for ***all*** participants to do preparation, even if the educator tells them it is essential. Roll with that and work with the majority of the group.

Preparation can be especially helpful for more introverted members who may have Reflector or Theorist learning styles. Activists may enjoy doing something or be content to "wing it" on the day. Pragmatists will be selective and identify something they think will work best for them. The point is to have some choices.

Explanations/timings

Apart from the debrief, the time used is in advance of the session. Educators must consider how much time they think is feasible, realistic and acceptable to spend on preparation and to take into account that different learners may have different levels of engagement with the preparation. Identifying suitable preparation or reading in advance is also a way to use educator time more effectively because the participants are doing some of the work in their own time.

The debrief: maximising the benefits

Bear in mind that participants may have done some, all, or none, of the preparation. Participants' reflections on what they gleaned from the preparation can be incorporated into the ENGAGE Hopes and Fears and ENGAGE Establishing learning needs at the outset parts of the session.

Allude to the preparation in advance:

- next week we will be covering…
- preparation could include…

and refer to it at the beginning of the topic:

- what did you make of the links to … that were in the preparation?"

Then, even if some participants have ignored the preparation they know that the educator will be addressing it and bringing up the relevant issues. This may increase motivation for next time.

Preparation can be labelled in the programme as **"preparation and further reading"** so that participants can fill in gaps after the session, as their needs dictate.

Equipment/resources needed

It is helpful to use a variety of preparation methods over time. Online sources, books, articles or activities such as diary keeping, thought experiments, or simple audits, can all find their place, so that there is variety in the nature and intensity of potential preparation, so that participants will be able to find something that suits their personal approach.

Skills to make this work even better

It can be useful on occasions to make some preparation "essential", for example, bringing case notes of a patient with a specific problem or a diary of experiences. In this case it is essential to refer to and use that material during the session. If this is omitted participants will become demotivated.

Some topics are intrinsically difficult; talking about errors, ethical dilemmas, or controversial matters such as Assisted Dying. Anonymised preparation can make discussion of sensitive subjects easier and less threatening. For example, each participant types a brief account of an error or upsetting incident to bring to the session. These accounts are then gathered together and mixed up. Each participant then receives an anonymised, random account for discussion. This means that the issue is discussed without the specific person having to account for themselves (Reference 5, page 9).

ENRICH Speed dating sessions require specific preparation or else they do not work properly. Participants need to know this expectation in advance. In some situations the group can be divided to prepare specific aspects (for example part of the group might bring information from the clinicians point of view, another sub group from the patients point of view and a third sub group from a commissioning point of view). If smaller sub group Action Learning sets already exist (see ENERGISE Creating action learning sets), they might be tasked with preparing different aspects of the topic.

Pitfalls/when NOT to use this method

If the participants are not known beforehand it can be hard to allocate preparation appropriately, so this will not work for a conference. If participants are expected to be too busy to do preparation, giving it will only induce a demotivating sense of guilt if it is not done, (so that people may even fail to turn up at the session). Offering preparation as an "optional extra" is one way round this. Preparation works best if it is feasible and realistic in quantity.

Applications in other areas of the session

Depending on the subject matter and the type of preparation, participants can be invited to share their prepared contributions at different stages of the session. This can be one way to maintain engagement throughout the session.

How does this help to build relationships?

Creating preparation options, even if not all participants do them, demonstrates that the educator recognises the agency of the learner outside the session and reinforces that they are seen as active participants, not passive recipients of information. This demonstration of respect may help to build relationships and also implies that the educator is "bearing the participants in mind" between sessions, which also help to reinforce the learning relationship.

How does this help to structure the education?

Preparation can help to bring everyone up to the same level before the session starts. This offers weaker participants the opportunity to become familiar with some material beforehand, which is likely to enhance learning. If the preparation is structured with some simple, and some more complex options, learners will be able to access material at different "Blooms taxonomy" levels, suitable to their own learning needs. Weaker participants will also be alerted to the possibility of "deeper issues" even if they are not *currently* engaged at that level. When stronger participants do the preparation they contribute at a higher level during the session, which acts as subtle peer pressure/role modelling. Having "preparatory" material available in the programme can act as a resource, to help participants identify where to look for future learning.

References and resources

1. More information about the flipped classroom concept is available here: https://www.heacademy.ac.uk/knowledge-hub/flipped-learning-0 and there are of course many other sources of information online.
2. *What doctors feel; how emotions affect the practice of medicine* by Danielle Offri, ISBN 13 978 0807 33302
3. A basic introduction to Bloom's Taxonomy is here: https://en.wikipedia.org/wiki/Bloom%27s_taxonomy
4. There is a good introduction to the concept of Miller's Pyramid here: http://www.gp-training.net/training/educational_theory/adult_learning/miller.htm and more information in *The Essential Handbook for GP Training and Education* by Ramesh Mehay ISBN 978 1 84619 593 8
5. This method is described in Educ Prim Care. 2014 Mar; 25(2):114-8. *Medical error: a dirty little secret or a great learning opportunity?* Lea A, Danczak A.

2// USING TAXONOMIES OF LEARNING 1 – KSA AND MILLER'S PYRAMID

This method is used to enhance the **planning** of educational sessions. Educators can consider different types of knowledge and understanding, so that participants can engage with "enriched", more advanced, content.

When to use it

The educator offers new approaches to thinking about the subject matter, so that participants can grapple with complexity, so that new ideas come to the fore and so that participants who are reflecting at deeper levels, gain opportunities to explore issues more fully.

> "When the pupil is ready, the master appears." **Mabel Collins**

Planning that goes beyond a straightforward analysis of the "knowledge, skills and attitudes" required, can unobtrusively enrich the educational process so that learning can be a transformative experience for those who are ready to take their *professional development* to the next level. Planning in this way moves further away from the "fill up the bucket" educational approach and helps participants to develop their learning skills.

The set up: how to use this method

When planning educational session the educator refers to a taxonomy of learning to help identify the areas in which the education can go beyond "knowledge transfer". A "taxonomy of learning" is simply a way of classifying and subdividing different aspects of what is to be learned.

A very familiar example would be learning to drive; there is a "theory component", **knowledge**, including the Highway Code, which is normally learned by private study, and is tested with a formal, computer based examination. This knowledge is insufficient on its own. A learner will only become a successful driver if they get supervised practice in an actual car, in actual traffic. The **skills** for driving a vehicle need to be learned at the wheel. Moreover, appropriate **attitudes** to driving, for example, agreeing to drive only when sober, or, being considerate of other road users, will require both practical experience and the opportunity for reflection, discussion and feedback.

This example shows how different types of learning need different educational approaches.

An educator can consider knowledge, skills and attitudes in planning, so that educational sessions cover all these aspects, using appropriate methods.

However, there are other taxonomies that can be used to enrich and develop learning further.

Many educators will be familiar with **Miller's Pyramid**. This way of thinking about **skills** proposes that there are stages in skill development: different educational (teaching) methods work best at different levels of learning.

Miller's Pyramid describes skill acquisition proceeding as participants "know about, know how, show how, and actually do" the skills. These stages can be used when assessing skills. However, this approach is just as useful in planning education, so that skill acquisition is approached in a methodical and structured manner. The stages are described in detail here:

1. **Knows about** the skill in question: participants first have to recognise skills, and see them as being "learnable". This includes naming the skillset, (for example, "driving a car safely") and this includes many subskills, such as steering accurately, changing gears smoothly, and obeying traffic signals correctly.

   In a clinical context, this could mean knowing about the skillset of "performing an appropriate physical examination". Examination includes many subskills. A few examples could include, deciding which examination is required, explaining it to the patient and answering any of their concerns, ensuring the patient's comfort during the examination, discussing and providing any chaperone that is needed, using the examination techniques correctly. Initially, recognising the nature of the skill to be learned may be achieved in a classroom, using a "knowledge transfer" approach, accompanied by a practical demonstration or simulation.

2. **Knows how** to perform the skill in question: practising the skills of manoeuvring a car safely to the satisfaction of the instructor, could happen away from real traffic, on a private road or car park, for example. The learner could explain to the instructor how those skills could apply when driving on public roads.

   In a clinical situation, a learner could develop their examination skills using simulated patients or real situations, but very closely supervised, with opportunities for feedback and improvement. The educational method here is experiential: the learner actually does something, experiences it and reflects upon it with feedback and discussion. Effective skills development needs to go even further.

3. **Shows how** to perform the skill in question: a learner driver develops their skills, and shows what they can do, by driving under supervision, in real traffic, being in control of the vehicle themselves. The driving test uses the principle of "shows how" in that the examinee is driving independently, in a real traffic. However, the learner remains under the direct supervision of the examiner or instructor, who also may have access to "dual controls" in case of danger.

   In a clinical situation, learners "show how" by performing real clinical examinations in "live" situations, while being responsible to a senior who may check or repeat their findings, and who may give feedback where required. Most clinical examinations use "shows how" as a method of assessment.

   However, passing a driving test is only the start of a driver's developing experience on the roads. What needs to happen next?

4. Does do the skill in question in usual circumstances: the driver now demonstrates their skills daily, even when not under supervision. This may be the time when their attitudes are tested too. Do they drive carefully all the time? Or do they break speed limits if they think they will get away with it? The awareness courses that speeding drivers are offered include attitudinal issues as well as increasing formal knowledge.

   In a clinical situation, a qualified practitioner is expected to perform the skills in question, as a matter of course. This is assessed using work place based assessments such as direct observation or video assessment of real situations, 360 degree appraisal using the observations of patients and colleagues, and by techniques such as audit. The educational methods here tend to relate to appraisal, reflection methods, mentoring or "deep" CPD such as Balint groups. These are not aimed at "knowledge transfer" but rather are intended to encourage self-awareness and increase the motivation of practitioners to appraise and improve their own practice.

How can educators use Miller's Pyramid to enrich the sessions they are offering to participants?

Firstly, in planning, educators can decide which of "knows about, knows how, shows how, or does" is the most important level to be aiming at, so that they can choose an appropriate educational method. In postgraduate education, educators will be aiming to move rapidly from "knows about and knows how", to using methods that enable participants to "show how" they perform skills, in a protected environment or simulation, so that participants can get feedback to improve their skills. It follows that the methods used will be experiential, and provide opportunities for feedback and repeated practice. See ENERGISE Energisers for consultation skills education and ENRICH Making skills rehearsals effective.

The development of skills in formal postgraduate educational sessions is arguably more important than "knowledge transfer". Postgraduate participants should have sufficient private study skills to acquire the formal knowledge required in their curricula. In the age of the internet, the acquisition of information has never been easier. However, participants may lack the skills to implement knowledge in practice.

At one level this requires effective consultation skills, which can only be acquired experientially with appropriate feedback. However, other skills are needed for effective clinical practice. These include clinical reasoning skills, so that diagnosis and management plans are approached methodically, critical appraisal skills, so that new evidence can be understood and used judiciously, ethical reasoning skills, so that clinical decision making is underpinned with sound moral and ethical principles and shared decision making skills, so that patients can be true partners in their own care. Using the "knows about, knows how, shows how and does" can assist educational planning for all these important skills areas.

An incremental approach, which proceeds to practical skills practice and feedback, is needed so that participants get beyond basic levels and apply and use their skills in practice.

Maximising the benefits of this approach

Educators can use this method as described above to carefully select the content of skills training and to select methods that will encourage participants to the higher levels, i.e. "shows how, and does". This means incorporating experiential methods and feedback. The benefits of this approach are increased if the educator shares this approach overtly with participants, so that they understand what experiential methods are, and why they are used, so that they understand how experiential methods will help them develop their skills. Focusing on the development of a wide range of skills, using appropriate methods, is more use to participants in the longer run. Knowledge gets out of date. Skills once learned can be continuously developed through practice and reflection.

In spite of many years of this approach in postgraduate GP training, the message is not always clearly understood by many participants. When they seek CPD they often continue to seek disease-based knowledge transfer approaches ("what are the new drugs available for x diseases") rather than a skills-based approach such as "what skills do I need to critically appraise the usefulness of new drugs", or, "what new skills do I need to manage my time more effectively?" or "what new skills do I need now, to ensure that my team can implement change effectively."

Educators can facilitate the long term CPD of their participants by sharing their thinking and planning methods explicitly.

3// USING TAXONOMIES OF LEARNING 2 – BLOOM'S HIERARCHY OF EDUCATIONAL OBJECTIVES

Sometimes we need to change the language we use and the paradigms we are thinking with, to really enhance learning.

When to use it

This method is used to enhance the *planning* of educational sessions. Educators can consider different types of knowledge and understanding, so that participants can engage with "enriched", more advanced, content. This method of planning can be very helpful when dealing with groups where participants are at different stages of training, or when participants vary a lot in their current level of achievement.

Planning sessions that include learning of different forms and levels, can enrich the educational process unobtrusively, so that learning can be a transformative experience. Including material of varying levels of complexity means that every participant is likely to be able to take their *professional development* to the next level.

Planning in this way moves further away from the "fill up the bucket" educational approach. The educator can be explicit about the changes in the nature of the learning on offer, so that participants understand how learning evolves, so that they, in turn, develop their own learning skills.

> "A linguistic contour may be in use, which no longer matches the landscape; this signals a paradigm shift is needed."
> Brian Friel

The set up: how to use this method

When planning an educational session the educator refers to Bloom's taxonomy of learning to help identify the areas in which the education can go beyond "knowledge transfer". A "taxonomy of learning" is simply a way of classifying and subdividing different aspects of what is to be learned.

There a variety of ways of describing Bloom's taxonomy (Reference 1) and a short video summarising it, (see Reference 2).

Briefly, Bloom's approach proposes different levels of learning, the domains of cognition, emotion and actions. In the cognitive domain the levels are:

- **Knowledge, in which information is defined, memorised, duplicated,** but may not be fully understood or applied.
- **Comprehension in which ideas are described, discussed explained or classified.**
- **Application in which concepts are demonstrated,** used to solve problems or use concepts in novel situations.
- **Analysis involves understanding the component parts and relationships** between them, making inferences, finding evidence for generalisations.
- **Synthesis involves combining, compiling, modifying or re-organising,** putting things together to make a new whole.

- Evaluation involves constructing or designing something new, forming judgements in relation to evidence and external criteria.

An example of this in action is given in ENERGISE Creating action learning sets.

How can educators use Bloom's taxonomy to enrich the sessions they are offering to participants?

Firstly, in planning, educators can use the different levels to plan different kinds of activity at different parts of the session, or series of sessions. This approach can also be used to tailor sections of the session to the needs of different participants.

Participants who are more advanced could be asked to define an area to be considered and transmit knowledge about this to participants at an earlier stage. This is revision for some participants (which reinforces learning) and new learning for others.

Then Comprehension can be tested by inviting the application of new knowledge to solve problems defined either by participants (using problems they have encountered) or by the educator (who proposes "typical" or illustrative problems or scenarios). Putting component parts together in new ways, or to create a new whole allows Synthesis and Evaluation. This is summarised in more detail in the Resources section below, with a practical example.

Skills to make this work even better

Educators commonly ask participants to prepare short presentations for other members of the group. Teaching others is an excellent way to learn, as many educators will attest. Educators can direct participants towards a formal method of deciding what to "teach", (such as the Knowledge, Skills, and Attitudes framework, Miller's Pyramid or Bloom's Taxonomy), so that they begin to understand educational approaches more fully. This is so that their planning will be improved, and also so that their skills in learning will be enhanced for the long term. Anything educators do to promote skilled, lifelong learning will potentially enrich participants' professional development long after they have completed training.

Applications in other areas of the session

Some familiarity with taxonomies of learning is useful for educators during sessions. It can make questioning more effective, by taking the discussion to a higher level, (So now we are familiar with applying audit skills in practice, how could we use audits in different ways?), or to change the emphasis, (How useful are the audits we routinely do? How well do they relate to the concerns of patients?).

How does this help to structure the education?

Good educational planning skills can help education to be suitably incremental, developmental and develop deeper understanding and skills over time. Taxonomies assist the educator, in that they highlight a structured approach, so that elements can be prioritised, so that planning is easier and more rational. Taxonomies enumerate different elements of learning, so that, if uncertain of how to approach a particular topic, an educator can ensure that all aspects are covered, or select those aspects which will take participants to a more advanced level.

References and resources

1. https://en.wikipedia.org/wiki/Bloom%27s_taxonomy
2. There is an amusing video summarising Blooms taxonomy using examples here https://www.teachthought.com/critical-thinking/blooms-taxonomy-according-to-jerry-seinfeld/
3. An example of how to use Bloom's taxonomy in practice to enrich a session, see also ENERGISE Creating action learning sets for another example.

Here is an outline of a session considering respiratory infections in General Practice.

(Bloom's Taxonomy levels given in brackets in **bold**)

1. Assess Learning needs/hopes and fears about RTI in clinical practice.
2. What RTI are the ones most commonly dealt with in GP? (**Knowledge** – revising previously learned information). What are the difficulties posed by making a diagnosis in GP? (**Comprehension** – discuss, give examples, classify).
3. What consultation skills are required to assess an RTI correctly? (**Knowledge** – revising previously learned information and also **Application** – use knowledge and skills in new situations).
4. What are the principles used to develop hypotheses about RTI symptoms and what clinical reasoning is employed? (**Analysis** – breaking into parts, justifying generalisations, critically considering and discriminating amongst models of thinking
5. What skills are needed to explain and justify treatment plans to patients, ensuring safety? (**Application** – use knowledge and skills in new situations and **Synthesis** – bringing component ideas into a whole, propose new solutions to the problems identified earlier.
6. During the next session, after new skills have been tried in practice:
   - How did "Breaking good news" go?
   - What effect did changes to positive language and increased active listening have?
   - What further explaining skills would you like to develop now? (**Evaluate** – assessing, comparing and evaluating)

4// MAKING ROUNDS EFFECTIVE

Clinical care is a team game. In education we can ensure that everyone gets to contribute, and that everyone stays awake during a "round" that everyone is invited to join in.

When to use it

There are times in a session, when the educator aims to have a brief contribution from everyone, so that the "state of play" of the whole group is shared, so that the educator can be sure that they can move on to the next section of the session appropriately.

This could be an introduction, it could be when assessing initial learning needs, it could be reporting back on experiences after a skills rehearsal or other exercise. By using the variety of methods described here, everyone gets involved.

The set up: how to use this method

Explain the task (this might be introductions, feedback about the task or learning points from the day). Options to complete that task include:

- **Doing a "sweep"**. This approach means asking everyone in turn. This risks participants near the end of the round failing to listen, while they decide what they are going to say themselves, and risks participants near the beginning of the round switching off, once they have contributed. It can work with a smaller group.
- **Talking stick**. Explain that everyone will contribute. Everyone will listen without comment until the speaker has finished. The speaker will then throw/pass some kind of "talking stick" object on to the person who is going to speak next. The next participant to speak is asked to begin by repeating something the person before them has said, building on that when adding their own contribution. This enhances listening, and can link contributions together.
- **Ideas bring and buy**. Ask participants, by themselves, to identify the key learning points from the task under discussion. Then ask them to walk around, talking to other members of the group so that they share their own learning and so that individual can acquire new learning points from others, until everyone thinks they have the full set of key learning points

Explanations/timings

Explanation should only take less than a minute. Introductions many only need a short time. If debriefing an activity say there will be one (or two minutes maximum) minutes per person. The time taken will then depend on how many participants there are.

The debrief: maximising the benefits

Have a clear question and ensure that everyone does the task accurately. Debrief might be a short summary for a sweep/talking stick," A lot of ideas came out there". For Ideas bring and buy ask one person to read out their list of points; then ask if anyone has any extras to add.

Equipment/resources needed

Any small object that can be used as a talking stick type token (see ENGAGE talking sticks). This approach usually works better if the group is in a proper circle, as this embodies that contributions from everyone are valued.

Skills to make this work even better

Consider using this method to trigger reflections afterwards about the group process. In a think, pair, pause, share sequence (see ENERGISE using questions effectively for details), or in simple buzz groups, ask participants to consider questions like:

- How well did the outcome link to the aims of the session agreed at the start?
- What input did you have to the outcome of the discussion?
- What were the valuable inputs others made?

This helps participants to reflect on the **process** of learning and will help them to anticipate what will help in future, how they might use such methods for future learning.

Pitfalls/when NOT to use this method

Rounds are rarely fully effective in very large groups (over 25) although can be used very sparingly in groups of around 25 to 30 in the context of introductions. In larger groups, the bring and buy method or a pause, pair, square, share method works best.

Applications in other areas of the session

Summarising in this way can be useful to punctuate a session, to reinforce learning and signal the way into the next part of the session.

How does this help to build relationships?

Listening to each other and sharing learning, explicitly encourages conversations, which builds relationships. Seeing how other people take different things from an exercise can help open up participants to relishing and cherishing differences within the group, seeing differences as resources rather than sources of frustration. Being exposed to the learning of stronger participants (which may be more detailed, deeper or more nuanced) can help to raise the learning ambitions of weaker participants.

How does this help to structure the education?

Reinforcing learning acts like a summary in the consultation, it brings things together and can then be used as punctuation and a signal that another section of the session is going to start.

5// MAKING EXPERIENTIAL LEARNING OF NEW SKILLS EFFECTIVE

This section describes techniques to make training in specific skills both effective and enjoyable for participants.

When to use it

In General Practice, this will most frequently be in the context of developing consultation skills. When discussing what participants dread most about practical training, (see ENGAGE Hopes and Fears), role play often crops up as an issue: many participants dislike, or fear, "role play" and are resistant to its use. Yet, educators know that skills training, away from patients, offers a safe place to experiment, in a kind of "skills laboratory". This enables practice, without any patients being subject to early attempts, so that skills can be gradually improved in the company of sympathetic peers.

So why is there such a disconnection between what educators know, and what participants feel, about "role-play"?

Effective approaches to setting up and debriefing skills training are explored below. However, it is worth considering the "dreads" that participants have about these experiential methods of learning. Here are some commonly expressed concerns from participants, with an educational perspective and some suggestions about how to overcome these particular fears. The basic approach is to have an accepting response, then an explanation of possible benefits, followed by discussion with participants about how that particular concern can be overcome.

- **It is not realistic**. This is of course completely true. Practising a skill, such as shared decision making, with peers is not realistic. However, realism is not the point. What we are aiming for, when learning practical skills, is to break them down into component parts, understand and practice those subskills in isolation, so that when those skills are needed in a clinical situation, the clinician has had some basic experience of recognising the skill needed, practising it and getting feedback to help them improve. Ask participants if they know of any other "unrealistic" situations that are used in training. CPR training is one such. Although simulated CPR is not like the panic driven "real thing", it helps to have done it in training, so that some aspects are second nature when the emergency happens.
- **I cannot act**. It is true that most people are not great actors, which is why we pay good money to go and watch actors on the stage and screen. However, fortunately, when we practice skills in a training context we are not "acting". We are being *ourselves* throughout, developing an interpersonal skill that will be useful to us when we are doing our daily clinical work. We all encounter difficult situations, such as the patient who responds to every suggestion with "yes, but". Ask participants if they have encountered such a difficulty. Would they now be interested in learning a few different ways to overcome that particular consultation problem? Are they interested in learning new skills to help with the particular issue that is your topic for the day? When choosing the "set up", it can also be useful to ask *both parties to be themselves*. Further details of suitable exercises for this are given in Resources at the end of this section.

- **It feels clunky**. Indeed, this is true. Practising new skills does feel very clunky. We can probably all remember learning a new skill that seemed artificial and weird at first, only to become second nature once learned properly. Can participants remember what it felt like the first time they changed gear in a car? The first time they put on skis? The first time they tried to cook or play a musical instrument? Ask participants what made those skills get better over time. Usually it is a combination of repeated practice PLUS effective feedback. Feedback could simply be that when we get it right, the gears stop crashing and the car accelerates smoothly. Having the clunky part of skills development away from patients is a bonus: we get to make our early mistakes amongst friends, rather than in front of patients or impatient colleagues. Of course, it is essential that the relationships between participants have been built into a solid foundation, to enable this. That is why most of the methods described in this manual consider the impact on building educational relationships.
- **It is embarrassing**. This is an important point, and often raised. It can be linked to other concerns, for example, **it was humiliating in the past**, or, it was an **awful experience at medical school**. These concerns are important, must be taken seriously, and require educators to "spend time to make time". Thank the participants who have raised this key issue. Emphasise that humiliation and embarrassment are not helpful at all, because such emotions impede learning, and that as the educator, you will be wanting to avoid this. Ask the group to explore their previous bad experiences, (perhaps in pairs initially). Explore the behaviours shown by the group or the educator in the past, so that these can be shared with the whole group, so that the whole group can find solutions to these issues in this present, different, situation.

  Perhaps mistakes were laughed at. Can the group agree to respect mistakes as part of the learning process? Indeed, Japanese quality improvement gurus say **"every defect is a treasure"**. This is because when we identify something that goes less well, we can also start to develop ways to do it better next time. Mistakes are to be welcomed, we never develop if we stay in our comfort zone of performance. As Nobel Prize winning writer Samuel Becket said **"Try. Fail. Try again. Fail better."** Ask participants to identify better alternatives to any unhelpful behaviours that they have seen in the past. Consider recording the helpful behaviours on a flip chart as a guide.

  What behaviours can participants adopt if they see their colleague struggling? Can they agree to be supportive (rather than laugh)? Can they agree to give helpful feedback about behaviours which worked well or less well (rather than attacking the person)? Can a participant have another go after feedback to see if they can make things go better?

  Convey the expectation that the group as a whole will be responsible for creating a supportive and helpful atmosphere.
- **I hate doing role-play in front of everyone**. It is understandable that this approach can feel exposing and uncomfortable. Agree that no one has to "perform" in front of *everyone* if they do not wish to do so. Explain that the benefit of practising skills in very small groups of two or three, is that it is essentially private. This makes it less anxiety provoking and makes learning more effective. Ask the group how they would like an observer in a group of three to behave towards them, if they are clinician practising a skill. Ask the group to abide by those principles. A respectful non-judgemental approach, specific feedback about behaviour, not about the individual as a person, making helpful suggestions rather than making critical comments, are all approaches that usually pay dividends.

While it might seem that these discussions will take up valuable training time, this can be an essential way to help participants "buy in" to the concept of experiential learning for new skills. See this as an investment at the start. When fears are allayed, the payoff will be enthusiastic participation. The educator must remain calm, and able to explain the benefits of this approach clearly.

The set up: how to use this method

Before setting up the exercise the educator needs to have done some preliminary planning.

Firstly, is the proposed exercise actually a "role play" at all? A role play is where the party being the clinician behaves as themselves (i.e. they are not "acting"). The situation being worked through is a whole scenario/consultation that will include a number of subskills. For example, participants could be practising "Breaking Bad News". This includes many skills. Here are just some of the skills required to Break Bad News; building rapport with the patient, establishing an agenda for discussion, checking how much information they need and their responses to information as it comes along, and so on.

However, in many situations the educator will be aiming for participants to practice specific skills, rather than practicing a whole consultation. For example, the emphasis could be on skills for gathering information, or skills used in explanations, or the skills needed to perform "safety netting" effectively. When undertaking this kind of practice it is more properly referred to as a "skills rehearsal". Using this term may help some participants to feel more comfortable, seeing the exercise as briefly practising a discrete skill, rather than a prolonged experience.

Explain the exercise and the nature of the skill to be practiced before splitting the participants into groups of three. If you do this after smaller unit formation, it is much harder to get everyone's attention. Ask the group to identify behaviours that can be observed when the skill in question is done well, and have a checklist (see Resources at the end of this section for examples). Give everyone the checklist of behaviours required to perform the skill. This will be used to guide feedback so that it is objective (Was that behaviour observed?) and SMART (specific, measurable, achievable, realistic, timely)

1. Use any suitable group sorting method (see ENERGISE Group sorting methods) to divide participants into groups of three. Tell them to designate each person as A, B or C.
2. Ask person A to be the clinician, person B to be the patient, person C to be the observer. Ask the observers to use their checklist and note which helpful behaviours are shown by the clinician. Tell participants to start the skills rehearsal on your cue so that everyone is doing it together. This makes noise, and makes each person's skills rehearsal more private to their group.
3. Time the exercise strictly. Skills rehearsals normally only require up to five minutes. If a role play is being done, then allocate 10 to 15 minutes for a whole consultation.
4. At the end of the designated time, ask the participants to feedback in their groups of three, commenting in the following order. Firstly, the clinician comments on what went well and what else they would have liked to have tried. Then the patient comments on what they experienced that was helpful or could be done differently. Finally, ask the observer to give them SMART feedback, using their checklist as a guide to specific behaviours.
5. Then ask participants to change roles so that B becomes the clinician, C becomes the patient and A the observer.
6. At the end of the designated time, ask the participants to feedback in their groups of three, commenting in the following order. Firstly, the clinician comments on what went well and what else they would have liked to have tried. Then the patient comments on what they experienced that was helpful or could be done differently. Finally, ask the observer to give them SMART feedback using their checklist to guide the feedback
7. Ask participants to change roles so that C becomes the clinician, A becomes the patient and B becomes the observer.
8. At the end of the designated time, ask the participants to feedback in their groups of three, commenting in the following order. Firstly, the clinician comments on what went well and what else they would have liked to have tried. Then the patient comments on what they experienced that was helpful or could be done differently. Finally, ask the observer to give them SMART feedback using their checklist to guide the feedback.

Explanations/timings

Depending on how comfortable the participants are with each other, and with experiential methods in general, the introduction to the exercise may take a few minutes or up to half an hour if there are fears to be discussed. Educators will normally only have to explore fears once with any given group, saving time on the next occasion. Allow at least five minutes for feedback and discussion after each round of skills rehearsal. This means that even a simple rehearsal of one skill (say, safety netting) will take at least 35 minutes; five minutes explanation at the start, five minutes for each rehearsal and five minutes debrief in small groups. Allow a further five to 10 minutes to do a whole group debrief with open questions such as "which behaviours were most helpful? Which was the most difficult?

The debrief: maximising the benefits

The benefits of a skills rehearsal are maximised if clearly seen in the context of the whole consultation, and if the skill in question is one that participants recognise as being of value. Starting the process with adequate discussion of the difficulties posed by particular aspects of the consultation (see ENGAGE Assessing learning needs at the outset) will ensure that the importance of the skill in question is highlighted. Skills development should be done systematically, starting with the skills required at the start of the consultation, and moving on to those required nearer to the end. Using a curriculum for consultation skills (see The Calgary Cambridge Process Guide in Resources at the end of this section) can help educators plan ahead.

Educators who are very confident that they can teach any skill, any time, could work in a more improvisatory style, asking participants to describe a real difficult situation they have encountered. Then the educator can "generalise away" from an actual situation, create a suitable scenario for a skills rehearsal, set up the ABC groups as above and draw out the key behaviours, using appropriate facilitation. However, this demands high order skill and considerable confidence from the educator. Most educators will plan ahead!

More complex skills such as Shared Decision making, Breaking Bad News are described in more detail in ENRICH Developing complex consultation skills. Participants should be confident in basic consultation skills before moving on to these more complex tasks.

Equipment/resources needed

This approach works best if there is space for each ABC group of three to be a little way away from the others. Having a checklist of behaviours to look for, (examples in Resources, below) prepared as a handout gives observers something to focus on and helps them to be objective.

Skills to make this work even better

If the group remains anxious about learning in this experiential way, then the educator can model possible approaches first, (see ENERGISE Consultation skills what do you say after you say hello). It can work well if the educator deliberately mixes up some helpful behaviours and some unskilled less helpful behaviours and invites feedback.

If there are willing volunteers, educators can modify the skills rehearsal using a "phone a friend or ask the audience" approach.

Participants are divided into two teams. One will be the clinician, the other the patient. One willing participant from each team starts the skills rehearsal. If either of them feel it is not going as they wish they can put a hand up and ask for a time out. They can then ask a friend on their team to take their place, or, ask the audience for advice about what to do next. This means no one has to do role play in front of everyone, unless they are willing, but the whole group gets to participate by helping the members who are doing the skills rehearsal in front of everyone.

Participants sometimes think that doing the rehearsal three times wastes time because "we know what is going to happen". However, the reverse is true. Participants being the clinician tend to get better over time, because they have seen what works and have been reminded of effective behaviours when using the observer's checklist. This means that participants get to see improving practice (thus demonstrating that skills can be learned). Watching examples of good practice helps weaker participants to understand what is required. The effectiveness of skills rehearsal can also be increased if it is permitted for participants to stop if they feel it is not going well, ask for advice and feedback from colleagues and then "have another go". **Feedback makes perfect; practice makes permanent.**

Working with this approach consistently, over several sessions will increase participants' confidence and skill in using this learning method. Using the final debriefing time to summarise key points and the key behaviours that get results can be followed up by asking each participant to note down "what they will do differently" this week in their clinical work. Making time to ask about this in a subsequent session will reinforce learning and enable discussion of any difficulties encountered. In the latter case, invite the participants present to say how they coped with a similar difficulty. Hearing other participants' solutions creates powerful learning.

The Calgary Cambridge Curriculum for consultation skills is a very useful guide when planning
skills rehearsals and when creating checklists of helpful behaviours to guide the observer feedback.
It can be found here:

http://www.skillscascade.com/handouts/CalgaryCambridgeGuide.pdf

RESOURCES

Examples of experiential skills practice

A skills rehearsal after the group/educator have clearly identified the skills required

CLOSING SKILLS for a consultation

Patient; you have been diagnosed with Shingles, on your chest wall. The doctor has explained the treatment and follow up plan to you (tablets for the Herpes virus, tablets for pain, a follow up appointment in one week and a blood test) and will start the END part of the consultation with the words: "Before you go, can we check that you are up to date with everything that will happen now?

SKILLS CHECKLIST for observers to look out for

- End summary – i.e. doctor summarises briefly and clarifies plan of care
- Next steps – checks that the patient knows the next steps for patient and physician
- Safety netting – possible unexpected outcomes, what if plan doesn't work, when and how to seek help.
- Final checking – that patient agrees and is comfortable with plan. Asks if any final corrections, questions, concerns at that point.

A role-play example to be used for "Shared decision Making"

Here is the patient information. You are a 56 year old woman, who consults with these questions in mind.

Is breast screening compulsory? Do I have to go? I hated the last one, it hurt a lot and I feel scared and anxious all the time now, thinking I have to go through all that again. My partner says I HAVE to go, but am I allowed to opt out, what would happen? I find thinking about screening preoccupies me a lot. What if I get something in between? To me it is much, much more important to live life as it comes, free of worries. If I get a lump I will act straight away then. I read in the newspaper that treatments for cancer are way better than they used to be, so screening not so necessary anyway

You will start the consultation by saying "Is breast screening compulsory?" The other thoughts will only be shared if you think the doctor is taking you seriously.

Information for the doctor.

Your next patient is a 56 year old woman. You have never met her before and she only has minor illness in her notes.

Your background information

Principles of shared decision making:

- Identify clearly the decision to be made.
- Clarify how much the patient wants to be involved.
- Identify the patient's own priorities and preferences, as well as what information they have already.
- Find out what other information they might need e.g. a Cates plot, side effects
- Summarised as TEAM TALK/OPTION TALK/DECISION TALK.

Continued overleaf

An observational study of the effects of screening in the United States suggests that 50 per cent of screen-detected cancers represent over-diagnosis, and that while early stage cancer diagnoses have doubled, advanced stage breast cancer is about as common today as it was before mammography was in widespread use.

Screening mammography saves some number of individual lives in the sense that there are almost certain to be women whose breast cancer is amenable to curative treatment at the time it is identified by mammography, but not amenable to cure at the time it is identified by physician examination or self-examination. However the number of cancers for which the window of curative potential exists exclusively during this time is likely to be small. Potentially one in two women could be harmed by a false positives, over 10 years of mammograms, one in five were harmed by an unnecessary surgical procedure over 10 years.

Observers notes – look out for:

TEAM TALK – recognises the existence of alternative actions or options, the patient's preferred ideas; seeking the patient's point of view using open questions, identifying that the decision is to be shared not imposed

OPTION TALK – Identify advantages/disadvantages/benefits/harms from the patient's point of view. "What would be your reasons to say "yes" to this option? What would be your reasons to say "no" to this? Clinician explains their reasoning and clarifies the patient's understanding of the reasoning. Benefits and harms; thinks widely including impact on relationships, self-image, other constraints or values.

DECISION TALK – the patient's preferences are articulated and integrated into the final decision. The clinician does NOT say "you decide", but helps to weigh things up. The clinician has a responsibility to help the patient recognise what impact the benefits and harms could be for them. Simply giving people information and asking them to make an "informed choice", risks abandoning them to indecision or poor decisions, if factors are not weighed up appropriately.

A suitable system for recording feedback could look like this Observer's chart

Type of chat	Phrases	Checked patient's responses?
TEAM talk		
OPTION talk		
FRAMING talk How important is making this change/taking this step for you? How confident are you that you can make this change/take this step?		
DECISION talk		

6// ENHANCED EDUCATIONAL SPEED DATING

This method is helpful when the subject has quite a lot of knowledge to be covered, has some "knowledge transfer" components, and the educator is looking for an approach that maintains engagement throughout.

When to use it

This method is especially suited to topics that cross several curriculum areas, (for example, nutrition has a part to play in many aspects of clinical care), or when the focus is on applying knowledge in a specific context, (for example, eye disorders in primary care). The power of preparation by participants is harnessed here, so that the material is reinforced when they teach it to others, (see ENRICH The power of preparation).

Each individual is challenged to prepare a short topic, so that they can "examine" other participants' knowledge, so that it can be updated if necessary. Participants often have more prior knowledge than they realise, and this method helps them to access and deploy that knowledge in unexpected contexts.

This method also offers experience of "thinking on your feet", so that participants learn the skills of using the knowledge they already have, by applying it and extending it in new ways. This method also gives participants insight into how others tackle problems, so that they can learn other ways of thinking. Finally, they even get some insight into the minds of their examiners so that they can perform better in practical examinations such as Clinical Skills Examinations or OSCEs.

The set up: how to use this method

Before the session, the participants need to be divided into small groups of equal numbers. It probably works best if the total group of participants is 12 or more. Existing action learning sets can readily be used for this method (see ENERGISE Creating action learning sets). The method works in several stages. Stages 1, 2 and 3 happen ***before*** the actual educational session stages 4, 5 and 6 happen ***on the day*** of the session.

Stage 1

The educator prepares one question relevant to the overall subject, for each participant, in advance. Each action learning set is given a set of questions, one for each member of the small group. Each small group has *different* questions i.e. there is one unique question for each participant. By choosing questions carefully the educator can ensure curriculum coverage and highlight likely "unknown unknowns" in a way that also uses the existing strengths of participants. This also reduces the work for educators: they control the content and ensure relevance while not having to know all the answers themselves. Examples of potential questions are given in the Appendix, below.

Stage 2

In advance of the session, (say two weeks before), all the questions are discussed in the action learning sets. The members pool their existing knowledge, so that they come up with the best answer they can make as a group. The "owner" of the question notes down the information pertaining to "their" question.

Stage 3

After the group session, each participant researches their own question, and circulates the full answer to all the members of their own action learning set. This is so that, before the session, participants will have fully learned the material allocated to their group. The aim is to get about 10 key points per question.

Stage 4

On the day of the session, the educational speed dating takes place in "rounds". The description here is based on the assumption of three action learning sets. Groups are designated as A, B or C.

Arrange the chairs so that Group A sit in a circle, facing outwards. They will be the "examiners" and should have their questions and researched answers ready. Each "examiner" should have two chairs opposite them, one for a Group B participant, (who will be the "examinee"), and one for the Group C participant, (who will be the observer and record the marks obtained by the "examinee"). Ask each observer to have a piece of paper on which they can note the examinees scores.

Stage 5

Using strict timing, allow each examiner three minutes to ask their question and for the examinee to answer it. Use a bell, or similar noise, to signal that time is up. Then allow a further two minutes for the examinee to get feedback from the examiner, who teaches the examinee about any points they may have missed. The examiner and the observer then agree a mark out of ten, which the observer notes on the examinees score sheet.

Then the examiners change seats, moving on to the next examinee, where the process is repeated. This continues until the examiners are back with the examinee they started with.

At the end of this round, the material, already familiar to the examiners, is known to the examinees also.

In subsequent rounds the roles of examiner/examinee/observer are rotated between the groups ABC so that at the end everyone has undertaken all the roles, and all the material, known only to a third of the participants *before* the session, has been transmitted to everyone. The observers learn alongside the examinees.

See the diagram (Reference 1, page 28) which shows the layout.

At the end of each round, ask the observers what the highest scoring question was, and what the overall highest score for the whole round was. Another option, if some competition between the action learning sets is thought desirable, (not necessarily), ask the observers to tot up the total marks scored by every examinee, to get a "group score". At the end of the round, it can be helpful to identify any outstanding learning needs, so that this can inform subsequent private study.

Stage 6

When all the rounds are complete, invite reflection from the whole group on their experiences, perhaps using a "pause, pair, square, share" approach (see ENERGISE Using questions effectively).

The speed dating method is also discussed in References 2 and 3 (page 28).

Explanations/timings

As this is a staged process, it works best if participants are given instructions in stages. First, the educator gives each group instructions for the preparation phase, and one question for each individual in the group.

On the day, the educator explains how to lay the room out for the "examination stations", and explains the process. Moving the room can take five minutes or so and explaining the process another few minutes. The educator need to time to stations equally.

The debrief: maximising the benefits

Debriefing at the end is useful, so that the power of prior preparation is explored and emphasised, and so that participants can reflect on how they often "knew things" that they did not readily transfer to other contexts. For example, everyone knows that insulin lowers blood sugar and that when you have a low blood sugar you feel hungry and eat more. However, participants may not link this together to explain the benefits of reduced carbohydrate intake for patients with diabetes, who need to lose weight. Other educational benefits may come to light in the discussion; see the section "skills to make this work even better" below.

Equipment/resources needed

The educator needs to prepare questions in advance. These need to be rich enough to generate (say) 10 points in the answer, and yet not so complex that three minutes is not enough time to respond properly. Ideally, the questions are all of similar difficulty. The room needs to have enough space for the layout required. The educator needs to bring paper for score sheets and a hand bell or something similar to signal the timings.

Skills to make this work even better

It can be very useful for the educator to sit in the circle with the examiners, providing an "educational reflection station". The educators question is "What are your reflections on this method of learning". This invites participants to consider preparation, the value of learning before the session and the value of sharing ideas in a small group. Examinees often benefit from the experience of "thinking on your feet", so that they practice applying knowledge to the specific context of the question.

The observers benefit from watching a colleague grapple with a question, so that they learn that others think in similar, or different, ways when tackling the challenge of the question. Observers and examiners start to understand the process of making judgments about colleagues.

Examiners may relish having mastery over one particular question and are able to see how different examinees approach things very differently. This sometimes helps them to be more systematic in their approach, or to see how other participants can creatively use their existing knowledge, in unfamiliar contexts. Many participants find this is useful examination practice, although that is not the primary purpose.

When the participants are familiar with the method, they could be invited to choose a different topic and write the questions themselves, researching the answers in the same two stage way.

Pitfalls/when NOT to use this method

This method requires a stable group of participants, who can work over a period of time to discuss and research the subject matter ahead of the session itself. Participants who are unwilling or unable to do this will mean that the session does not work. It works best if participants already have a commitment to working together that has been built in previous sessions, using techniques from the ENGAGE/ ENERGISE sections.

Sometimes, participants may feel that the rapid fire format is too fast and that some questions need much longer to answer/feedback on. Educators can use such responses to encourage participants to see this as a way of identifying knowledge gaps, so that their private study is appropriately directed afterwards. Emphasise that the aim is to reproduce the quick thinking and creative use of knowledge that is required in many clinical situations. Was Einstein correct when he said "imagination is more important than knowledge?"

Applications in other areas of the session

A similar approach can be used during sessions to discuss other questions or controversial issues. For example, examiners could prepare questions and answers about the work of a CCG or practice manager, or could present situations, asking "examinees" to articulate which ethical principles are involved, or which regulatory frameworks apply. This can help participants to think on their feet more quickly, as happens during real life consultations.

How does this help to build relationships?

When participants work together ahead of the session they build their relationships. During the session, participants engage with nearly everyone in the group and this promotes mixing as they get to know each other. Quieter participants get to participate fully, which increases their confidence in talking with other participants and this can increase their ability to contribute to the group over time.

How does this help to structure the education?

This method sets out the benefits of preparation clearly, and the session itself has a structure that participants can follow. It enacts the idea that we build on existing knowledge all the time, and shows how skills and knowledge can develop with feedback.

Resources and references

1. Diagram to show the movement of group members around the question stations. There are just four illustrated here for clarity, although in practice there could be up to eight or ten examiner stations.

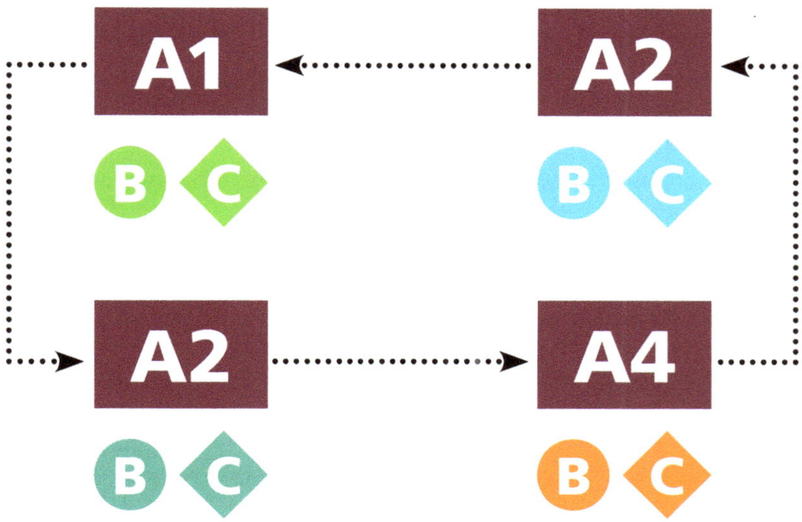

2. Speed-dating: a novel approach to GP education. *Education for Primary Care 2010* Nov: 21(6):392 by D Lashbrook
3. Teaching Exchange Enhanced educational speed dating: making education more "nutritious" *Education for Primary Care Teaching Exchange* by A Danczak 2012 https://doi.org/10.1080/14739879.2012.11494154

APPENDIX

Examples of questions that could be used for a nutrition session

There are some answers for the first two questions to illustrate the principle. When giving questions to action learning sets, including one completed question/answer set will help them to get the idea of what is required.

- What are the benefits/risks of a low carbohydrate diet and what might it consist of? Where could patients get good quality information about this?

  (Example answers could include; weight loss in those who tolerate carbohydrate poorly, better blood sugar control especially in Type 2 Diabetes, reduced requirement for glucose lowering medications and or insulin, if weight loss sufficient Diabetes may go into remission, better blood pressure control, improvements in non-alcoholic fatty liver conditions. Diet could consist of protein sources such as meat, eggs, fish, with green vegetables, low starch vegetables and low sugar fruits (not bananas or pineapples for example) and no sugary foods including many low fat foods such as yoghurts which have sugars added. Diabetes UK has an online course explaining how to follow this with online support from others)

- Which ethnic groups may have specific nutritional problems and what kinds of problems might they face?

  (Examples could include: higher rates of G6PD deficiency in certain groups with consequent restrictions on eating fava beans, red wine, various berries, and the use of many drugs is contraindicated especially some antimalarial drugs, aspirin. Lactose intolerance is more common in some black populations who need to avoid dairy produce, milky formulations of nutritional supplements and products, some people may find the lactose filler in some tablets affects them also, coeliac disease is said to be more common in those of Irish descent, and requires avoidance of gluten in all forms, including processed foods which often contain gluten from wheat flours)

- What are the nutritional requirements for a patient with acute copious diarrhoea?

  Explain how to make a suitable rehydration fluid at home and how much should be given. What advice about drug treatments should be given?

- What dietary advice would you give to someone wanting to reduce their cancer risk?
- What is a BMI and where do "normal" reference ranges come from? How did **29 million** Americans get to become overweight overnight in 1998?
- What are the potential benefits/risks of a vegan diet?
- What nutritional support is required for patients who have had Gastric bypass/banding operations? Who should pay for that?
- How can food /eating interact with the treatment of patients with depression or pulmonary embolus?
- What are the dietary needs of a breastfeeding mother? Any specific nutritional issues for the baby?
- What are the obesity "paradoxes"? How would you respond if a patient says "I am fat but healthy so stop harassing me to lose weight".
- What nutritional advice could you give someone who wants to maintain bone health/ who has arthritis?

Questions about "Eye disorders in Primary Care"

- Starting anteriorly, what are the layers of the eye?
- What eye testing equipment should a GP have at their disposal and give examples of how they might be useful in practice.
- What are the ways in which acute glaucoma might present?
- Can you list some, commonly used, drugs which may cause side effects affecting the eye or vision?
- What are the main likely causes of an acutely red eye? How can you use simple history and examination techniques to distinguish between them?
- What information should be given to patients starting Hydroxychloroquine treatment?
- How can a practice use its IT system to ensure that patients on Hydroxychloroquine get appropriate follow up checks?
- Which eye conditions tend to run in families? What actions should a GP take when a patient gets a new diagnosis of one of these conditions?

7// USING A FILM TO TEACH PROFESSIONALISM

A film called The Doctor starring John Hurt (Touchstone Pictures) is a useful way to teach professionalism/fitness to practice/practicing ethically in bite sized, enjoyable chunks.

What it is for?

Professionalism and Fitness to Practice are two crucial, yet not directly clinical, aspects of what it means to be a clinician in general, and a doctor in particular. Clinicians have to cope with the pressures of clinical work and the emotional strain of death and suffering, while meeting the requirements of Regulatory organisations.

Can we teach these aspects of clinical practice? Often, this is not actually taught; it is simply learnt on the job. Clinicians bring their idealism, their intelligence and their years of training to bear, and get on with their daily work.

- They watch other doctors and choose role models – people they would like to emulate
- They also choose negative role models –people whose behaviour repels or appals them.

These are some of the ways that the hidden curriculum is transmitted (See General Introduction, page 2).

Initially, I used an extract from a film called The Doctor, to illustrate a caricature of doctor centred consulting. This helped to identify some simple ways towards more effective behaviour. One participant, being very interested in the film, said "can we watch the rest of it?"

Using good ideas from participants increases their engagement in learning. So, we started using the film like a soap opera. Every week we watched another section, so that it could be used as a trigger to short discussions about the issues arising. There are natural breaks/cliff-hanger moments, so it can easily be seen in segments. This could happen over the course of a single session, pausing at breaks for discussion. An alternate approach is to show about 10 to 15 minutes of the film at the start of every session, using it as a warm up activity over a period of weeks.

Watching the film joins the group in a shared experience, so that they have a punctuation mark from their busy clinical time, into the more reflective space of the Study Release Course. It focusses their attention on the wider issues of medical practice, beyond guidelines or passing their exams, so that many interesting reflections result.

Watching a drama directs attention to that which could otherwise go unnoticed, or be taken for granted as "how things are". Fitness to Practice issues arise insidiously, at the same time the need to support colleagues is emphasised. Emotions are portrayed sympathetically; diagnoses and adverse events trigger fear and angry responses, which need to be met with kindness. Through facilitated reflection, a rich picture of appropriate and sensitive behaviour builds up, as we see all aspects of illness. "Cum Scientia Caritas" as the RCGP motto says, is shown in action.

Explain that reading a relevant book or watching a film and writing a reflection on what you have learned that will help you be a better doctor is a **valid form of CPD** and can be put in your ePortfolio or Appraisal Portfolio and will be accepted and welcomed as long as you can relate it to what you need to be learning about at work.

When to use it

Using a film is usually most effective when participants have had some experience of independent practice. This approach can be used for a single session/whole day or shown in sections like a serial or soap opera over the course of a few weeks.

> **Discussion question:** is part of a doctors job, to contain and manage individuals and society's fears and anxieties, about death and dying?

The set up: how to use this method

The educator needs to prepare by watching the film beforehand, (nice cup of tea in hand?), deciding on where to stop and have discussions. Having the word pictures from the competency descriptors for Fitness to Practice (see Appendix page 36) to hand can help to create effective, focused, questions.

Show the section of film to be discussed; then pause and ask the group individually to consider their response to what they have seen and what they think is the most significant or interesting part. Then, in pairs, ask them to discuss a trigger question(s). A full description of the film and possible segments is given in the Appendix to this section (page 35). Select the aspects that make most sense you and your participants.

Practice the IT set up beforehand; nothing is more frustrating than finding that the DVD does not work or the sound is off.

Explanations/timings

Start by explaining that the film is about a senior surgeon who finds himself facing cancer. It is an adaptation of a book called *A Taste of My Own Medicine: When The Doctor Is the Patient* by Edward Rosenbaum (see Resources and references, page 34), also worth a read if you have time. Explain that you will be watching, then discussing, the film in sections. Sections of about 10 to 15 minutes work best. Shorter sections can be hard for participants to "tune into" and longer segments can mean they get too involved in the story and feel a bit disorientated when you stop the film to talk.

Decide how long the discussion should be, usually five to ten minutes is enough to raise interesting questions and ideas. The total time is then about 20 minutes – ideal for a warm up activity as a prelude to the rest of the session.

The debrief: maximising the benefits

Have one or two clear questions for the participants to discuss. After the pairs discussion, ask a more open question such as "what issues have you been talking about?" or "what kinds of things are coming up in your discussions?". This avoids repetition of what each group has been saying in discussions, so that the educator you can "generalise away". This is so that the educator can introduce general principles, or professional standards, or further challenging questions, according to what comes up. You can ask each pair to report if the group is small enough or ask a general question to everyone if the group is larger. In the latter case, to draw out other contributions: explicitly call on pairs who have not reported back by saying something like "what were other pairs talking about?" or "let's hear from other people now?" or "anything else that came up?". This ensures widespread engagement from all members of the group, even quieter members and this increases commitment to the learning process. Sometimes key contributions come up very late, as reflectors and theorists get their thoughts together, after activists have initially plunged in.

Equipment/resources needed

A copy of the film The Doctor, a suitable player and projection facilities with good sound. The room needs to able be appropriately darkened, although total blackout not required.

Skills to make this work even better

Referring to the competency framework and descriptors can help educators create interesting discussion questions. Participants could also use a competency framework, so that they reflect on "Excellence" criteria, as this is what they are aiming at.

This method could be strengthened by asking one participant to summarise the issues discussed, so that they relate ideas to the competency framework. This is so that after sharing this with all members of the group (via an email or similar link), all participants can create effective log entries, providing evidence of learning for their ePortfolio.

Watching a film can also be used to sharpen participants' observation skills. For example, in the scene when the surgeon comes home to a kitchen in the middle of refurbishment, the ruins of the old kitchen act as a sort of metaphor for the upset in his life. When he and his wife talk through a hole in the wall, the wall symbolises the barrier that has sprung up between them because of his illness. Ask participants to describe what they see in a still frame, and to reflect on what this is telling us about the couple at that moment.

Play very short segments of just a minute or so, (for example the row with his wife in the den). Then challenge participants to repeat the dialogue verbatim, so that they develop their ability to listen intently, and remember everything that is said, (a crucial consultation skill, often lacking). Challenge participants to notice every single thing they see in one image (for example in the same scene in Jack's den), remembering that all the objects have been deliberately placed by the director/designer. How do they interpret the meaning of these objects? What do they tell us about Jacks life/state of mind? Such skills in observing the environment are very useful on home visits too!

More information about using film is given under Resources and references (page 34), with some other possible films to use.

Pitfalls/when NOT to use this method

There are few downsides to using film as a trigger for discussion; it may not work so well if people are already familiar with the film, although I have seen it many times with groups and see new things every time. If participants miss some sessions they may worry about picking up the thread. In fact, the narrative skill in a Hollywood movie, tends to make any segment readily understandable.

Applications in other areas of the session

If something crops up later, refer back to the Fitness to Practice, Ethics or Professionalism issues raised. This "looping" helps to link learning together and reinforce it.

How does this help to build relationships?

Watching a film in a shared space is a bonding experience in itself. Sharing the issues raised in the discussions also brings participants together. Consider using a variety of ways to form the pairs (see ENERGISE group sorting methods for ideas) because this can also help people talk to everyone in the group, even those they know less well or who have different ideas. Try to avoid Buzz groups that are always "who I usually like to sit next to".

How does this help to structure the education?

Linking the discussion to the competency framework is a useful way to fit learning into a bigger structure. Using the film as a "warm up" for as session in short segments breaks up the day and gives participants a reassuring sense of starting things off together as a group.

Resources and references

1. *A Taste of My Own Medicine: When The Doctor Is the Patient* by E Rosenbaum ISBN 0 394562828
2. *Cinemeducation: A Comprehensive Guide to Using Film in Medical Education* by Matthew Alexander Patrician Lenahan and Anna Pavlov Radcliffe ISBN 1 85775 692 4
3. *Signs of Life: Medicine and Cinema* Graeme Harper and Andre Moor. Wallflower Press. ISBN 1 904764 16 9
4. *Medicinema: doctors in films* by Brian Glasser. Radcliffe ISBN 1 84619 157 2
5. *Existential Psychotherapy* by Irvine D. Yalom. Well written, if long, book full of fascinating stories that illuminate the common life problems that patients have and the underlying realities they are avoiding.
6. Watching a film attentively improves generalist "Biographical" skills see JRSM Short Rep. 2013 Dec; 4(12): 2042533313510155. Published online 2013 Nov 21. doi: 10.1177/2042533313510155 *Examining the practice of generalist expertise: a qualitative study identifying constraints and solutions*. Reeve J, Dowrick C F, Freeman GK, Gunn J, Mair F, May C, Mercer S, Palmer V, Howe A, Irving G, Shiner A, Watson J

Other films that have been used with GP participants to good effect include:

The Arbor

This film shows life on a deprived estate, using the words of real people, spoken by actors. It is dramatic, disturbing and can be used to give new insights into the hardships faced in some communities.

See *The Arbor: a film that brought new insights to 'community orientation'* by Avril Danczak and Paul Westhead. Br J Gen Pract 2016; 66 (650): 479. DOI: https://doi.org/10.3399/bjgp16X686893

12 Angry Men

This is a gripping tale of how a jury deliberate on what verdict to give in a murder case. Starring Henry Fonda, this film provides an effective demonstration of how evidence and reasoning can be subject to serious biases. Could be used as a prelude to any teaching on clinical reasoning (see also ENERGISE Warm up Critical Reasoning) and refers to the competencies of Maintaining Performance Learning and Teaching, illustrated by the criterion "Judges the weight of evidence, using critical appraisal skills and an understanding of basic statistical terms, to inform decision-making ".

How to die: Simon's Choice

This is a documentary about one man's journey through Motor Neurone Disease and how his family and friends respond to his determination to go to Dignitas when he wants to end his life.

Made by Minnow Films who very kindly made a DVD available when I requested it – info@minnowfilms.co.uk See http://www.minnowfilms.co.uk/contact.html

A very powerful film that can be used as part of ethics teaching, using the subject of assisted dying as a trigger to reflection on ethical principles.

APPENDIX

Summary of the film The Doctor and links to Ethical, Fitness to Practice and hidden curriculum themes (Jack as a role model).

A cardiac surgeon, Jack McGee, develops laryngeal cancer, taking him on a journey from health and success, into vulnerability, illness, loss and death. In a parallel story, his colleague, Murray, faces litigation. Jack's thoughts and feelings about health, disease, and his relationships, change and he questions his values, and attitudes to patients; each section triggers discussions about ethics, fitness to practice and the different world view of doctors and patients. Watching a film attentively improves generalist "Biographical" and observational skills.

Ethical themes

Initially, we identify with Jack, a decisive surgeon, but his sexist, racist and judgemental behaviours to colleagues and patients become increasingly apparent, unchallenged because of his high status. Jack consults an ENT surgeon who is efficient, quickly making an accurate diagnosis, but she shows no kindness or compassion. After watching the extracts, discussions flow easily, considering whether all doctors behave like this at times, whether patients' feelings matter if the correct diagnosis is made quickly and what our behaviour towards less powerful people should be.

Hospital processes, by which Jack "becomes" a patient, compromise his autonomy, his confidentiality is breached, he mistakenly receives an enema intended for another patient and he is subjected to procedures with little explanation or consent. The casual lack of dignity, helplessness and frustration imposed on our patients by our systems is exposed; participants sometimes find it painful to reflect on their own unwitting collusion in such behaviours.

When Jack faces decisions about his treatment, we discuss the impacts of patient choices on resource allocations. Another patient is refused a scan on cost grounds, highlighting issues about justice and fairness. Jack is discomforted when a fellow patient describes her "missed diagnosis" and his colleague wants him to lie in court and alter notes. Uncomfortable questions arise about our responses to error, and whether we are willing to expose poor practice or criticise others.

Fitness to practice themes

Jack's relationships at home are strained by long working hours and his lack of attention to family life. Discussion could centre on how to honour both work and family and extends to consider our ethical duties to family members. Jack escapes the city with a patient who is dying, betraying his wife's trust. His angry rejection of care and concern from family and colleagues is rendered understandable, if not ideal, as Jack continues to work while having radiotherapy. He is grumpy with clinic staff, expecting to be fast tracked because of his high status.

These scenes raise difficult issues; how should a doctor protect patients from the effects of his own poor health? Do we offer support to sick colleagues, or exclude them? (See also ENRICH When the doctor becomes a patient).

A senior person might expect to be seen ahead of other patients, although we see the potential for harm when Jack gets his test results in a locker room. One colleague's caring approach is initially mocked by Jack; why does he then value that approach when he becomes a patient himself? As his friend worsens, we confront universal questions about how to live and die well, and whether we can be compassionate, while remaining effective clinicians.

Being a role model

Jack learns to show empathy to patients, understanding their concerns and fears, sitting instead of standing in clinic. He chastises students for being impersonal and makes them dress in patients' robes and use bedpans to improve their empathy. Discussions could consider whether it is acceptable to hug a patient, and whether Jack's teaching method is another abuse of his power, or an acceptable way to promote learning. Do we risk giving a doctor's personal experience more importance than patients' accounts of their indignities and difficulties?

Film Title THE DOCTOR starring John Hurt Touchstone Pictures

Here is a summary of the story and links to RCGP WPBA competency framework. Each of these sections could be broken into shorter 10 minutes sections for discussion. The total duration of the film is 118 minutes.

The story begins

We see a senior cardiac surgeon operating and doing his rounds. He says a surgeon should be detached, decisive, direct and is contemptuous of "a great deal of caring". He is sarcastic to his patients, a man who had attempted suicide and a woman whose husband is terrified by her enormous chest wound.

The doctor is seen driving in his sports car up the hill to his home; he races an attractive woman who turns out to be his wife. He tells her he will not be coming to the event she is speaking at as promised, as he has double booked another event, to raise money. She is disheartened "not again Jack".

Later he coughs while laughing and spits blood on his wife accidentally. His colleagues recommend a young ENT surgeon. In the consultation she appears cold, doctor centred, doesn't make much rapport and bluntly breaks the bad news that he has a cancerous growth on his vocal cord.

Possible discussion points

- Whose commitments are more important – the doctor or his wife?
- What is it like when the doctor steps into the shoes of a patient and experiences a brisk surgeon himself?
- Is what he metes out to others OK when he is on the receiving end?
- His child is summoned to say hello and picks up the phone – he is not used to his father being at home. How do we integrate our home and work lives to honour both?
- Is his behaviour towards women, people from ethnic minorities, and his students ethical or acceptable?

Competency framework word pictures

- Anticipates situations that might damage their work-life balance and seeks to minimise any adverse effects on self or patients. Reflects on how their values, attitudes and ethics might influence professional behaviour.
- Anticipates situations where indirect discrimination might occur. Demonstrates equality, fairness and respect in their day-to-day practice
- Values and appreciates different cultures and personal attributes, both in patients and colleagues

The story continues

The doctor has a biopsy which confirms cancer and he starts treatment. Initially he throws his weight around, not wanting to fill in the forms, not wanting to be kept waiting. He is gently reprimanded by another doctor, his oncologist and also by a fellow patient who says "don't shout at June, it's not her fault". We see him helpless strapped to a table having scans and DXT.

Possible discussion points

- What is it like when a doctor becomes a patient? (SEE ENRICH When a clinician becomes a patient).
- We see him being treated with indifference. When have we behaved like that or seen others do that? (It happens to all of us – why and how and how can we change that?)
- How do we come to be indifferent to the needs of the patients, failing to explain what we are doing, or being cold or unkind like the people in the scan room?
- What is the emotional labour of caring?
- How do we help each other to maintain warm approaches and attitudes to each other and to our patients?

Competency framework word pictures

- Encourages an organisational culture in which the health of its members is valued and supported.
- Encourages scrutiny of professional behaviour, is open to feedback and demonstrates a willingness to change.

The story continues

The initial treatment fails and Jack has to have surgery. His friend in chemo takes him up to the roof like Jesus being tempted by the devil and says, well kill yourself if you want to… He has to make a choice. He also has to decide what to do about a colleague who has acted fraudulently. As Jack faces decisions about his treatment, he hears about a patient is refused a scan on cost grounds, highlighting issues about justice and fairness. Jack is discomforted when a fellow patient describes her "missed diagnosis". His colleague wants him to lie in court and alter notes.

Possible discussion points

- Does a doctor have to have personal experience of illness to exhibit compassion?
- How do we cope with the spiritual/existential challenges of life:
  - that we have to discover what our life/work really means
  - that we have to make choices
  - that we suffer and die for ourselves (no one can die for us or suffer on our behalf)
  - that death is inevitable (See *Existential Psychotherapy* by Irvine Yalom in reference list).

Competency framework word pictures

- Reacts promptly, discreetly and impartially when there are concerns about self or colleagues.
- Provides positive support to colleagues who have made mistakes or whose performance gives cause for concern.
- Reflects on and discusses moral dilemmas encountered in the course of their work, able to analyse ethical issues with reference to specific ethical theory. Anticipates the potential for conflicts of interest and takes appropriate action to avoid these.

The story continues

Jack takes his friend for a trip without telling anyone and has some important experiences. He then has to undo the damage he has caused to others and face the death of his friend. He has to reconcile with a colleague and undergoes difficult surgery. Afterwards, he literally "loses his voice" and we start to hear more from others as a result. He listens more too. He makes important changes at work.

Possible discussion points

- What does it mean to open up to others?
- What changes has Jack made at work? How do we live with integrity and honesty?
- What are the limits of loyalty to family/colleagues/friends?

Competency framework word pictures

- Uses mechanisms to reflect on and learn from complaints or performance issues in order to improve patient care. Actively seeks to anticipate and rectify where systems and practice may require improvement in order to improve patient care.
- Reflects on and discusses moral dilemmas encountered in the course of their work, able to analyse ethical issues with reference to specific ethical theory. Anticipates the potential for conflicts of interest and takes appropriate action to avoid these.

Jack as a teacher and role model.

We initially see Jack as the top surgeon, dominating his students and expecting them to "know the right answers". One colleague's caring approach is mocked by Jack; how does he come to value that caring approach when he becomes a patient himself? Jack learns to show empathy to patients, understanding their concerns and fears, sitting instead of standing in clinic. He chastises students for being impersonal and makes them dress in patients' robes and use bedpans, to improve their empathy.

Discussions could consider whether it is acceptable to hug a patient, and whether Jack's teaching method is another abuse of his power, or an acceptable way to promote learning. Do we risk giving a doctor's personal experience more importance than patients' own accounts of their indignities and difficulties? If we "move towards" patients could this help us be more resilient? Fighting against human connection takes a lot of energy. How do patients give back and help their clinicians? (see also ENRICH Weaving in resilience techniques)

8// WEAVING IN RESILIENCE TECHNIQUES

This topic can be introduced in small chunks, in a small strand of a session that offers some techniques for increasing resilience.

What it is for?

Some topics or competencies can be daunting or difficult to "teach". Educators and trainees alike think resilience cannot be specifically taught or learned. A variety of experiences build resilience and the links should be made explicitly in sessions that harness creativity, encourage new ways of looking at things and greater understanding of the stress response. See also ENRICH Artist in residence, ENRICH Creative writing, ENRICH Using a film to teach professionalism. Resilience can be increased throughout training.

When to use it

During a study release course or in tutorials a "bite sized" opportunity to consider and reflect on different aspects of resilience can be useful. This can be used as a warm up to any activity/ session, or used as punctuation if an issue comes up in discussion. There are resilience issues involved in many aspects of clinical care. When the main discussion is about "teamwork" or "managing chronic disease" discussing ways to achieve sustainable practice includes resilience in a natural way and in digestible pieces.

The set up: how to use this method

In this section there are some examples of techniques that improve resilience. There are all brief and can easily be "woven into" sessions, either as warm ups, or when discussing a variety of difficult issues. Try using just one of these in a session. In a longer session on resilience, several of them could be combined.

Infusing positivity

1. **Three Good Things**. Ask everyone to stand up and move around the room. Greet each person you encounter and then share three good things that happened to you in the last week. Even better if this is "three good things that happened at work, or because of work".(for example, a pay cheque could be a good thing!)
2. **Be positive about the benefits of gratitude**. Ask participants to write down three things that they were grateful for yesterday. Share with participants on either side of them. Encourage them to do this daily at work, it improves mental health (Reference 1). Even better if participants focus on three things at work that they are grateful for. It's a good way to end each day before you go home. Discuss what would happen if this gratitude was sincerely expressed at work. How would relationships change if we said "thank you" more often?
3. **Balancing strengthening activities and draining activities**. The educator begins by drawing a simple bucket on a flip chart. Create a small hole in at the bottom, draw drops of water constantly trickling out. Ask the group if this is what work feels like, the energy in their bucket constantly draining out as the demands of the day drain away their inner resources. Usually everyone nods, sometimes a pause is required, for enthusiastic agreement to be ventilated.

Ask participants to consider what fills up their bucket with energy when they are **at work**. Ask some participants to consider what they do for themselves to "recharge their batteries" when at work. Ask another group to consider what our colleagues do to help us, and what we do to help our colleagues to "recharge the batteries". Another group could consider how interactions with patients can also recharge our batteries at times. This simple exercise can help people recognise the re-energising effects of the support and help that is around us. Even better if we remember to thank our colleagues for what they do and ensure we do our bit to re-energise them too.

Personal strategies

1. **Be aware of your surroundings**. In his book "Attending", Epstein describes a number of ways to re-centre and calm oneself in the middle of a busy day (Reference 2, page 41). My favourite is his advice to find one moment of exquisite beauty every day. This could be a spectacular sky glimpsed through a window, a lovely smile when a patient gets better, or the beautiful colour of someone's scarf. **Even better** if participants then make suggestions as to how they could bring beauty into their workplace, and what beauty they might notice as they do their work.
2. **Use your breath to build up your energy**. The simplest breathing technique to is breath in for a count of four, hold the breath for a count of four, breath out for a count of four and hold the breath for a count of four. Repeat this "Square breathing" four times to re build energy between patients or at the end of a clinic. **Even better** if participants identify ways to do this regularly through the day, to relieve stress and provide moments of calm. Similar methods can be powerful for patients too, as Venetia Young so eloquently describes in her article (Reference 3, page 41).
3. **Use the Positive Mental Training resources**. Alastair Dobbin and Sheila Ross have developed useful relaxation, pain relieving and weight loss meditations that patients find beneficial and which are just as useful for clinicians to use for stress, sleep issues and to develop resilience. Play one of the short relaxations and or meditations to the participants and let them experience the benefits, in real time (Reference 4, page 41). **Even better** if participants are invited to use one such meditation every day and to report back on the effects at a subsequent session.
4. **Using non-work time for "Re-Creation" of our energy**. Non work time is for relaxation, leisure activities, private study and TV or sleep. Getting the balance right is important. The burn in "burnout" requires fuel and we often provide this by ruminating and stressing about difficulties after work. Ask participants to share what methods they use to **let go** of work stresses at the end of the day, to **rebuild their energy** ("Re-Creation") in their leisure time, and how **they promote good sleep**. Good sleep improves academic performance, work performance and creativity (Reference 5, page 41).

Explanations/timings

The explanation for each exercise needs to be succinct and precise. Choose your words carefully to be positive in tone, with the expectation of benefit. Words can have a placebo effect when chosen carefully; equally, tentative or negative language can have a nocebo effect too.

The debrief: maximising the benefits

Debriefing these exercises need only take a few minutes. Ask what the experience was like? How might the exercise might change their thinking? How could these insights/exercises be incorporated into daily work?

Equipment/resources needed

None, except for facilities to play the relaxation/ mindfulness audio tracks. Most postgraduate centres will have suitable audio-visual equipment in place.

Skills to make this work even better

Plan ahead so that these resilience exercises are slotted in comfortably amongst other material. Sometimes participants are resistant to the idea that resilience should be taught. They blame all stress and difficulty on external factors such as understaffing, lack of resources, difficult patients, too much work….It can be stressed that we all need to care for ourselves during the day. These approaches refresh the mind in the way that coffee, or lunch, or a stroll, refresh the body. When the mind is calm and relaxed, clinicians are more likely to talk to each other and build good relationships so that they can work together to develop solutions to problems in their own workplaces.

Pitfalls/when NOT to use this method

This works best with a group that will meet regularly. It could work in a conference or one off session if there is time to follow up and discuss the experience, or if the participants are already experienced in this type of educational method.

Applications in other areas of the session

Refer back to what points come out when covering other topics are relevant. This reinforces that professionalism and Fitness to practice are involved in all aspects of clinical care and are not a separate entity.

How does this help to build relationships?

Widening the view of the sessions on a study release course to take a more holistic approach can develop resilience, so that the skills to create a sustainable practice are seen to be learnable, so that the benefits to relationships in study sessions and in practice teams are highlighted. This is likely to strengthen relationships between the group and the facilitator. Relationships between participants improve, as they share some of their own successes in managing their energies.

How does this help to structure the education?

Having brief warm up exercises helps to give the session shape and interest. Planning ahead can mean that these exercise slot in comfortably between other sorts of material. They can be used at the beginning as a warm up activity, between topics to signal a change of pace, or perhaps at the end of the day to send participants away refreshed and relaxed.

References

1. https://www.psychologytoday.com/us/blog/what-mentally-strong-people-dont-do/201504/7-scientifically-proven-benefits-gratitude
2. *Attending: Medicine, Mindfulness and Humanity* Ronald Epstein ISBN 978-1501121722
3. Reflections on Medically Unexplained Symptoms in Older People. Venetia Young Br J Gen Pract 2016; 66 (649): 423. DOI: https://doi.org/10.3399/bjgp16X686317
4. see http://www.foundationforpositivementalhealth.com/ for resources that can be used for clinicians and patients alike. There are examples of muscle relaxation and three-minute mindfulness audio tracks here: http://www.foundationforpositivementalhealth.com/listen-now/audio-tracks/

   These can provide short, but extremely refreshing breaks during the busy working day.
5. *Why we sleep: The new science of sleep and dreams* by Matthew Walker ISBN 13 978-0141983769 and *The Business of Sleep; how sleeping better can transform your career* Vicki Culpin ISBN 13 978-1472936578 Both these books offer compelling information about the benefits of sleep and the best times to sleep, for effective study, learning and performance.

9// TEAMWORK STYLES – RED, GREEN, YELLOW AND BLUE

This is a method to help groups investigate and understand teamwork in more depth.

When to use it

This is a method to help groups investigate and understand teamwork in more depth. It is based on the work of Merrill and Reid (Reference 1, page 44), using an abbreviated version of one of their team style questionnaires. This is a useful way to deepen participants' appreciation of other people's styles of working and interacting. This approach is best used when they have already had some experience of working together, in action learning sets, perhaps, (see ENERGISE Creating action learning sets) or in their regular professional teams. By setting a task in which participants with similar styles work together, the features of that style are highlighted, so that the value of diversity in teams can be explored.

The set up: how to use this method

The educator needs to set the scene of the session, which is to explore and understand teamwork in greater depth.

Part 1

Participants are first asked, as individuals, to respond to some scenarios and predict their responses. Then they classify themselves into four groups based on their typical responses. These groups are **red, green, yellow and blue**. The scenarios, and the method of sorting participants into their "colour" is set out in detail in the Appendix (page 45).

Then ask all the members of each colour group to gather in one part of the room, so that they can work together on the next task. This means there will be a **red** group, a **green** group a **yellow** group and a **blue** group. It does not matter if the groups have unequal numbers in them. In any given group of participants all "colours" will be represented, but groups vary a lot as the actual distribution. This method can work well, even if there are only two people in a sub-group.

Part 2

All the sub-groups are given the same task. This works best if it not a clinical task, so that participants are less likely to consider that there is a "correct" answer, and so that the content of the task enables them to work in their preferred style.

> A suitable task is:
>
> *The Queen is very impressed by the work of your part of the health service (for example, Primary Care or a Gastroenterology team). As a reward she has instructed that you must have a day off clinical work in the NHS, the other sectors/teams will magically look after all your patients.*
>
> *This will give you a full "awayday", to develop your team. Your task is to* ***plan*** *a great team development day, working with the other people who share your teamwork "colour".*

Alternative tasks are listed in the Appendix (page 45).

During the planning stage, the educator should move between the groups, noting down behaviours or phrases that correspond to "typical" colour styles (more details in the Appendix, page 45)

Part 3

Ask each group to feed back their plan in the order **green, blue, red, yellow**. The educator can then add a strictly non-judgemental description of any typical activities or phrases used by group members. For example, in the **blue** group, the educator might report back hearing phrases like "Will we need more than one coach to transport everyone?". In the **green** group they might hear something like "This will bring everyone together". More details are given in the Appendix, page 45).

Part 4

Invite reflection and discussion about how the different groups approached the task. Educators may like to facilitate discussions that include:

- What attributes did the different groups bring to the task?
- Which groups had the "big idea"?
- Which groups had an "action plan"
- Which groups considered the interpersonal relationships?
- Which groups had considered accurate costings/numbers/timings?

Explanations/timings

The initial explanation of teamwork exploration need only take a few minutes. The process of assessing individual team work "colours" takes about five minutes. Allow 15 to 20 minutes for the planning meeting and up to 30 minutes for the feedback and debriefing discussions.

The debrief: maximising the benefits

After giving the participants the scenarios, and telling them which "colour" each quadrant corresponds to, allow a small amount of discussion about how they chose their answers. The setup is that individuals choose their own preferences, knowing that there is no "correct answer", so that participants discover that other people may make quite different choices to themselves. This insight alone can help participants begin to recognise that variations in "style" are inevitable in teams, and that other people may have ***different thought processes***.

Equipment/resources needed

A PowerPoint presentation of the scenarios and how to "score" the teamwork style makes the separation of participants into groups much easier. Having the task on a screen during the discussions can be a helpful aide memoire.

Skills to make this work even better

The purpose of this exercise is not to create "perfect" plans, nor to put across the idea that people can only behave in certain stereotyped ways. The purpose is more to demonstrate that variations in preferred style of working exist, so that participants can recognise that all the styles can work together in effective team working. Indeed, different styles and strengths are needed so that teams work effectively.

Big ideas can be essential. To make them happen, ideas people need to work with those who develop good relationships, so that work proceeds smoothly. Those whose strengths lie in making suitable lists/detailed plans need to be able to recognise and work with those team members who are good at keeping on track and getting things done, so that projects do not get bogged down in detail. The educator can bring all these points out with skilled facilitation of the debriefing, picking up on the comments and actions that support this line of thinking.

Pitfalls/when NOT to use this method

This method may not work if the participants are not used to working in an experiential way, or where participants have not had experience of working with others in teams. It will usually work best where groups are working together over a period of time and have built up some trust in each other.

It could work well as a standalone half day session or as part of a team training day if care is taken to introduce the purpose carefully and to do the debriefing in a supportive and non-judgemental way. Care must be taken to "generalise away" from individual people to the behaviours that are part of that colour. For example, this may mean saying "Often people with a **blue** style will contribute detailed planning, for example, about menus" rather than saying " I heard M spend ages talking about how many people might be allergic to any nuts in the buffet".

Clearly, many participants will have skills that serve in several styles. The purpose of this exercise to generate thought about how teams ***benefit from diversity***. The person who irritates you the most in the team is probably a different "style" from you. They are likely to have something very useful to offer, that you may well have overlooked because it is "not your style".

Applications in other areas of the session

Not applicable as such. However, in subsequent sessions it can be helpful to refer back to teamwork styles as needed. "We need a good analyst to help us with this problem".

If taking participants to a conference (see ENRICH Conferences and how to make them into enjoyable and effective education) it could be useful to ask participants to organise the trip themselves, harnessing the different styles. **Blue analysts** are good at organising coaches, **green amiables** can get social activities working well, and so on.

How does this help to build relationships?

Understanding how other people have different attributes, strengths and preferred styles is a good step towards more effective working relationships, both amongst participants and in the clinical teams they work in. Participants who feel their particular strengths are welcomed feel more valued. Understanding the strengths they lack, can help participants positively seek out those strengths in others, which also helps to build stronger relationships.

How does this help to structure the education?

This approach demonstrates that effective team work benefits from diversity and that team members can learn to value the styles of others. This approach shows that this approach is a learned skill, so that participants understand that they can develop these skills systematically over time. The educator can link this learning to the curriculum and to relevant competency statements, so that participants see how their educational experiences are related to what is required in a clinical context.

References

1. Merrill DW, Reid RH. *Personal Styles and Effective Performance: Make Your Style Work for You*. London: CRC Press; 1999
2. Other useful reading about teamwork and management styles:
   - *The 7 Habits of highly effective people* by Stephen Covey
   - *Eat that frog!: Get more of the important things done today* by Brian Tracey
   - https://www.businessballs.com/
   - The *One Minute Manager* series

APPENDIX

How to divide participants into a teamwork style "colour".

Participants are asked to draw a box on their notepad, dividing it into four squares like this:

Ask them to consider these scenarios in turn, noting whether they prefer to answer A or B, L or R.

If you are late for a group or team meeting:

- Do you get upset, rush there as fast as possible, apologise to everyone there when you arrive? (A)
- Don't panic, call ahead to say you are a few minutes late, feel bad about keeping people waiting? (B)

When speaking in front of a whole group:

- I am entertaining, humorous, or maybe relatively quietly spoken (A)
- I am clear, concise, direct, specific possibly loud (B)

My own space (work, office, home spaces):

- Looks disorganised, piles of stuff, arty, family photos, sentimental things on display (A)
- Looks tidy, organised, has to do lists, calendar, (B)

After these scenarios ask participants who mostly get A to shade in the two lower boxes in their square, those with mostly B to shade the upper two boxes

If I need help with a problem from someone:

- I explain the problem in as much detail as possible, and how the problem makes me feel (L)
- I explain how I see the problem being solved, sometimes making my point by exaggerating a bit (R)

When I am setting goals I choose

- Things I can realistically attain, make me feel good when I achieve them (L)
- Are challenging or exiting to achieve, perhaps part of a bigger objective (R)

When I am at education/meetings/presentations

- I get bored if it is too slow, I want it interesting as well as informative (R)
- I support the speaker as it's a hard job, and look for the logic behind what they are saying (L)

After these scenarios ask participants with mostly L to shade in the left hand two boxes (top and bottom) and those with mostly R to shade in the right hand two boxes (top and bottom).

When this has been done ask participants to note which of the quadrants has been shaded twice. This corresponds to their "colour" as in the box here.

BLUE	RED
GREEN	YELLOW

Possible Alternative Tasks

- Your group has to organise a fundraising event to raise money for your society/club/school or faith organisation.
- Your group has to organise a day of activities for the non-clinical partners, of a group of visiting clinicians from another country, who want to learn about our local culture.
- Your group has to organise a one day outing, for a family reunion of 35 family members of all ages.

Summary of the Characteristics of the colour types to share with participants AFTER the task debrief and to facilitate discussion of diversity in teams.

GREEN sometimes called AMIABLE

Strengths – calm, team player, seek harmony, encouraging, sharing, caring, relaxed, get on with the job in hand.

Drawbacks – will submit to avoid making waves, avoid hassle, may become passive.

BLUE sometimes called ANALYTICAL

Strengths – formal, measured, systematic, seek accuracy, precise, deliberate, formal, cautious, and questioning.

Drawbacks – get over-focused on detail, may withdraw themselves from participation if overwhelmed.

RED sometimes called DRIVER

Strengths – business like, fast, decisive, seek control, purposeful, determined, demanding, and energetic

Drawbacks – assertive can feel controlling, may become ruthless

YELLOW sometimes called EXPRESSIVE

Strengths – flamboyant, fast, spontaneous, seek enthusiasm, demonstrative, persuasive, expressive, sociable and dynamic

Drawbacks – rise to the challenge at first, but can get stressed, may flip and become ruthless drivers

10// USING SCULPTS

This is a good method to introduce any session that is concerned with the relationships between people, in particular between team members, between organisations or between different parts of an organisation.

When to use it

It could be helpful when education is about partnerships or clinical teams, or when considering the relationships between primary care and secondary care, or between different component parts of a larger organisation like a CCG or even a hospital. The aim is to use a variety of non-clinical objects to create an image which describes the organisation and its relationships.

> "It is the artist who tells the truth and the photographer that lies." **Auguste Rodin**

The set up: how to use this method.

The example described here is used to help participants in training reflect on the team they work in, and how the relationships are structured.

Before the session the educator gathers together a large number of random objects, ensuring that there at least ten potential objects per participant, maybe even more. Suggestions are given in the equipment/resources paragraph below. These should all be placed at random on a large table or tables at the side of the room.

Ask participants to arrange their chairs in a circle, with the seats facing outwards. If there is insufficient room for this, ask participants to arrange their chairs in two equal rows, back to back. If they sit in the chairs they should be looking outwards.

Ask participants to look at all the objects and choose some of them to represent the people in their team. Then the objects should be arranged on their own chair, so that they demonstrate what the team is like and how people relate to each other. When complete, participants will take turns to talk through their "sculpt".

Explanations/timings

First, before moving any chairs or explaining the specific task, ask participants, individually, to reflect on all the professional teams they have ever worked in. Then, with a partner, ask them to discuss the differences between those teams. Were some friendly, or merely efficient? How did the newer or more experienced members of the team relate to senior members? What was the overall feeling of the team like?

Then, ask them to reflect on their *current team,* again individually.

Then, explain that the objects on the table are to be used to create a representation of their current team, using their chair as the frame. Emphasise that there are no right or wrong ways to represent a team, that no one will be asked to reveal anything that they do not wish to discuss, and that the sculpts that result are *private to the group*. Explain why you have chosen this approach (to illustrate what teams feel like, and as an introduction to the topic of the day, to do with teamwork skills).

Ask them to move the chairs into a suitable arrangement. Then allow 10 to 15 minutes for participants to select their objects and create their "sculpt". Explain that objects must be used, **not words**, so that participants will use the holistic, integrating and emotionally aware right side of their brains, so that the image produced will be more true to life. As Rodin said, "It is the artist who tells the truth and the photographer that lies".

Allow one to two minutes for each participant to explain their team representation. If the group size is large, this may benefit from having two educators present and dividing the group into two for the debriefing.

The debrief: maximising the benefits

Model an accepting, non-judgemental approach right from the start of the debriefing, by thanking participants for their enthusiasm and the interesting sculpts they have produced.

Ask each participant to talk through, how they chose the objects, and how they chose the arrangement. Allow questions from other participants, asking them to avoid making judgements, but just to ask about matters of fact. Ask the participant if they have any thoughts about their team or sculpt that they would like to share.

It is useful to link the relationships of the "sculpts" to any other work that has been done on this relationship in the group beforehand. This might mean simply commenting on how varied the teams seem to be, or how many interconnections there are, (or not), using the same active listening skills as used in consultations to draw out any interesting thoughts.

Equipment/resources needed

This method works best if the room allows for the chairs to be rearranged, such that the whole group can walk round and see each other's "sculpts".

Suitable items for the resources table could include some, any or all of:

- **Natural objects** found lying around such as pebbles, leaves, flowers, twigs, feathers, (on one occasion when doing this exercise on a residential, the participants collected objects from the beach to do the sculpts with).
- **Objects that naturally come in multiples** such as playing cards, loose change, pens and pencils, chess pieces, jigsaw pieces.
- **Objects that can have many uses** such as string, straws, BluTak, sticky tape, sticky notes.
- **Tools** such as spoons, scissors, paper clips, bulldog clips, bags, wires, phone chargers.

Educators can use their imagination here, or just empty that drawer that everyone has in their kitchen where all these sorts of things migrate to! This is a good use for that pack of cards that has a few missing.

It works best of there are lots of things to choose from, so that every participant can find as many objects as they need to represent their team and its members.

Skills to make this work even better

Having completed a "sculpt", participants could be asked to consider what a "sculpt" of their previous team might have been like, and to reflect on any differences/similarities. When everyone has explained their team representation, ask participants to consider:

- How the team came to be that way?
- Who drives that?
- What team processes hold their team together?
- If they were to invent a totally new team, what would it look like then?
- How would we set about achieving that?

These kinds of discussions can lead into any session on aspects of teamwork, partnerships, or practice team development.

Alternative approaches could be to ask participants to model the relationship between their current team and all the other organisations that their team interacts with. This could include other parts of the same organisation, other organisations that impact on healthcare such as the GMC, NMC, CQC, or other parts of public service such as NHS England or the Treasury. This could help participants orientate to sessions on organisational matters.

Sculpts do not always require objects. Participants could be asked to "model" a particular relationship by asking fellow participants to represent the other parties. For example, a difficult clinical situation, with angry family members, frustrated team members and a complicated patient, could be represented by other participants, The person doing the "sculpt" moves the other individuals into the positions they occupy, (near to the team or far away), and their significance, (small and crouching down? Hiding behind others? Shouting from a distance?). This can illuminate the dynamics of a situation clearly.

Pitfalls/when NOT to use this method

This method usually works best if a group has worked together for some time, or who have gathered to consider team issues, such as participants on a leadership course. It could work well with a group who were meeting for the first time if they were wishing to discuss organisational issues, or if they had some previous experience of group working. It may not be the best technique to use if participants are only meeting you once, or if they are very unused to group work, expecting a formal lecture.

Applications in other areas of the session

A sculpt can be used spontaneously, perhaps asking participants to use other members of the group as the "pieces". This can illustrate a complex difficulty or facilitate a case discussion. Objects in the room could also be used. Educators can even ask participants to use the contents of their pockets or bags as the raw material for a representation. The more imagination used the better.

How does this help to build relationships?

Discussing representations that come from the participants imagination helps participants to see each other "in the round", accepting each other's differences. This helps to build more respectful and deeper relationships. Seeing how others understand things in different ways, is a powerful way to widen the view.

How does this help to structure the education?

This approach is a useful punctuation, whether used at the start of a session or later on. It can precede or follow ENGAGE Hopes and fears or ENGAGE assessing learning needs at the outset. This method encourages participants to use their imagination and to reflect on an issue, so that they consider their learning needs.

An activity of this nature naturally attracts the keen enthusiasm of "Activist" learners, so that their involvement acts to encourage and inspire those of a less forward nature. Theorists and Reflectors often find that this method is a useful way to start getting their thoughts in order. Pragmatists will usually go with the flow!

11// WHEN A CLINICIAN BECOMES THE PATIENT

Discussing clinicians' own health has perhaps become less of a taboo than in the past, when all too often clinicians own mental and physical health needs could be ignored or minimised.

When to use it

We all become patients at some point. Helping clinicians to think about themselves as the "patient" creates opportunities to explore important issues about caring for oneself and colleagues properly. Becoming a patient generates difficulties for a knowledgeable clinician, who is not used to being on the "other side of the desk". However, looking after a colleague who is ill can be challenging too!

> "The physician who looks after himself has a fool for a patient."
> **Sir William Osler**

This session is best used towards the end of training, or in situations where a team regularly cares for other clinicians. It is helpful to face these issues in a training environment, so that when participants become ill themselves they will be better prepared, and so that they will be more skilful in managing some of the difficulties that can occur when they are caring for sick colleagues.

The set up: how to use this method

Tell participants in advance that the session is coming up and ask them to do some preparatory reading. Some possible reading is suggested in the References and Resources section below, some of it readily available online (References 1 and 2, page 52). This enrichment session is usually best done in small groups of six to eight participants, facilitated by a colleague who has experience of caring for colleagues. Most GP Trainers will be able to fulfil this role admirably.

Ask participants to familiarise themselves with the GMC guidance on practitioner health, or any guidance from their own professional body, if clinicians from other disciplines are present (see Reference 3, page 52).

Introduce the topic and share the GMC guidance. There are two parts to this session.

Part one: invite participants to consider these questions:

- Have they had to care for other doctors/ doctors families in their role as a GP?
- What was that like?
- What problems did they encounter?
- How were they tackled?

Part two: invite participants to examine issues from the other side with these questions.

- What happens if you are ill yourself?
- How do we behave as clinicians when we are ill?
- What do we need from our doctors?
- How can we help them?
- How can we avoid making things worse?
- Which part of our professional guidance on health is the hardest to follow? Why?
- Do we all have GPs of our own?
- What are the barriers to getting effective health care for clinicians?

Explanations/timings

The explanation need only be brief, and could be preceded by a brief ice breaking introduction round, (acknowledging that this is an uncomfortable topic for clinicians) and ENGAGE Establishing learning needs at the outset. If participants are already familiar with each other, introductions need only be brief, but enough to ensure that the educator facilitating feels that they have developed some relationship with the participants. This encourages discussion of potentially difficult material.

The debrief: maximising the benefits

The key points to explore are the challenges of caring for other clinicians. This includes examining the assumptions we make about clinicians knowledge, finding that there are issues around maintaining appropriate boundaries while also acknowledging the special vulnerability of clinicians, and negotiating appropriate care without simply yielding all clinical control to the clinician themselves.

When discussing the impact of sickness on clinicians themselves there may be many emotive issues including clinicians' concerns about whether their treatment is correct, and being unsure how to approach seeking help, yet wanting to be "cared for". There can be difficult issues for the sick clinician to face, including loss of power and identity, shame, stigma and loneliness. Allowing free discussion will normally allow these issues to be ventilated. The educator could summarise these at the end.

Equipment/resources needed

Participants can benefit from looking at the resources, there is an information sheet for clinicians seeking help in the References and resources section to give as a handout at the end (Reference 4, page 52). The group needs a private space to meet in, as sometimes discussions can become emotional.

Skills to make this work even better

Groups may begin by talking in generalities. Sharing specific experiences can often be more helpful. The educator should regularly ask for specific examples, or ask what direct experiences participants have had themselves. Asking if anyone feels comfortable sharing a bad experience can be fruitful. Allow participants to talk with each other across the group, not just in dialogue with the educator. Aim to let at least two or three participants speak before adding facilitation. If there is a short silence, it is OK to stay with it for a while. Participants will soon jump in without specific encouragement.

Educators will make careful judgements about what they share about their own experiences of illness; the educator's role is to facilitate the group discussion, not necessarily to be part of the discussion itself.

Finally, the group may wish to consider to what extent it is acceptable for a clinician to share their own experiences of illness with patients. What are the pros and cons of doing so?

Educators can also extend the discussion to prevention:

- How could participants look out for their colleagues and provide support when needed?
- What are the best ways to ask for support and help?

The scope of the discussion could be extended by considering these questions where relevant:

- How would we tackle it if one of our partners was:
  - Drinking too much?
  - Suffering from depression?
  - In constant pain because of arthritis?
- How would we know?
- What can teams do to maintain awareness of each other's needs?

Pitfalls/when NOT to use this method

Small groups discussing potentially difficult topics work best when there are experienced group members who already know and trust each other, or if participants already used to group working methods, such as those who may have attended a Balint Group.

Care needs to be taken if the educator knows that some participants are vulnerable because of existing health issues and negotiating some "group rules/expectations" may also be helpful. Participants should always have the possibility of "opting out", if things become too painful for them.

Applications in other areas of the session

N/A

How does this help to build relationships?

Discussion of sensitive subjects such as illness means that participants give of themselves and this deepens relationships. If participants go away with the idea that we need to support, and be supported by, our colleagues in an atmosphere of mutual concern, then working relationships could be improved also.

How does this help to structure the education?

A serious subject like this can signal that training is coming to an end and that participants need to prepare themselves for being full members of the workforce.

References and resources

1. Articles that shed light on the challenges of caring for fellow clinicians include:

   Domever-Klenseke and Rosenbaum in Fam Med 2012 Jul Aug 44 p 471–7. *When doctor becomes patient: challenges and strategies in caring for physician patients*. A good abstract is available here: https://www.ncbi.nlm.nih.gov/pubmed/22791531 and describes difficulties with boundaries, avoiding assumptions and negotiating care.

   Jonathon Tomlinson's article in the BMJ has much useful information and insight based on clinicians own experiences, see *Lessons from "the other side": teaching and learning from doctors' illness narratives*. BMJ 2014; 348 doi: https://doi.org/10.1136/bmj.g3600 (Published 02 June 2014) BMJ 2014; 348:g3600

   This interesting blog from abetternhs.net which covers important issues including shame, loss of identity and stigma, while having many useful links and resources, see *When doctors become patients* https://abetternhs.net/2014/01/27/dr-patients/

2. A comprehensive account is in *When Doctors become Patients* by Robert Klitzman ISBN 9780195327670
3. GMC information about managing one's own health is available here: https://www.gmc-uk.org/concerns/information-for-doctors-under-investigation/support-for-doctors/managing-your-health
4. A potential handout to be given at the end of the session as an aide memoire.

   Key GMC points from Good Medical Practice.

   77. You should be registered with a general practitioner outside your family to ensure that you have access to independent and objective medical care. You should not treat yourself.

   78. You should protect your patients, your colleagues and yourself by being immunised against common serious communicable diseases where vaccines are available.

   79. If you know that you have, or think that you might have, a serious condition that you could pass on to patients, or if your judgement or performance could be affected by a condition or its treatment, you must consult a suitably qualified colleague. You must ask for and follow their advice about investigations, treatment and changes to your practice that they consider necessary. You must not rely on your own assessment of the risk you pose to patients.

Handout for after the session. Many thanks to Dr Tim Greenaway who produced this.

Being a good patient and getting the best from your doctor

- Register with a GP who is not one of your partners
- Avoid treating yourself or those close to you with prescription only drugs (GMC and BMA guidelines). N.B. Chemists will now question this if it is obvious.
- Doctors tend to worry about their health! Checking out problems and fears with close friends can help get things in perspective before a formal consultation.
- Avoid formally referring yourself to non-emergency secondary care where ever possible. If you feel for some reason that it is necessary then inform your GP, i.e. "Do as you would be done by."
- Consider an initial phone or email consultation with your GP: "I have got a problem I would like to come and talk to you about ..." may lead to a more timely appointment and a more effective consultation.
- Respect your GP's time and privacy – e.g. avoid ringing at home or in the middle of surgery if at all possible.
- Follow the convention of the consultation – allowing your GP to maintain routines will prevent error and lessen risk.
- Ask questions – don't forget you need to share your ideas, concerns and expectations,
- Explore management options and agree treatment plans like everyone else.
- Don't feel foolish if you don't understand something but ask for more information.
- Talk to your colleagues as seems appropriate and remember to provide support to other colleagues if they are the ones suffering illness.
- If you have a problem you are uneasy discussing with your usual doctor, consider contacting:
  - BMA advice line: 0330 123 1245 (you can remain anonymous)
  - The Doctors Support Network (www.dsn.org.uk) is a self-help group available to doctors
  - There is now a practitioners support service and there is full information available at http://php.nhs.uk/

12// ENDINGS

This section is not so much a single method, so much as an invitation to educators, to consider that how we finish off training and training programmes, requires attention in the same way as how we begin them.

When to use it

The need for induction to a training programme or placement is generally accepted. What happens at the end of training programmes?

Groups and teams who work together over time go through the stages of "Forming, storming, norming and performing" as discussed in the General Introduction to this manual. The final phase, "mourning", can be understood as the means by which participants gain a sense of completion, so that they understand it is "OK to say goodbye", so that a change in the relationship between the participants and the educator, (who may have worked with them for some time) is recognised. Informally, many groups will arrange some kind of social event to mark this process. However, not all participants may attend, and there may be celebrations, with little opportunity for reflection.

What can educators do to highlight the important closing moments of a course or programme? Psychologists have studied the planned "endings" of therapeutic groups and recognise several components.

- Denial – participants may "forget" that this is the last session, or "arrange to do something else". Participants may simply agree to carry on meeting and focus on reunions or ongoing meetings outside the formal programme. While this can be an extremely useful facet of Continuing Professional Development, the existing group also needs to be attentively disbanded, as any future group will not be the same group.
- Regression – while this may apply more to therapeutic groups, some training groups will exhibit regression by pointing out how much there is still left to learn, or asking for "extra sessions".
- Flight – participants may leave the group early, or seek to join another CPD programme. Sometimes, they may express frustration or anger about the perceived shortcomings of their training, although this may not always be brought to the attention of educators.
- Reviewing – participants go over past, shared experiences and use them to make sense of where they are going next. Reminiscence or evaluation can also prepare the participants for the weakening and breaking of their bonds with each other, as they say goodbye and move on. These processes help to fully integrate the learning that has been shared, into the minds of the participants (Reference 1, page 56).

The set up: how to use this method

It is worth planning ahead for the end of the course. One way to orientate participants towards "endings" is to arrange visits to other places where education can be obtained. For example, visits to conferences, or to alternative providers such as Art Galleries, (see ENRICH Conference and ENRICH Artist in residence).

Build in activities that help participants to focus on their next workplace, (such as career planning, interview preparation, considering the management or financial skills they will require), so that participants are already thinking about "what happens next?".

When planning final sessions, ensure that the title for the day promises interesting content, so that as many participants as possible actually attend. I have found that if the programme says "Evaluation and close", participants may not bother to turn up. This may represent a mixture of "denial" and "flight" as above.

Labelling a session as, "career planning", or, "the future of your place in the NHS", or, "how to survive and thrive in your career", is more likely to get everyone's attention. Having a high profile visiting speaker for part of the session can also increase motivation to attend.

The end of a course should also offer time for evaluation and reflection on the content and process of the course. There are a variety of methods to help achieve this in the EVALUATE section of this manual. The aim will be to invite reflection on changes that have occurred in individuals and in the group. The kind of questions may be triggered by questions, such as, "where did we start from, what have we been experiencing together, where are we now and where are we going next?" In effect this invites a "look how far we have come!" response, so that participants can more readily accept that "our work here is done", while also acknowledging that there will always be more learning to do in future.

Having some a formal process or ritual can also be helpful. Creating opportunities for everyone to formally shake hands and say goodbye, to produce a work of art commemorating their work, or, perhaps, having a gift or certificate giving ceremony, can all highlight the importance of ending the group well.

Explanations/timings

Explaining that the group is nearing its end, and whatever process is chosen to highlight this, may only take a few minutes. Participants may require considerable time to express their understanding of what they have learned, and where they will take it next. This could be facilitated though a creative writing exercise (see ENRICH Creative writing).

The debrief: maximising the benefits

Much as in a consultation, the educator will need to use sophisticated listening skills so that the participants are enabled to express, fully and freely, their thoughts and feelings about the ending of their work together. The educators own feelings and thoughts need to acknowledged (perhaps privately first), and expressed appropriately. If the main feeling is of relief at never having to see these participants again, then that is best discussed with a senior colleague rather than participants themselves! It is legitimate to acknowledge what the ending of this group will mean, and what the educator themselves has learned/gained from being with that particular group of participants.

Equipment/resources needed

There sources for endings will depend on the educators chosen method, and could include "gifts", objects or pieces of writing developed during the session.

Skills to make this work even better

Some groups reach a stage of maturity, such that, they themselves can contribute to the organisation and planning of the endings session or sessions. Being able to articulate the life of the group and the boundary that marks the end of the group, can actually be helpful to participants, who will benefit from the clarity that the educator brings.

Pitfalls/when NOT to use this method

Ending and mourning methods can only be used with groups that have met regularly for at least some weeks. These methods are not applicable to one off sessions as a rule. There may be elements of this approach that are applicable where groups of participants at different stages of training attend a "rolling programme". This may mean that participants do not all complete the programme at the same time. However, when participants in such groups reach certain stages, pass specific hurdles or reach the end of their training, then having some kind of marking process will help all participants to feel that their progress is valued, and that their achievements are recognised.

Applications in other areas of the session

N/A

How does this help to build relationships?

Although these approaches may seem only to signal the end of relationships, respectful partings are the reverse side of the coin of respectful beginnings, discussed in the ENGAGE section. Helping participants to realise that working together means introductions and other engagement strategies, helps them to understand that leaving requires attention too. Nobody wants to leave a team without anyone taking any notice at all! This approach models appropriate team behaviour for the future.

How does this help to structure the education?

Having an explicit ending process provides a containing and boundaried structure to the programme, where appropriate.

References

1. Jarlath Benson. (2001) 'Work at the ending stage of the group: separation issues', chapter 7 in Benson, J., (2001) *Working more creatively in groups*, pp. 145–54, Abingdon, Routledge.

   https://www.open.edu/openlearn/ocw/pluginfile.php/465018/mod_resource/content/1/e118_ol_reading_2.pdf

13// CONFERENCES AND HOW TO MAKE THEM ENJOYABLE AND EFFECTIVE

If you stay inside your comfort zone it will just get smaller and smaller … and more and more uncomfortable: find ways to stretch your comfort zone.

When to use it

This method is about helping participants to seek out conferences as part of their Continuing Professional Development (CPD), by taking them to a conference as a group during training, so that they are offered education about how to get the most out of a conference.

Educators use enrichment methods to help participants learn in the here and now, and also to enable them to have effective learning skills lifelong. Thinking of learning as a skill that also needs to be "learned", is not self-evident. However, by offering different kinds of learning opportunities and reflection afterwards, educators can help participants choose the best educational opportunities in the future, after they have left formal training.

In evaluations, participants often rate experiential methods quite highly, and appreciate opportunities to discuss and explore. After training, those same participants often choose CPD that involves lectures, disease focussed learning and what is already familiar. However, staying inside your comfort zone can mean it just gets smaller and smaller. Seeking out a conference, or meeting, about something less familiar can be a challenge. Some conferences seem rather intimidating to attend: many (apparently confident) people bustling around, complex programmes hard to navigate through, queues for coffee or lunch, the great and the good of one's professional group greeting each other effusively in corridors (making the rest of us feel a bit insignificant).

This educational method offers participants ways to overcome these issues, to develop confidence in attending a conference and to get the most out of attending in future.

The set up: how to use this method

During training the educator identifies a conference that could offer suitable interest and challenge to participants, especially if they are not used to attending conferences. This could be a national conference of a relevant Royal College, or a smaller conference centred on a particular area of interest. The conference is offered to the group as part of the educational programme that all participants can attend together. For suitable one day conferences, organising a bus to take everyone can be a relatively cheap and convivial way to travel. Travelling together also increases the enjoyment.

Most conferences offer cheaper rates for clinicians in training, or for group bookings. The educator can negotiate with organisers if this is not obvious on the promotional material. Most conference organisers (especially of smaller conferences), love to have groups of younger participants there. Participants can be encouraged to get involved in the organisation themselves; organising the bus, arranging meeting up times and places and so on, increase engagement with the conference experience. Before the conference educators should offer participants the opportunity to discuss their approach.

Explanations/timings

Initially, when offering conference attendance explore participants' expectations using the ENGAGE Hopes and fears method. A conference may seem too high powered, too difficult to get to or too intimidating.

Then using the issues below as a guide ask participants to consider how they might organise themselves, as individuals, or as a group, to get the most out of a conference, perhaps using a "pause, pair, square, share" approach (see ENERGISE Using QUESTIONS effectively), or perhaps by allocating smaller groups different issues to consider.

- **A conference seems intimidating** – what approaches could be used to overcome that?
- **Will it be too difficult** – what will participants look for in the sessions, to help them choose which they want to attend?
- **I will not know anyone there** – how can we work as a group to overcome this?
- **The other people will be more knowledgeable than me** – what approach could participants take to have some interesting conversations with those people?

The debrief: maximising the benefits

The debriefing needs to be skilfully facilitated to ensure that positive approaches are highlighted. These could include having a "conference buddy" system, so that everyone knows they will have at least one person to talk to, using gamification approaches (Reference 2, page 59), so that, for example, everyone has the challenge of saying "hello, my name is" to one new person they sit next to, saying hello to one younger person and one older person, having an open question to ask people in the coffee queue (for example, "what has been your best moment? Or how did you come to be here today?), choosing their own personal top three posters. It is worth considering having specific meet up locations for lunchtime or the end of the day, or agreeing what social evening events to attend at multi-day conferences, so that participants always know that they can find a familiar face at certain times.

This could be summarised at the end as "Top Tips" for making a conference enjoyable and educationally valuable. Remember to emphasise that often the best bits are the unexpected conversations with new people. These can lead to fruitful ideas or even new collaborations.

Equipment/resources needed

The educator should have the conference programme available for consultation and discussion in advance and talk participants through how it works. Educators need to be keeping eyes and ears open for suitable conferences which could include a suitable Royal College national conference, a one day conference on an unusual subject or a conference considering a different aspect of a common subject.

Recent suitable examples have included a conference on the subject of Overdiagnosis (an unusual subject), a conference considering how Lifestyle Medicine could change our approach to Diabetes care (a new approach to a common subject), a Deep End (Reference 1, page 59) conference on the "Exceptional Potential of General Practice" (examining the Inverse Care Law) and a BJGP research conference (Royal College driven and offering the opportunity to consider some new ideas).

In many training contexts, participants will have some kind of study budget to support attendance. If this is not available, participants could be invited to consider how they will set money aside as an investment in their future learning, an investment in their "thriving not surviving".

Skills to make this work even better

After the conference, make sure to offer some evaluation and debriefing time. Focus on what was new, interesting, challenging or inspiring and on the effects of networking and meeting new people. Ask how this approach might help them "thrive not just survive" in future.

Another approach might be to ask participants to do some research in advance on the most unusual, interesting, different or easily accessible conferences going on in the next three to six months, so that they can choose a conference to try out within the training programme. This could be an interesting task for action learning sets. Also ask them to set themselves some aims and objectives for the potential conferences they might attend in future, so that the skills of using a conference for effective education are reinforced.

Pitfalls/when NOT to use this method

Try to avoid "conferences" that are really "courses". They will have titles like "A one day update on Hypertension". These will tend to be didactic and lecture driven in content and will be aimed at knowledge transfer. Conferences are more fun if they challenge attitudes, offer new skills, a chance to meet and network with new people, or offer the opportunity to work in well facilitated small groups.

Participants need to have at least some study budget available to cover registration costs and transport. This may mean that not all participants attend the conference. However, even if only some participants attend, discussing how they made the most of it afterwards may inspire others to try something new in the future.

Applications in other areas of the session

Referring back to conference experiences and benefits can be useful in future sessions, when considering what CPD participants plan for their future career.

How does this help to build relationships?

When educators take concerns about conferences seriously, participants' relationships with the educator will benefit. Attending together helps build relationships between participants and if they start to learn networking skills, their relationships with other professionals will also develop.. This can help build a sense of "belonging" and of connection to others doing similar work. Isolation is a potential driver for burnout. Good quality CPD that connects clinicians to others can be very important in building resilience.

How does this help to structure the education?

This approach further emphasises that training is for life not just examinations. Attendance at a conference can be a highlight in a programme, offering a variation in the approach to learning.

References

1. **"Deep End"** refers to a network of General Practices that work in the most deprived areas of the country, and who have developed support and resources to assist those working in such areas to be effective and to thrive. See:

   http://www.rcgp.org.uk/clinical-and-research/resources/bright-ideas/deep-end-group.aspx

   https://yorkshiredeependgp.org/

   https://twitter.com/deependgp?lang=en

2. **"Gamification"** This is a concept borrowed from interactive video games. It means structuring learning in a way that has playful elements (including aesthetics) and also "levels" that participants can aspire to. In this context it could mean participants get "points" for speaking to new people at a conference, for attending a session on a subject that they know nothing about beforehand, for introducing themselves to someone whose work they are interested in, (for example, someone whose poster they enjoyed), or for the degree to which they have learned a new skill (networking, critical appraisal of conference posters). The aim is to increase motivation to try new things, capturing interest and inspiring them to continue learning, perhaps in new ways.

14// ENRICH WITH A GIFT

We all love a party bag; offering a "gift" for participants to take home can be life enhancing.

What it is for?

Giving participants a "gift" means giving them something (literally "some thing", an object of some sort) that they will take away from the session to reflect on, use or keep at home. Gifts can be of various kinds, (suggestions below) and should be in some sense personal to the individual recipient. Having something to take away at the end of the session offers the opportunity (not the guarantee) that the session will live on in the mind, helps to make it more memorable and can also signal that the participants are in themselves valued, if they are presented with something that will have personal meaning.

When to use it

This approach is useful as a way of punctuating the end of a session, or the end of a term, or of whole course/programme, so that the content is personalised, so that the individuality of participants is recognised. This can help to increase the sense of "belongingness" in a group that can really increase educational effectiveness, especially for those who are unsure of their welcome.

The set up: how to use this method

"Gifts" may be literally that – presents given to participants to mark an occasion; Christmas perhaps, the end of a session, the end of a course. Depending on budgets it can be helpful to give participants a present of a book, or a DVD which will expand their understanding of the role of the clinician. Most bookshops will offer discounts for larger orders so costs can be kept down. Suggestions for possible books to give are listed at the end under RESOURCES.

However, gifts can also be things which are created during the session, which can be taken away either as a literal objects, or, as photographs. Examples could include the outcomes of team building exercises that involve construction (see ENERGISE Teamwork skills using constructions), or personal feedback, (described below, in detail) or the outcomes of using the arts such as drawings, collages, pieces of creative writing.

Explanations/timings

If giving a book or similar, explain the occasion, why this was chosen and hand over at the right time, usually at the end of the session.

Give gifts with intention and directly to the individual person, make sure it has their name on the wrapping.

If creating something during the session, explain that they will take that away with them as a reminder (see ENRICH Artist in residence).

To give participants a gift of very personal feedback divide the group into groups of about eight to ten (it takes too long if the group is larger). Give each person an A4 envelope containing a sheet of A4 plain paper. Give everyone some sticky notes. Then ask each person to write their name on the outside of the envelope in big letters and pass the envelope to the person on their left.

Then each participant will use the sticky notes to write about the person whose envelope they now have (i.e. not their own). On one note they should praise the person, writing something they have appreciated about that person, something that they brought to the group. On a second note they should write something they think the person could do less often, or do more of. For example, someone might write:"you always say humorous things that lighten the atmosphere when we are struggling with difficult topics – you could encourage others who are quieter to speak more in the group".

When complete, the sticky notes are stuck on the A4 paper inside the envelope. Then the envelope is passed to the left again and the process repeated until everyone gets their own envelope back – this is their "gift" of feedback to take home with them. This can be a useful way for the educator to get personal feedback about their style too. Participate in the group or add an envelope with your name on to the process. It takes about 15 to 20 minutes to do this exercise.

Evidence shows that personalising an advice sheet for patients (by adding their name, highlighting the parts that may be especially useful to them, removing irrelevant parts), increases effectiveness. Transferring this same consultation skill to an educational context suggests that educators who personalise gifts, and even handouts, will increase their impact. A personalised handout, highlighting strengths and future learning needs could be the outcome of a one to one discussion with participants, scheduled into a programme (see ENRICH One to one discussions).

These are just some examples, educators will surely be able to devise interesting "gift" ideas to suit their own particular group of participants.

The debrief: maximising the benefits

If giving a book/DVD come back to it later and have a "Programme book club" in a future session. Referring back to the content and having a discussion about it will reinforce that reading a book is valid learning, will reinforce the reflection implied in the book and demonstrate how engaging in an arts-based activity can help us process difficult aspects of our work as clinicians. This is because the artist has, in a sense, done some of that processing for us.

If personal feedback is the gift, refer back to it later. What was helpful about the feedback? What kinds of feedback were less helpful? How did they use it? What did they put in their appraisal or other portfolio?

Educators using a personalised handout hand out or similar, can ask participants at a subsequent session to discuss what was most useful for them, so that participants can reflect on their individual learning needs, and how education is helping them to focus on their needs in particular.

Equipment/resources needed

- Gifts of books obviously need planning and are even better if individually wrapped and labelled, for example, by putting it into a coloured envelope or by attaching a personal note to the person receiving it.
- For the feedback exercise, A4 envelopes and paper, pens and sticky notes need to be available.
- For other "gifts", the resources will depend on the educator's choice of activity.

Skills to make this work even better

Educators could encourage participants to think about and gather the various "gifts" they receive from their education programmes, and also the various "gifts" they give themselves, in the form of contributions to the educational process and to the learning of others. Making a collage/ construct, image or sculpt of such "gifts" could be a valuable part of EVALUATION.

Pitfalls/when NOT to use this method

Even if everyone gets the same book, giving a gift needs to be personal, so avoid just leaving books in a pile and saying "help yourself". The method is probably not appropriate if there is no ongoing relationship between educator and participants.

Are handouts "gifts" in this sense? I would say not – a handout is a generalised, generic object given to everyone, and therefore more public, less specific and more utilitarian. A gift is better if it has an extra, personal, quality. A handout could become a gift if it is individualised and personalised in some way.

Applications in other areas of the session

N/A

How does this help to build relationships?

Giving a gift or helping the group to create "gifts" for each other personalises the educational process, so that relationships develop and deepen, based on acceptance of who the participants really are. Acceptance and belonging are powerful motivators for learning.

How does this help to structure the education?

Giving a gift such as a book, then having a discussion about it at a later session can give shape to a course, and helps participants to get a better sense of things unfolding and developing. It helps the educator in planning, as some sessions will naturally follow on from others.

Resources

Here are some suggestions for possible books to give participants in General Practice Education settings (other specialities may have different ideas of course)

The *Country Doctors Notebook* by M Bulghakov. ISBN 978 0 099 52956 9

This book describes the experiences of a young Russian doctor who is posted to the countryside to work in what is effectively a primary care centre. He describes the intensity, the uncertainty, the doubts and triumphs as well as his often dysfunctional ways of coping. Short and well written.

***The Suburban Shaman; Tales from medicine's front line* by Cecil Helman ISBN1 905 14008 9**

Helman also wrote the book "Culture Health and Illness" which is well worth a read for any GP (but is rather long). He brings a wealth of understanding of different cultures and approaches, humour and sensitivity to this collection of short stories from GP land. Accessible and interesting and can be read in bite sized chunks.

***The Citadel* by A J Cronin**

A book from the inter-war period that describes the struggles of a pre national health service doctor and how he finds his integrity when faced with various conflicts of interest and tradition.

***A Fortunate Man* by John Berger**

A thought provoking book with an accompanying photo essay describing the complex life of a single handed practitioner in the Forest of Dean. Although few doctors work in this way now, the book does raise important questions about the GPs role in the technical and non-technical aspects of the job, how the GP deals with suffering and his failures, and to what extent a doctor is in the community or part of the community.

15// CREATIVE WRITING

This technique is useful for exploring difficult areas such as resilience, the difficulties of clinical practice or tricky subjects like angry patients.

When to use it

This technique is useful for exploring difficult areas such as resilience, the difficulties of clinical practice or tricky subjects like angry patients. Used as a prelude to other discussions it can free up participants to talk about a wider range of issues, or enable them to talk about their own emotions connected with their (difficult) clinical work.

> "Imagination is more important than knowledge." **Albert Einstein**

Many clinicians feel that they "cant" do art or writing, and this method uses an approach that means everyone can produce something worthwhile, without having to share it with the whole group, unless they want to. It is essential to emphasise that there are no "right answers" or "proper pieces of writing". The aim is to allow our right brains to do the work for us and select what is important, interesting or significant. Afterwards we can reflect on that, without judgement.

The set up: how to use this method

There are two phases to this exercise: an initial "free writing part" which is kept completely private to the individual, (unless they feel they want to share it), and a second phase when they use a little bit of their initial writing to create a poem, using a formal method explained by the educator.

Phase 1

Everyone needs paper and pen, (one dyslexic participant told me she preferred to use a writing App on her phone – this is also OK).

The task is to spend five minutes writing about their last day in clinical work, (yesterday, perhaps). The aim is to put pen to paper and **write without stopping to think at all** continuing until the five minute bell goes. This may mean writing sentences or words, about one patient or about logging on, or about **anything at all that pops into their heads**.

"Just write about what pops in, do not worry about spelling or punctuation at all. If you get stuck you can write "I am stuck now" until any new thought that comes into your mind, and then write that thought down without thinking about it, without judging whether it's a good thought or not. This writing is private to yourself. It will only be shared if you choose to do that"

It is pretty much impossible to think about nothing (it takes years of intense Buddhist meditation training, apparently), so all that's needed is encouragement to write the thought down even if it is "I hate writing about myself, it is silly, nothing much happened yesterday except...". Time the writing very strictly, with a bell or similar, stopping after five minutes. Keep encouraging people to keep the pen on the page and to write anything, trusting their unconscious mind to bring up something. You can model writing in this way yourself.

At the end of five minutes, ask participants to stop and read what they have written privately to themselves, noting anything they find interesting or important.

Phase 2

Again working alone, ask participants to underline the words or phrases that they think are most interesting to them, most significant to them or even most surprising to them – the aim is to underline things that "catch their eye". Again, emphasise that the unconscious will do the work, they can let go and just see what comes up. There are no right or wrong answers here. Some participants need to hear that said overtly.

Explain they are now going to write a poem whose lines have syllables arranged like this:

- Line one has two syllables – this could be a phrase, or, one word
- Line two has four syllables – this could be a phrase, several words, one word
- Line three has six syllables This could be a phrase, several words, one word
- Line four has eight syllables – this could be a phrase, several words, one word

It works best if they do this line by line, so start by asking them to write two syllables, then when everyone seems to have finished, the next line of four syllables and so on.

Finally, ask them to repeat the lines in reverse, i.e. eight, six, four, two syllables, to complete the poem.

Here is an example for clarity:

Widow
Weight loss, bleeding.
I meet her eye, she knows,
I will care for her until death.

I will care for her until death.
I meet her eye, she knows,
Weight loss, bleeding,
Widow

Ask participants to form pairs, perhaps with someone they are used to working with. Ask them, if they are willing, to share their poems with that one other person. Allow sometime for them to discuss with each other what they have been writing about.

Then debrief with the whole group.

Explanations/timings

Explaining the free write and getting everyone to have a pen and paper takes about three to five minutes. Allow five minutes for the free write and then five minutes to go through the poem syllables, like by line. Allow a few minutes for discussion in their pairs, stopping when it is clear the room is going quieter or participants are changing the subject. Allow a few minutes general discussion.

The total time needed for this exercise alone is about 20 to 30 minutes.

The debrief: maximising the benefits

The initial debrief happens when participants write and read their poems to each other in pairs, allowing them to express themselves and share their thoughts and feelings in a safe situation. The discussion with their partner may be the most effective debrief for some participants.

In the large group debriefing could cover questions like:

- What was it like to write knowing you could not get it wrong? (Because any writing was fine)
- What kinds of thoughts came up?
- What kinds of feelings came up?
- How did your partner respond to your poem? (Helps to emphasise that participants can trust their colleagues to take them seriously).

Equipment/resources needed

Pen and paper. Watch or phone to time the free write.

It can help to put the arrangement of syllables on a slide, however there are disadvantages to this. If it is on a slide it immediately becomes formal, structured, implying a "correct approach". It works better if the educator simply describes what participants need to do, so that they will become absorbed in remembering and acting on that. This approach tends to make participants become less self-conscious, so that they use their "holistic" right brain skills, which will help them pick out the right words. The automatic element, when the lines are simply reversed is extremely easy to do, and often unexpected for participants. This reduces their stress at doing an unfamiliar task, because success is guaranteed. There are no bad poems here.

Skills to make this work even better

There are many way to use creative writing in education: this method is a "starter for 10" as they say on University Challenge! Educators who wish to venture further could enlist a local poet, writer or member of the Society of Medical Writers to help them do a more extensive writing workshop (see Resources and References below). The Curators of Art Galleries or museums are keen to engage with all kinds of groups and may have suggestions about local writers who are used to doing workshops in this way. They are readily contacted via their institution's web pages. Writers or poets need careful briefing beforehand, to discuss what they propose doing and how best to work with your specific group of participants (see ENGAGE Preparing an educational brief).

There are some other suggestions for writing tasks in the Resources section below. This approach can be used on different occasions with a different focus.

The arrangement of lines suggested in the setup is not the only one. A **Haiku** could be suggested instead: this is a poem of just 17 syllables arranges in three lines of having five/seven/five syllables. Usually Haiku are about natural subjects, but adapts itself well to the "natural subject" of the clinicians own state of mind.

Pitfalls/when NOT to use this method

This method is best used with groups who are used to working together and who have developed enough trust in the educator to try something "out of the box". Groups of experienced educators, or participants who already have some group skills, can do this effectively, even if they have never met before, provided some attempts have been made to engage them using suitably chosen ENGAGE techniques.

Applications in other areas of the session

If a session throws up and emotive or difficult subject, the educator could use this method as a way to allow some non-judgemental exploration of the issue, prior to more extensive discussions.

How does this help to build relationships?

Writing can feel odd or exposing to clinicians and yet at the same time, it can enable them to reflect on what their work means for them, in a safe and helpful way. Sharing builds relationships over time, and can make the education more effective. There is evidence that practitioners who share this approach with others feel better, less stressed and get less burnout. Feedback after one workshop included comments like:

- "Life changing"
- "Creativity in writing can be helpful for resilience".

How does this help to structure the education?

It can be used on its own as a stress reliever, or as a prelude to talking about resilience, or other less clinical subjects. It can be used as part of a longer session of writing when other methods are also used.

References and resources

Reflective Practice by Gillie Bolton
ISBN 978-1848602120 gives an interesting over view of this kind of approach, with lots of more complex ideas that could be applied to portfolio entries or appraisal, with helpful comments on how to avoid difficulties.

The Artists Way by Julian Cameron
ISBN 978-1585421466 This book has some interesting ways to enhance reflection and creativity, especially with the use of "free writing".

Alternative tasks for a free write could be:

- My last patient yesterday was …
- My youngest patient this week came with …
- The team I work with …

Or start by saying one of these "stems"

- Write about what passes through your mind if the situation is …
  - When people say thank you
  - When I cry
  - When I stay awake at night
  - When I first became a doctor
- A good doctor is …

The Society of Medical Writers may be able to put you in touch with a local writer who would be willing to do a workshop.
See: http://somw.org.uk/wp/

16// ARTIST IN RESIDENCE

This method is best used with a group that has an ongoing life, for example a GP ST3 group who have been working together for a while.

When to use it

The aim is to find an artist who can work with a group over time, say three sessions, so that their artistic insight into the clinical world builds up and so that the group of participants develops a relationship of interest and trust in the artist and their perspective. Some notes on how to find such a person are given in the Resources section below. The work of the artist needs to be integrated into the programme and into sessions that may, overtly, be about other subjects. The example given here is of one such piece of work, so that educators can have a rough guide to some of the possibilities. Working with the artist you choose will inevitably throw up other possibilities. Discuss the process together, perhaps using ENGAGE Preparing an educational brief as a guide. Working with an artist can explore issues of what we pay attention to, how we represent things and what images we use, how we are affiliated to each other and how we can develop and harness our creativity in working environments.

The set up: how to use this method

Here is just one possible example. Working with artist Matt Worden, we devised a three session "Artist in residence project".

First session

The artists was introduced to the participants and he facilitated a "quick draw" exercise for them, collecting the images on a board to inform his work.

That day we had a session working with a GP in how to motivate patients towards behaviour change, illustrated by his work on improving diabetes care, which was focussed on helping patients to understand and implement low carbohydrate diets. While the "usual work" of the session was going on, the artist painted and sketched alongside, responding to the issues coming up visually and artistically. At natural breaks in the session he then showed his work and explained his thinking and his responses. This helped to highlight the "unseen" issues that both patients and clinicians feel: the "weight" of responsibility and experience of illness, the "helplessness" that we sometimes share when nothing is improving, the "hopefulness" that came from working alongside and with patients, rather than trying to do things "to them or for them". This illustrated many of the issues about positive language that the speaker was concerned with. Alongside this I noted many of the exact words used by speaker and participants and summarised the session's work in a poem (see Resources, page 69).

Second session

This session took place at the Whitworth Art Gallery, which promotes strong links between Arts and Health (see Resources section), so that the participants have an experience of working and learning in a totally different environment, so that they can be exposed to different ways of understanding health, and also have some creative experiences of their own.

The programme for the session was devised by the artist and the gallery staff and included a life drawing class and responding to the pictures on display in the exhibition areas.

During previous visits participants have been able to have close up private viewings of prints and objects from the museum which are not usually on view. This has include artefacts from ancient Egypt which were used by ancient physicians, (which provoked discussion about how many preoccupations of doctors and patients are just the same now), a series of Hogarth prints about the ravages of alcoholism, (no changes there!) and objects relating to rites of passage (such as naming of children or funerals), so that participants could discuss about these important matters in relation to their own contributions and experiences. A series of pictures about the work of medics in the first world war provoked reflections on the nature of suffering, what it is like to be exposed to people in pain as clinicians, and how the arts help us process difficult experiences.

Third session

The final session with the artist, was also the final session of the whole Study Release Course. All the methods in the ENGAGE section help participants to FORM, NORM, STORM and PERFORM as a group. When such a group comes to a close it is important to recognise and enable the group to MOURN, so that the experiences of the group are recognised and valued, and so that the participants can see their way forwards after the group has ended.

The artist did an upside down drawing exercise with the participants (providing the materials required). This helped them to see the value of non-judgemental focussed attention. What they produced astonished them all.

Then, being able to use a large variety of media (collage, pencil, paint, felt tip) each participant produced a personal image on the theme of

"What the Study Release Course has meant for me". Plenty of time was allowed for this, and the artist was available for advice about materials and managing the images.

Finally, we held an "exhibition" and everyone talked about their image. Each participant was formally thanked for their contribution to the Study Release course by the educator, who shook hands and said goodbye to each participant individually wishing them well in the future.

Explanations/timings

- In the first session the artist stayed all morning, while the usual work of the group went on, with a few minutes at intervals when he explained his work.
- The Art Gallery session was a whole afternoon.
- The final session was about two hours long and took place after evaluation and feedback processes.

The debrief: maximising the benefits

Allow participants time to reflect on their own about the question: "what did art bring to the session today?" Then ask them to share their reflections in pairs. Ask if someone has something, or has heard something they wish to share with everyone. Be accepting and non-judgemental about all such contributions.

One benefit was summed up when a participant said: "It has already changed how I look at things during consultations. I look to see what is there without making a judgement first, and I see more".

Another commented: "I have already signed up for a life drawing course; drawing was so relaxing to the mind I want to do more of it as way of staying sane".

Equipment/resources needed

The artists will need a table and some space and perhaps some noticeboards to display things on. These resources are usually readily available in postgraduate centres. Discuss with the artist in advance what the arrangements will be for materials/paper and agree who will provide/pay for them. In our St3 course we use a limited number of external speakers so we were able to use our speaker budget for the artist. Some Galleries have small budgets for public engagement work which you may be able to tap into.

Pitfalls/when NOT to use this method

It is likely that some participants "get" the artists role completely and find it a truly enriching experience. It is possible that some participants will not "get" some or all of what their contribution is about. This is OK. Enrichment activities are about making an offering that participants can take and develop, in a way that meets their needs.

This means that not all enrichment activities help everyone all the time. The aim is to have a variety of such methods on offer, so that participants can pick up what works best for them. When it does work for them it can have a massive impact. Accept puzzlement or criticism of this approach in a non-judgemental, accepting way.

Sometimes the impact is felt far down the line. When I meet participants years later they often say: "I did not get why you did such a thing at the time – now I have been in practice for five years I see how it matters".

Applications in other areas of the session

Once familiar with quick drawing techniques educators can call upon this in other parts of other sessions. For example, asking participants to draw "how they felt at the end of the day" so that they are orientated to a discussion of how to make recreation time more effective can work. Drawing can be used to clarify current views so that discussion opens up to new understandings.

We asked participants in groups to "draw a picture of the typical alcohol abusing patient". Then used the caricature, (red eyes, big liver, bottle in hand, fag ash dropping from mouth, smelly, unkempt) to reflect on ways that we make judgements, how we may miss alcohol misuse in those functioning well and how we need to widen our view about alcohol problems. This was the prelude to a useful session using other methods to develop participants' understanding about alcohol in clinical care.

How does this help to build relationships?

Educators can create a non-judgemental atmosphere, so that sharing the arts and creativity happens with no "wrong answers", so that participants relax and are able to be themselves, allowing many different perspectives to come out This increases sharing of thoughts and feelings, increases a sense of "belongingness" which helps to strengthen relations between participants, and between the group and the educator.

How does this help to structure the education?

The arts can be used as a commentary on what is happening, as punctuation or trigger to the next set of ideas or as a way of signalling ways that participants can enrich their own education after formal training is completed. Using the arts, in whatever form, signals that the whole of our minds are useful in clinical work, and enlarges the view.

Resources

Working with an artist

One artist who is able to do this work is Matt Worden, who has done work with the arts in mental health and is used to working with clinicians. He can be contacted on matt@art-social.co.uk

See also: https://www.facebook.com/mattworden66/

It might also be worth contacting Art Therapists in your local Mental Health Services. Contact your local Art Gallery or commercial space where art is sold, they will have contact details for local artists who may be interested in this kind of work.

Working with an Art Gallery/Museum

The Whitworth Art gallery has a strong outreach programme see their websites at:
http://www.whitworth.manchester.ac.uk/learn/healthandwellbeing/
http://www.healthandculture.org.uk/
and contact:
http://www.healthandculture.org.uk/contact/

info@healthandculture.org.uk – Wendy Gallagher is their current coordinator for this.

If you are working outside Manchester, check out your local Art Gallery or Museum. They would be delighted to hear from you.

Poetic summary of the artist's first session

What kind of doctor do you aspire to be?

Pin drop silence in the room.
"I am a cheerful, old, GP", he said.
"Starting out, it dragged me down.
Either I die or they die.
Patients reduced from people to
One, two or three Jaffa cake problems.
But, I did not want to be lonely".

After all why do we care?
What would be the difference that I could make?
I discovered the power of hope,
The older I get the straighter I get,
Honesty led to collaboration.
Let's risk it for a biscuit.

I am hopping mad!
Flip the consultation and pay attention.
Moaning diminishes us,
All this talk of killing, sleeping, weeping.
Make every word count.
You are a tough cookie,
You have dealt with a lot,
What was your best day?
Your daughter is brilliant,
She has hopes.

I did not want to be lonely.
I'm still here, after 32 years.

Books

Drawing from the right side of the brain by Betty Edwards ISBN 978-0285641778. This book has many ideas for enhancing creativity.

The Artists Way by Julian Cameron ISBN 978-1585421466

17// ONE-TO-ONE MEETINGS

Educators working with a group of participants over time can use this method to help individuals recognise their strengths and weaknesses, help them identify how best to work with their group, and help them to identify effective learning strategies.

When to use it

Educators working with a group of participants over time can use this method to help individuals recognise their strengths and weaknesses, help them identify how best to work with their group, and help them to identify effective learning strategies. I have used this method mostly with participants in their final year of training, and where time permits, it could be used at any stage of training with benefit.

The set up: how to use this method

The aim of this method is to meet each participant individually, for a short conversation (say, 10 to 20 minutes) to help them use their training time most effectively and to identify ways in which the educator can assist that particular individual in the context of a training course.

The basic outline of the conversation is planned in advance, and recorded in real time, so that the participant and educator agree and share the outcomes of the meeting immediately. The focus is on strengths, learning methods and what strategies could help that participant's learning become even more effective. One suitable proforma is included in Resources (page 72).

Explanations/timings

Early in the programme the educator explains the process, so that participants know that very short meetings will be arranged with each participant, usually in the coffee or lunch break. The explanation to the whole group need only take a few minutes. The length of the meeting should be kept brief. If a major problem emerges, that requires detailed attention, the educator should schedule a longer, more thorough meeting at another time.

The debrief: maximising the benefits

The notes taken should be openly shared with the participant and agreed with them, inviting any extra comments. The record can be scanned or photographed by the participant for their e portfolio entry (normally in General Practice, under "professional conversations"). The educator can also seek agreement to add a short educator's note recording the fact of the meeting and any key suggestions or comments. Again this should be kept brief and specific. There is an example of an educators note in References and Resources below.

Equipment/resources needed

A sheet to record the conversation is all that is required, together with a suitably private space to share a cup of coffee and a conversation, such as the postgraduate office. The record should be taken at the time and a copy immediately available to both parties.

Skills to make this work even better

Participants can be given the format of the conversation in advanced to help them reflect on what would be helpful for them. The skills needed to make the conversation effective are the same as those used in a consultation; active listening, the ability to pick up and react appropriately to cues and clues about participants' views, the ability to summarise and share a plan. This is another example of the overlap between consultation and educational skills.

Pitfalls/when NOT to use this method

This method is not really applicable of the educator is not in an ongoing relationship with the participants through a group process. It must be clear that this is a process for all participants, and is seen as a formative, encouraging process. Preparation of an appropriate structure is essential.

Applications in other areas of the session

N/A

How does this help to build relationships?

This helps build the educator/participant relationship. This may enhance the use that participants make of sessions, and also increase the likelihood that they will seek appropriate advice for any problems arising.

How does this help to structure the education?

Reflecting on educational strategies and techniques can help advanced participants consider how to develop even further and can help weaker participants make the most of their learning opportunities.

Resources

One possible proforma for a one-to-one meeting

One-to-one meeting between educator *(insert name)*

And *(insert name of participant)*

Date *(Educator reaffirms that this is a planned one to one meeting, arranged for all participants to create an opportunity to discuss how training is going)*

How is your training going?

What is your biggest worry about training?

What has been the most useful bit of feedback you have received? How did it change things? *(Note: ensure the participant is specific about feedback, referring to a specific occasion and a specific thing that changed. This helps to focus their attention on the power of good feedback. Practice just makes permanent; only feedback makes perfect.)*

What resources are you using to help? For example which books, 14 fish, audiobooks, online? *(Note: this helps the educator to direct the participant to sources of learning they may not be exploiting fully. The educator can also help to ensure that methods to identify learning need, such as multiple choice tests, are not being used as a substitute for learning.)*

How can I help you to succeed this year?
(Note: many participants are pleasantly surprised to understand that someone is keen to help them succeed. Being recognised as worthy of being helped to succeed, can be extremely motivating for some participants.)

Note to participants: you can add this to your portfolio as Professional Conversation. Can I have your permission to add a brief educator's note to your portfolio also?

Example of an educator's note in the e portfolio

It was a pleasure to meet Dr P today for a one to one meeting, as part of a series of scheduled meetings with all participants on the … Course.

DR P feels that training is going well, has passed all the examinations so far, planning to take the final CSA examination in march.

The biggest worry Dr P has about training is completion of their portfolio, caused by Dr P having a period of time off, due to family problems, in the last 12 months. Dr P is planning to overcome this by setting aside 20 minutes after each shift, to complete their portfolio.

Their most useful feedback was being made aware that they frequently ask patients the same question more than once, which irritated some patients. It appeared that this was because Dr P was thinking about the next question, rather than focussing on what the patient's answer was. Since changing their approach, and deciding what to ask, only after the patient has finished speaking, they have found their consultations to be shorter and easier.

Dr P is using appropriate textbooks and online resources for study, they will consider using Skills for Communicating with Patients to enhance their consultation skills.

Dr P is a fairly quiet person and thought **I could help them succeed** by encouraging them to contribute more actively during discussions on the course, perhaps by asking them directly. Dr P agreed to volunteer to be the rapporteur in the next small group session, to practice speaking out more.

18// INVOLVING PATIENTS IN EDUCATIONAL SESSIONS

Having patients involved in teaching sessions can bring new layers of understanding to participants and remind them of the humanity of the patients they work with every day.

What it is for?

Having patients at teaching sessions alters the way participants behave and can change their thinking; it brings clinical learning to life.

When to use it

Having patients present during sessions works best if the session is directed towards a specific illness or issue that patients can give a personal and unique insight too.

The set up: how to use this method

Preparation is key. **Firstly,** as the educator the exact purpose of having the patient there needs to be clear; is it to discuss their experience of the illness, their experience of healthcare, or their views about what doctors do? Is it to encourage specific understanding in the participants or to identify specific behaviours in the participants that could be helpful or unhelpful?

Secondly, the educator needs to prepare with the patient so that they agree on the purpose and thrust of the patients involvement. The patient may be asked simply to give an account of their experience, the educator can "interview" the patient using a Question and Answer format, or, participants could be asked to send questions in advance to be discussed with the patient. The patient also needs to be asked if they are happy to be asked questions on the day, and if so whether there are areas they would prefer not to discuss. The educator can then steer any discussion appropriately.

Some patients will need time to see questions written down in advance, so that they have time to consider them, especially if they are not used to public speaking type situations. Discussing it in advance means any specific agendas that the patient may have can be considered and incorporated appropriately.

The educator's questions need preparation; obviously avoid closed questions that can only be answered with yes or no. Equally, entirely open questions can go off track ("Tell me about yourself…"). Open directed questions can be very useful, followed up with specific probing questions to clarify detail (just as in the consultation). For example:

"How did your illness first start?" (Open directed question), can be followed up by "How did things go when you went to the doctor?" (Probing question but linked to what the patient has been talking about)

Thirdly, participants need to be aware that a patient will be present, and to be encouraged to behave professionally.

Robust arrangements need to be made to meet and greet the patient, ensure they are comfortable, have access to a drink/the loo, etc. Usually a dedicated person needs to be available for this. Always invite patients to bring a family member or friend if they want to (not all do), and offer practical support such as arrangements for car parking or travel expenses, making sure the venue is appropriately accessible.

Explanations/timings

Introduce the patient at the start and explain the purpose of their attendance and how they are going to interact with the group. Ensure they have a microphone if needed. Timing will depend on the purpose. Decide in advance if they are going to stay throughout the session or leave once their part is done. Sometimes participants need time away from patients to discuss and digest their thoughts. Sometimes the patient may wish to debrief with an educator. Plan this advance if needed. If the session continues after the patient has finished their contribution, ensure that there are suitable arrangements for thanking them and offering any assistance needed. Sending a formal "thank you" letter afterwards is essential. Postgraduate administrative staff are often extremely helpful in these matters.

The debrief: maximising the benefits

Careful planning as above will increase the benefit by directing attention to the relevant issues. Inviting questions or responses from participants before the patient leaves can offer opportunities to enrich the discussions.

Equipment/resources needed;

Appropriate seating and microphone if needed.

Skills to make this work even better

The educator must really focus on the purpose of having the patient there, so that the benefit to themselves and to participants is maximised. Try to identify patients who have some insight into the medical world or who are not too starry eyed and admiring of clinicians. Conversely, avoid those who are furious with their care, or who bring a particular axe to grind.

Patients can also be helpful participants even if they do not come. Asking a patient who has a particularly helpful or interesting story if it is OK to discuss their situation anonymously can also be a helpful way to get the patient's view of things integrated into the session.

Seek feedback from the patient as soon as possible after the session. What did they make of it? What suggestions do they have for improving the impact of their contribution?

There is an interesting report from the Health Foundation about involvement of patients in education (Reference 1) and Amanda Howe's article covers many practical aspects (Reference 2).

Pitfalls/when NOT to use this method

The patient needs to be carefully briefed and chosen for being able to articulate their situation in a helpful way. Clearly, this will go wrong and be potentially harmful to the patient if they are chosen inappropriately.

Applications in other areas of the session

Refer back to the issues brought up by the patient later in the session. This reinforces the benefit.

How does this help to build relationships?

This approach demonstrates that learning is two way and we can learn a lot from listening carefully to patients experiences and thoughts. Participants are usually extremely respectful and friendly to patients and this can facilitate them learning more via their questions.

How does this help to structure the education?

Having the patient's point of view first and foremost in the session, can help to provide interest, punctuation and a welcome reminder of why we do our work.

References

1. https://www.health.org.uk/sites/default/files/CanPatientsBeTeachers.pdf
   This report from the Health Foundation covers some interesting aspects of involving patients in education.
2. Involving patients in medical education, Amanda Howe BMJ 2003; 327 doi: https://doi.org/10.1136/bmj.327.7410.326 (Published 07 August 2003): BMJ 2003; 327:326 https://www.bmj.com/content/327/7410/326

19// USING POEMS TO PROCESS SUFFERING

The power of poetry can help clinicians process the impacts of their work in highly-charged emotional situations.

What it is for?

Clinicians spend their time with patients who are nearly always suffering in some way; in General Practice patients are never "discharged" as such and so the closure that a surgeon may get after a successful operation/discharging the patient may never be achieved. Even when a patient recovers well from an illness, they will consult again, when another problem arises. Increasingly, care of older populations will be dominated by long term, complex conditions which can be emotionally draining at times. Care of younger people can mean clinicians being exposed to trauma, premature death and deep emotional distress.

Making sense of this is hard. The practice of evidence-based medicine is all left brain; cold, precise, generalised. Reading poetry can use the "right brain" skills of integration, seeing the whole picture rather than focusing on parts, while experiencing deep emotional connections. This can help us process the suffering we work amidst. Poetry emphasises "emotion recollected in tranquillity" as Wordsworth describes it. When we read poetry, the poet themselves has done some of the work of processing powerful emotion. We can enjoy and appreciate that, and at the same time, the experience offers us ways to process our own experiences. This is helpful for clinicians in respect of experiences of suffering and even death.

When to use it

This method can be used a standalone section for example as a warm up, or as part of a larger session where themes such as our resilience, bereavement care, breaking bad news, or, palliative and end of life care are to be discussed.

The set up: how to use this method

Using a longer poem – Black Roses: the killing of Sophie Lancaster by Simon Armitage

This poem is in the form of a very short book, about 20 pages long. It describes the life and death of Sophie Lancaster, a gentle young woman who dressed in black "goth" clothes. She and her boyfriend were attacked in a park; he was badly injured and survived, she died later of multiple injuries.

Get two copies of the book. Divide it into sections of about a page long. Ask participants to sit in a circle. The poem should be read by taking turns, by each participant reading a page or so. The poem is not written in difficult language and the effect is greater if participants do not have time to prepare. Go round until the poem is complete; some people may need to read twice if the group is smaller.

As the story unfolds, the room tends to become very quiet. Often participants can become very sad, tearful and reflective.

Using shorter poems

Other approaches to using poems are described more fully in the Resources section (page 78). Taking poems that have death as a theme can work well if "serious" poems are contrasted with ones that contain humour. Black humour is often used as a coping mechanism in clinical work after all.

Explanations/timings

Using poems may seem unusual to some participants. Explain that we all experience emotionally charged situations and that reading poetry can explore this, so that, we can use the reflections to help us process and release the distress we encounter. This is an experiential method, so keep explanations brief. The benefit comes from the reading out loud and the reflecting. If having discussions in small groups, allow time for the poem to be read privately and out aloud; sometimes participants like to hear the poem again after the discussion.

The debrief: maximising the benefits

"Black Roses" by Simon Armitage; when the poem is finished, allow a few moments for the silence to settle and for participants to digest what they have heard. Some will be weeping, which is OK, Allow time for everyone to settle. A few short empathic comments along the lines of "This is a difficult story to hear", with pauses for the group to digest their feelings, will give everyone time to "return to the room". Simply commenting that the emotional distress in the poem reflects the intensity of the emotional distress we are constantly surrounded by as clinicians, may be all the debriefing required.

Educators may wish to invite participants to share their response to the poem. After that, one may consider asking how the various participants might present to the GP, whether they have known had any patients who died in traumatic circumstances…see where the discussion goes…it may be too emotional to do more than acknowledge how emotions surround us all the time. Participants may benefit from a walk or a coffee or lunchbreak after reading Black Roses.

Equipment/resources needed

Black Roses: the killing of Sophie Lancaster by Simon Armitage ISBN-13: 978-1904590293

If using shorter poems, it is usually helpful to have copies for each person or if the group is small to have them on a PowerPoint so all can see them. The shorter poems are attached in Resources (page 78).

Skills to make this work even better

After reading and listening to a poem, and initial discussion, another approach might be to ask participants to do a second reading of a poem "with the pen". This means reading the poem to themselves, using a pen to highlight any words or phrases that they particularly respond to or are curious about, by underlining them or using a highlighter. This is so that deeper meanings or connections are highlighted to a greater degree. Debrief this way of reading the poem with an open question like "what struck you this time around?"

Pitfalls/when NOT to use this method

This method is probably best used when a group have got to know and trust each other and the educator enough to try something new, that they may not be expecting from their medical education. Thus, it may be best done later in a programme. Experienced clinicians who are used to experiential methods could use this after a shorter time period of group work and getting to know each other. Be careful to use positive language when explaining the purposes. If unsure ask them directly for any "Hopes and fears" they may have for working in this way. Acknowledge that it may feel unusual and ask that they give it a try without expecting anything. Not every participant will get the same things, or indeed anything, from this approach; this is OK. The purpose is to provide an opportunity for those that are ready to take it.

Applications in other areas of the session

Using poems can be a good punctuation in a long or emotionally difficult session. Having a poem to read beforehand can be a good orientation to a session about Breaking Bad News (Seamus Heaney's Mid Term Break is one possible poem to use). Robert Frost's Poem the Road Not Taken or his poem "Stopping By Woods on a Snowy Evening" can be useful parts of a session on resilience. Many educators will have their own favourites; asking participants to bring a poem they have found consoling or helpful to a subsequent session may yield unexpected treasures.

How does this help to build relationships?

Hearing others respond to a poem often helps participants to realise both their commonalities and also help them to understand and respect the differences between people. This helps to build trust and interest between the group members, so that they can develop stronger relationships.

How does this help to structure the education?

Poems can be used as introductions and also make a useful ways to punctuate a session (by changing the tone and method of presentation). A well-chosen poem can make a good ending to a session on a difficult or emotionally laden topic. Poems can also make good introductions to creative writing exercises.

Resources

Some poems to consider with educators notes on how to use them.

Poems about death

Educators notes

The aims of this session of group work are twofold:

- To use non-traditional subject matter to help to break down barriers, so that group members get to know each other and can work together at a deeper level.
- To use the poems about death or resilience to help clinicians reflect on difficult issues in their work, so that they appreciate that different people, at different times, have different understandings, so they can develop greater awareness of cultural and other differences. Divide the group into smaller units of about four to six participants.

Tasks

- Each group has two poems, one that is quite serious in intent and a second which perhaps takes a more humorous view of death.
- Take each poem in turn (in what order the educator prefers). Ask the participants to read it carefully themselves.
- Then ask one participant to read it out loud. Explore the themes about death that arise, what meanings for death are given in the poetry, and what resonances this may have for us as clinicians. Themes to consider could be:
  - the fear or apprehension that death brings
  - what happens afterwards, can we be resurrected?
  - mechanical versus the psychological aspects of death, black humour about death.
- Finally, consider asking participants to decide what they will feed back to the larger group, the key reflections that they have had about these poems. Another option is to consider a second reading "with the pen", discussing any developing ideas.

Death be not Proud by John Donne

Death be not proud, though some have called thee
Mighty and dreadful, for, thou art not soe,
For, those, whom thou think'st, thou dost overthrow,
Die not, poore death, nor yet canst thou kill mee.
From rest and sleepe, which but thy pictures bee,
Much pleasure, then from thee, much more must flow,
And soonest our best men with thee doe goe,
Rest of their bones, and soules deliverie.
Thou art slave to Fate, Chance, kings, and desperate men,
And dost with poyson, warre, and sicknesse dwell,
And poppie, or charmes can make us sleepe as well,
And better then thy stroake; why swell'st thou then?
One short sleepe past, wee wake eternally,
And death shall be no more; death, thou shalt die.

The Dying Airman (anonymous)

A handsome young airman lay dying,
And as on the aerodrome he lay,
To the mechanics who round him came sighing,
These last dying words he did say:
'Take the cylinders out of my kidneys,
The connecting-rod out of my brain,
Take the cam-shaft from out of my backbone,
And assemble the engine again.'

The Hearse Song

The old Grey Hearse goes rolling by,
You don't know whether to laugh or cry;
For you know some day it'll get you too,
And the hearse's next load may consist of -- you.

They'll take you out and they'll lower you down,
While men with shovels stand all a-round;
They'll throw in dirt and they'll throw in rocks,
And they won't give a dam-m-m if they break the box.

The worms crawl in and the worms crawl out,
They crawl all over your chin and mouth,
They invite their friends and their friends' friends too,
And you look like hell when they're -- through -- with you.

ZEN Poems about death

Since time began
The dead alone know peace.
Life is but melting snow.
(Nandai)

Sixty-six times have these eyes beheld the changing scene of autumn.
I have said enough about moonlight, Ask no more.
Only listen to the voice of pines and cedars when no wind stirs.
(Ryonen)

Farewell ...
I pass as all things do
Dew on the grass.
(Banzan)

Omar Khayam verses from the Rubayat

XXVIII
Oh, come with old Khayyam, and leave the Wise
To talk; one thing is certain, that Life flies;
One thing is certain, and the Rest is Lies;
The Flower that once has blown forever dies.

XXIX
Myself when young did eagerly frequent
Doctor and Saint, and heard great Argument
About it and about; but evermore
Came out by the same Door as in I went.

XXX
With them the Seed of Wisdom did I sow,
And with my own hand labour'd it to grow:
And this was all the Harvest that I reap'd --
"I came like Water and like Wind I go."

XLIX
Strange, is it not? that of the myriads who
Before us pass'd the door of Darkness through
Not one returns to tell us of the Road,
Which to discover we must travel too.

LX
The Moving Finger writes; and, having writ,
Moves on: nor all thy Piety nor Wit
Shall lure it back to cancel half a Line,
Nor all thy Tears wash out a Word of it.

LXIII
With Earth's first Clay They did the Last Man knead,
And then of the Last Harvest sow'd the Seed:
Yea, the first Morning of Creation wrote
What the Last Dawn of Reckoning shall read.

Dahn the Plug'ole (Anonymous)

A mother was barfing her biby one night;
The youngest of ten and a tiny young mite.
The muvver was poor and the biby was fin;
'twas naught but a skelington covered in skin.

The muvver turned rahnd for a soap off the rack.
She was but a moment, but when she turned back
Her biby had gone, and in anguish she cried,
"oh, where is my biby?"– the angels replied:

"Your biby as fell dahn the plug'ole.
Your biby has gone dahn the plug.
The poor little fing was so skinny and fin,
He oughter been barfed in a jug!

Your baby is perfectly 'appy;
He don't need a barf anymore.
Your biby 'as fell dahn the plug 'ole
Not lorst, but gorn before!"

From Measure for Measure by William Shakespeare

Ay, but to die, and go we know not where;
To lie in cold obstruction and to rot;
This sensible warm motion to become
A kneaded clod; and the delighted spirit
To bathe in fiery floods, or to reside
In thrilling region of thick-ribbed ice;
To be imprison'd in the viewless winds,
And blown with restless violence round about
The pendent world.

The weariest and most loathed worldly life
That age, ache, penury, and imprisonment
Can lay on nature, is a paradise
To what we fear of death.

DEATH (Anonymous)

Do not stand at my grave and weep
I am not there, I do not sleep
I am a 1,000 winds that blow
I am the diamond glints on snow
I am the sun on ripened grain
I am the gentle autumn rain
When you awaken in the morning's hush
I am the swift uplifting rush
Of quiet birds in circled light
I am the soft star that shines at night
Do not stand at my grave and cry
I am not there; I did not die.

Poems about resilience

Educators notes

The aims of this session of group work are twofold:

- To use non-traditional subject matter to help to break down barriers, so that group members get to know each other and can work together at a deeper level.
- To use the reflective space of poetry to explore some of the challenging aspects of our work and careers going forwards..

Stopping by Woods on a Snowy Evening by Robert Frost.

His house is in the village though;
He will not see me stopping here
To watch his woods fill up with snow.

My little horse must think it queer
To stop without a farmhouse near
Between the woods and frozen lake
The darkest evening of the year.

He gives his harness bells a shake
To ask if there is some mistake.
The only other sound's the sweep
Of easy wind and downy flake.

The woods are lovely, dark and deep,
But I have promises to keep,
And miles to go before I sleep,
And miles to go before I sleep.

There is also a good recording of Frost reading this himself on YouTube.

The Road Not Taken by Robert Frost

Two roads diverged in a yellow wood,
And sorry I could not travel both
And be one traveller, long I stood
And looked down one as far as I could
To where it bent in the undergrowth;

Then took the other, as just as fair,
And having perhaps the better claim,
Because it was grassy and wanted wear;
Though as for that, the passing there
Had worn them really about the same,

And both that morning equally lay
In leaves no step had trodden black.
Oh, I kept the first for another day!
Yet knowing how way leads on to way,
I doubted if I should ever come back.

I shall be telling this with a sigh
Somewhere ages and ages hence:
Two roads diverged in a wood, and I –
I took the one less traveled by,
And that has made all the difference.

Debrief

Take each poem in turn (in what order the educator prefers). Ask the participants to read it carefully themselves. Then ask one member to read it out loud.

Explore the initial responses to the poem, and what the themes of the poem are, how does this relate to our work?

Themes to consider may be:

- the conflict in a moment of solace versus pending obligations
- the idea of the dark woods representing death, but also solace or release
- ideas about solitude and the thoughts of others
- choice and what that means for us, how do we decide on a direction?

Usually, simply listening to participants' reflections will release rich thoughts and reflections.

EVALUATE

INTRODUCTION

This section is about methods that help educators to **evaluate** the educational work they have been doing with participants.

The introduction considers the "What, why and when" issues and then the sections that follow are detailed descriptions of different **methods** ("how" issues).

What does "evaluate" actually mean?
Here are some definitions:

1. To form an idea of the amount, number, or value of; assess, put a value or price on, as in "the study will assist in evaluating the impact of recent changes".
2. Find a numerical expression or equivalent for (an equation, formula, or function) as in "substitute numbers in a simple formula and evaluate the answer".
3. The regard that something is held to deserve; the importance, worth, or usefulness of something, as in "your support is of great value". This also has connotations of merit, utility, practicality, desirability, benefit, gain, helpfulness, assistance, efficacy, significance, effectiveness.

The word "value" in itself, conveys some complex meanings:

1. Principles or standards of behaviour; one's judgement of what is important in life, as in, "they internalize their parents' rules and values". This also has connotations of codes or behaviours applying to moral issues, or rules of conduct.
2. To consider (someone or something) to be important or beneficial; have a high opinion of, as in "she had come to value her privacy" which also has connotations of holding in high esteem, appreciating, respecting, admiring or cherishing, setting great store by.

> "Questioning together begins to demonstrate that as individuals we have the capacity to become part of something larger than ourselves. Those in the conversation begin to share a concern for deeper levels of shared meaning[1]."
> **Juanita Brown and Sherrin Bennett**

Evaluating educational activities is obviously a good thing to do and yet the definitions above raise many questions. What is it that we are trying to evaluate? Who for? When is the best time to attempt evaluation and what different methods could be used?

Evaluation can be a very tedious business. At the end of a session, questionnaires are handed out and participants furiously, or languidly, tick boxes before they rush away, often leaving some boxes unfilled or free text comments that are illegible, monosyllabic, or rude. Wearily we hope that someone else will process the results or that there are enough "excellent" ticks to keep our morale up a bit longer. The frustration of this kind of tick box evaluation for educators is that it doesn't capture what happened, may give little guidance as to what to do next, or next year, and seems of little importance to the participants. They may mainly see it as an impediment to getting to lunch, or to the bus home.

However, evaluation can be done by many different methods, at different stages of training programmes, so that it yields useful insights. Educators can check that they are on the right track and have a source of EBI, ("Even Better If"), ideas. Evaluation can give participants opportunities to reflect on and reinforce their learning. To do this kind of evaluation effectively means thinking about the methods, timing and the purpose of the evaluation. Educators can let go of the guilt, if not every session is evaluated, every time, (yielding a pile of paper for the shredder and not much else?).

Evaluation can be complex. Evaluation could consider the experiences of participants. However, feedback and evaluation of the educator's skills is also important if improvements in education are to be achieved. Are educators trying to "form an idea of the amount or number" of activities, (see the definitions above), or are educators trying to enumerate the range of views expressed by participants? Perhaps educators are really trying to assess value in broader terms, to include questions such as "what was most important aspect" or "what was the impact" or "how useful" was the education? Educators may also wish to assess the extent to which participants' own professional values and attitudes have developed. After all, our professional roles include adherence to well defined "standards of conduct and behaviour". Can such judgements be expressed in a numerical way, or are there other ways to present the value of our educational endeavours?

Evaluation must also consider the "stakeholders"; those who have a legitimate interest in the outcomes. These can include the educator, the participants, the local educational hierarchy including Health Education England, and national standard setting bodies such as the GMC and the Royal Colleges. Evaluation may be part of the quality assurance processes for such bodies, as well as informing the personal professional development of educators. These stakeholders can be valuable sources of evaluation information, such as, examination pass rates.

The EVALUATE section covers what kinds of issues evaluation might address, why those are important and then considers how evaluation can be approached in a systematic way, to focus on the most important features of educational activities. This should enable educators to get useful feedback on what has happened, so that they can continue with activities that are working well and improve elements of the education that are not proving their worth. Effective evaluation will usually involve a variety of different methods, to seek information from several vantage points.

The key part of the word "evaluate" is the "value" element. Our educational activities are planned to include "values and attitudes" as well as "knowledge and skills" (see ENRICH Using taxonomies of learning 1). When educational activities aim at high levels of Blooms taxonomy (see ENRICH Using taxonomies of learning 2) this inevitably includes matters of analysis, comparison and judgement. Our evaluations should aim to capture and assess, (at least some of), the complexity of our participants learning experiences.

This may initially seem too complicated for routine evaluation, however, the methods described here offer opportunities to evaluate deeper learning as well as initial responses.

Evaluation can be thought of in two different ways. Firstly, evaluation can be seen as a kind of summative assessment for the educator; to what extent did the education on offer do its job? Secondly, the term evaluation can comprise more of a formative, feedback element, for the educator to use to improve quality, and to inform their own Continuing Professional Development needs.

Understanding the nature of evaluation and feedback raises important questions about what educators could be evaluating, against what criteria/standards, and when and how to get appropriate feedback.

These approaches are summarised under the following headings:

- Evaluation as a summative process.
- Evaluation as feedback on the educator's skills.
- The formal, informal and hidden curricula; which to evaluate?
- Fitzpatrick's hierarchy of evaluation.
- Constructing good questions.
- Tick box versus free text.
- Responding and working with evaluation findings.

Evaluation as a summative process

When considered summatively, evaluation can been seen as a form of audit. This helps educators to put a value on what they have been doing educationally, and measures the effectiveness of educational activities. In this sense, evaluation has to take place against expected criteria and standards, similar to the clinical audits that are familiar to all clinicians. Judgements have to be made about educational "value". However, evaluation does not necessarily lead to improved performance, unless combined with specific feedback about behaviours that need to be changed.

Educational outcomes have to be compared to something that is considered desirable by the educator, and whose value may or may not be shared or appreciated by participants. For example, the educator could consider evaluating a programme, focusing on the extent to which participants agree that they have "learned" enough, compared to the requirements of a defined curriculum, (usually set out formally by the relevant professional body such as the Royal Colleges). Success in examinations may be part of this assessment of educational activity, but clearly depends on many other variables, including the study habits of participants and their skill in taking examinations.

Educators may also want to assess the extent to which participants have developed "professional values" (such as an ability to think ethically, or an understanding of what types of behaviour are acceptable for professions). Such matters may be recognised as important by educators, while being "unknown unknowns" to some participants. Participants' assessments of their own learning needs can sometimes be rather narrowly confined, to matters of knowledge transfer initially; educators need to widen this view and assess the extent to which they have been successful. This kind of evaluation is often best done after the educational activity has taken place, has settled in participants minds, and coalesced into a whole. Thus, summative evaluation may occur at the end of a module, term or programme. It is difficult to evaluate educational activities when participants have departed into the next phase of their professional lives and are no longer in a training environment. However, this may be a valuable type of evaluation to attempt.

Evaluation as formative feedback on the educator's skills

Evaluation can also be seen as a form of formative feedback to the educator, being information gathered with the sole aim of improving performance, and usually confined to matters of observable fact. Feedback is not advice, praise or evaluation, but rather information gleaned with a view to improvement, irrespective of the current level of performance. While practice tends to make educational skills become *permanent*, it is **feedback** that will help educators to make those skills *perfect*. Feedback can happen informally, especially within sessions, when the educator will continuously monitor the "feel of the room", the relationships amongst participants and the progress that is being made towards the chosen educational aims and objectives.

There is again a link between Consultation Skills and Educational Skills here. In successful consultations and in successful educational activities, the clinician/educator will be continuously monitoring and developing the relationships in the room, and ensuring that the structure of the conversation proceeds towards achieving all the goals of the consultation/ educational activity, (see Table 1 below). The skills needed are very similar in education and in consultations: active listening, using empathic comments to build relationships, picking up clues and cues and responding appropriately, while keeping things on track and in a logical order.

Feedback can also be gleaned from formal post session information gathering processes such as questionnaires. However, participants may be skilled learners, but they are not necessarily skilled *educators*. To develop their own skills, educators will benefit from direct observation of educational activities by other, skilled educators, who can give feedback and suggest practical ways to improve educational delivery. Discussions with educational colleagues in meetings, conferences or appraisals can be useful *benchmarking* processes (how does my work compare to what other people are doing?), can be fertile sources of *inspiration* (that would be a good thing to try!) and triggers to *self-reflection* (how is my educational performance?). All these factors are potentially stimulating sources of evaluation and feedback for educators.

The formal, informal and hidden curricula; which to evaluate?

The content of the formal curriculum is transparent and available to anyone via the relevant Royal College or other professional body. When evaluating education, educators need to decide which elements of the curriculum they are planning to cover in formal sessions, which elements are expected to be covered in private study and which elements are likely to be picked up informally. Clearly, professional examinations are specifically designed to assess against the curriculum. If participants pass their examinations, that might be considered a "good enough" evaluation of whether the formal curriculum has been covered adequately.

However, educators may wish to address more difficult, more complex or deeper levels of the curriculum, especially if they have planned sessions that address the higher levels of Miller's Pyramid or Bloom's taxonomy of learning objectives. In that case, evaluation needs to go beyond finding out if participants enjoyed the session or had an initial positive response. The next section on using **Fitzpatrick's hierarchy of evaluation** can be used as a guide when planning evaluations. Testing the educational activity against its planned aims and objectives, revised at the start with participants and reviewed at the end of the session, will provide a good background.

What of the informal and hidden curricula, which by their very nature are less transparent, less likely to be understood directly by participants and less likely to be identified during examinations?

Table 1

	Stage of the educational intervention	
Develop the relationship with the participants	ENGAGE at the start to get learners and teachers working together and to establish the relevant agenda for the process.	Attend to the structure of the educational programme and make this explicit to participants
	ENERGISE throughout the intervention using techniques that maintain interest.	
	ENRICH the experience by using varied techniques that enable working at different levels, exploring knowledge skills and attitudes.	
	EVALUATE effectiveness during the intervention and afterwards using techniques to promote reflection and improvement.	

The **informal curriculum** includes all those things which are understood to be important to learn, but which are not necessarily written down formally. This includes all the behaviours that reinforce and transmit the attitudes, norms and beliefs about what being a clinician is all about. This type of curriculum is *imbibed* rather than taught. The informal curriculum may be transmitted by role modelling by seniors, via peer pressure, and via the implicit expectations that educators have of participants, (See General Introduction for more details about the informal and hidden curricula).

The **hidden curriculum** is not overtly stated either, but expresses the priorities, deeper beliefs and practices of the environment or institution. The aims of the hidden curriculum are not explicitly articulated and yet are woven through all the practical and educational experiences that participants have during their training. For example, a hidden curriculum could include the expectation that learners strive for, and that they are capable of, excellence. In contrast, the expectation could be that clinical practice is too difficult to do well and that "getting by" is all that is reasonable. Some clinicians may absorb a "hidden curriculum" which includes ideas such as "the main thing is to finish on time" or "patients do not really want shared decision making", or "we have to follow the guidelines all the time".

This quotation from Mahmood, (Reference 2) gives a flavour of one kind of "hidden curriculum":

"The hidden curriculum consists of what is implicitly taught by example day to day, not the explicit teaching of lectures, grand rounds, and seminars."

Hopkins et al (Reference 3) expand this by saying

"In essence, it is a set of ethical, moral, and value-based teachings communicated, often in a non-explicit manner, to doctors-in-training. It is a foundation for communication and influences future interactions with patients, peers, and colleagues. The hidden curriculum can be a negative, empathy-disabling curriculum."

Thus it seems that the hidden curriculum is usually "code" for the negative aspects of training, the imbibing by learners of harmful, or even unprofessional, attitudes, values or behaviours. However, in an educational setting we can turn this to its flip side and ensure that our "hidden curriculum" demonstrates **positive professional values**. Educators can evaluate these aspects formally so that we highlight the importance of a positive set of values and attitudes. In formal training programmes, educator values are manifest in their professional behaviours (turning up on time, being well prepared, attending to the welfare of their participants,) and in the assistance and support they give to the relationships that develop a community of practice. This may include helping participants feel that they belong, that intra group behaviours are appropriate, or that difficult issues can be raised and discussed. The hidden curriculum includes concepts of "professionalism", which includes acceptable professional behaviour and also recognises what Schön calls *"professional artistry"*: making judgements, having room to be wrong, going beyond protocol, developing yourself, understanding self-regulation/professional regulation (Reference 4). Such matters can be rendered explicit by the evaluation questions chosen by the educator.

Fitzpatrick's hierarchy of evaluation

When planning evaluations, it can help educators to use some formal tools, just as using taxonomies can be helpful in planning the education in the first place (see ENRICH Using taxonomies of learning). One such evaluation tool is called "Fitzpatrick's hierarchy" (see Reference 5). Fitzpatrick considered that evaluation has to go beyond exploring participants initial feelings about their education or training, sometimes dismissively referred to as "counting smiley faces". Rather the benefit of training is considered as a series of related benefits, which develop over time. These are benefits are summarised as reaction, learning, behaviour and results/outcomes.

1. Reaction

Reaction is considered to be what participants thought and felt about the education at the time, capturing their initial responses. While this type of evaluation often stops pretty much at the "how was it for you?" level, the immediate response to education is nonetheless important. Boring, irrelevant, rushed, or obscure inputs, will not enable participants to learn much effectively. They express themselves as not having enjoyed the session.

However, I am always a little anxious about sessions that are described in positive terms as "The trainees really enjoyed…". This is because no learning happens without change: it is rare that change has no downsides or is not painful. Some of our most important learning happens when we realise that everything we knew before was wrong, or that we have misunderstood something and now see the light; these are rarely comfortable experiences. Assessing immediate reactions goes further than exploring what fun people had; a trip to a comedy store can be fun, but may not be effective clinical education.

Immediate responses can be very helpful in considering organisational matters:

- Did participants know which room to go to?
- Did they waste time doing preparation that was not used in the session?
- Questions about the rooms/lunch/coffee might be answered by the educator taking a view, although participants may be invited to consider these matters if the educator considers that they are amenable to change. This is not always the case.

2. Learning

Learning must follow, if the education is to be of real value to participants. This can be evaluated in different ways and at different time scales. However, most educators soon learn (painfully at times), that teaching is not the same as learning. What you *teach*, however carefully prepared and imaginatively presented matters not a jot; what matters is what is *learned* by the participants. So methods of evaluation need to focus on what is actually learned and also to try and get at the learning that participants may not own up to. Participants love telling educators that they learned loads. However, sometimes participants struggle to recall or articulate any specific, actual thing, they learned. Evaluation questions are more valuable when they ask participants to spell out exactly what they learned. This type of evaluation can also reinforce learning, if participants are asked to rank, prioritise or ascribe value to learning points.

Participants also learn things you do not want them to learn such that "doing x seems like a lot of trouble don't think I will bother" or "this stuff is only for high flyers not me" or "I just refer every patient I am not sure about". These are examples of undesirable "hidden curriculum" outcomes. However, an evaluation that reveals this is very useful. The educator can address such challenges and difficulties in later sessions.

3. Behaviour changes

Behaviour changes are the result of translating learning and applying it in the workplace. This is usually evaluated sometime after training has happened, to allow time for changes to become established. Directly after sessions, it can be useful to invite participants to reflect on how they think their learning could change their behaviour in the workplace. The educator can invite reflection on factors that will help or hinder that behaviour change, so that participants develop realistic strategies for applying learning. Extending evaluation from Response, to Learning, to potential Behaviour change, helps to highlight higher levels of Miller's Pyramid or Blooms learning objectives in the education, (see ENRICH Using taxonomies of learning).

4. Results/Outcomes

Results/Outcomes reflect the highest level of evaluation and the most difficult to achieve. This level evaluates the impact of training on the end recipients. In a clinical context, examples could include effects on patients, teamwork, adherence to appropriate guidelines, the ability to work in novel or complex situations, or to the development of self-reflection and the skills of life-long learning. It can be extremely difficult to evaluate the longer term results of educational activities, as outcomes are the results of a complex mixture of training and education, personal engagement and environmental factors. Educators cherish any feedback they get from participants who have long moved away from training and into the workplace. Sometimes this comes from chance comments, from meeting participants later on in new contexts or from unexpected encounters. My most cherished piece of feedback came in an email from a participant who knew me from years before, and heard me speak at a conference; "You started me thinking and I have not stopped thinking ever since". I can only hope that the other participants got something a bit like this from their experiences! That type of long distance evaluation may not help educators to understand what "even better if" would look like, but it certainly helps to maintain commitment and morale.

The method and timing of evaluations can be guided by the Fitzpatrick level that is being targeted, and asking the right questions will facilitate this.

Constructing good questions

There is some information about using questions effectively in an earlier section of this manual (see ENERGISE Using questions effectively). The approach to using questions in an evaluation context is similar. Educators can plan suitable questions in advance, aiming for an appropriate questioning style. In evaluation contexts, questions can be used in nuanced way to help focus attention on important aspects of the education, and, in particular, on the aspects that the educator especially wishes to highlight. There are three components to this; the construction of questions, the scope of the question and the assumptions that underlie the questions.

The construction of questions is familiar to educators both from an educational point of view, and because the same concepts apply to questions in the consultation. Open questions are preferred for gathering a lot of information. For example, "what were the most worthwhile aspects of this training?" leaves the focus entirely to the participant. However, another approach uses "open directed" questions. These remain open, while narrowing the area of enquiry down appropriately. For example, "what aspects of training helped you to develop your professional resilience?" is an open question, and also directs attention to a particular aspect of training that the educator wants to evaluate. This question also helps the participants to recognise that training in a particular topic has occurred, and that it is of sufficient importance to merit specific evaluation and comment.

Another type of open question has been termed the "Grand tour" question (Reference 6). This could also be a useful approach in evaluations. Questions take the form "Describe what you got out of a typical day at the study release course", or, "describe a typical Action Learning Set Discussion and what benefits you got from it" (see ENERGISE Creating action learning sets).

The **scope** of questions can be varied in evaluations, easily adding nuance and complexity. The invitation to, "State three things you liked about the course", implies that "liking" is a significant factor in evaluation. This may be so, and educators may consider this a perfectly valuable question. However, if the wording is changed to say "State three activities that you found most practically useful" the scope of the enquiry is different; it is directed towards activities (rather than the whole course), it asks about utility rather than enjoyment (which directs thought to the purpose of the activity).

I may not like being sent for CPR training, but I may nonetheless be clear about the activities that will be useful to me. In a way, considering what the relevant evaluation question could be, is part of the *planning* of any session.

Educators can ask themselves:

- What value should this session give to the participants?
- How could my evaluation questions capture the scope of this session?

Finally, evaluation questions incorporate various **assumptions** about what might be happening during educational sessions, and what importance is to be placed on various outcomes. If educators ask about knowledge transfer, (what did you know after the session that you did not know before) participants may not reflect on other issues. Educators may want to ask about skills, (what did you learn to do, or what skills did you acquire, how did your skills develop?) or may wish to explore wider attitude or values development. Asking about issues such as skills for life-long learning, self-awareness, and resilience or professional behaviours, *assumes* that these are important matters for education to cover. Such approach to questions can help to reinforce a positive "hidden curriculum".

Of course, participants may legitimately value quite different things, (compared to their educators) in their educational activities. Participants may be focused only on examination success, or stress relief, or simply having a breathing space outside their workplace. Evaluation questions can address these issues too. This is why the "Everything with a purpose" approach is so helpful. Educators can relate learning to intended learning outcomes, using the phrase "so that", to link the learning to all kinds of desirable outcomes, including examination success (see ENGAGE Everything with a purpose). If the direction of the learning is signalled by the educator, (and jointly negotiated with participants), *during* the session, evaluation will be easier *after* the session.

Tick box versus free text

The sad fact is that some evaluation exercises are done because "we are supposed to evaluate things" and because various external pressures are on educators to provide evaluation of their programmes of education. Many educators would agree that as long as most tick boxes are in the OK area, the most interesting part of an evaluation on a tick box form, is the free text element, where you get to know what (some) participants are really thinking! Tick box type evaluations can be useful for very specific issues (Did you get the information about your course in time, was the room suitable?), which can be dealt with quickly. However, is this the best use of the limited time available for evaluation? Participants are often impatient about filling in forms of this nature: the risk is that they do it perfunctorily or lie. One participant said to me that he never ticked "excellent" for anything on principle. It is clear, when looking at forms, that other participants tick the same box for everything, as quickly as possible. Getting round these limitations means using other methods. The more tick box questions there are, the less accurate or reflective the answers will be.

One approach is to evaluate less frequently, but in more detail ("better fewer but better" as Lenin once said). This might mean evaluating a new session or module carefully, incorporating changes made as a result until it seems no further improvements are likely. This might be signalled by participants shrugging if asked to suggest improvements, or by feedback from a fellow educator observing. Then shift to evaluating another part of the programme, being careful to evaluate against the intended learning outcome and the relevant Fitzpatrick level (likely to be 1 and 2).

Another approach is to take a broader brush and evaluate a term/module or programme against the overall aims of the education and aiming to explore the higher Fitzpatrick levels (likely to be levels 3 and 4).

Responding and working with evaluation findings.

Inevitably, evaluations will reveal mixed messages. Participants will provide warm and positive feedback about some aspects of their experiences, and be equally scathing, dismissive or negative about other aspects. It is best not to over react or under react to the information. The educator needs to ensure that they are aware of and dismantle any defence mechanisms, so that negative issues can still be noted and acted upon. It always helps to start any reflection or conversation with an attitude of "Thank you for this feedback". Not all positive responses are because the educational activities were good, and not all negative views reflect true failings in the education on offer.

Educators can reflect on and analyse the sources of participants' comments so that any problems or issues can be identified. Some problems are clearly actionable and require attention. Some problems may be well recognised by educators, but not immediately soluble. For example, educators may have little control over the group size, the teaching venues available to them or what the course budget can be spent on. When feeding back the findings educators can be honest about the constraints they are working with.

The frequency and intensity of comments on particular issues can also be a guide to action. If ten participants all comment on the same deficiency or problem, then it is more likely to be worthwhile for the educator to try and solve that problem, than to try and solve ten different issues that only one participant is bothered about. Sometimes, small changes to how things are done can have big effects. This is especially so, if the changes allow for increased attention to participants own concerns, if changes improve and develop the relationships in a programme, or if changes address the structure and flow of the programme. The parallels with processes in the consultation are clear.

Evaluation information can also be helpful in identifying the development needs of the educator, and can be used to inform appraisal and professional development discussions. Having suitable plans for developing educational skills can help educators make significant changes, to their own and participants' satisfaction.

Finally, it is essential to "close the loop" in evaluation, just as we "close the audit loop" in practice. The information gleaned from evaluation should be shared with participants, and they should know in advance how and when this is going to happen. Any actions arising should be shared with participants also, so that they see the benefits of participating fully in evaluation processes. It can be useful to highlight specific changes that are made to subsequent participants, so that they understand why and how things came to be the way they are.

Some different evaluation and feedback methods that can be used are summarised under these headings:

Evaluation methods to use during sessions

1. Evaluation during the session
2. Feedback from colleagues
3. Participant driven methods

Evaluation methods to use at the end of sessions

4. All-purpose questionnaires for Fitzpatrick levels 1 and 2
5. Snowball evaluation methods
6. Reviewing the last session

Evaluation methods to use at the end of modules or programmes

7. World Café method
8. End of programme Fitzpatrick levels 3 and 4
9. Using key words and word clouds

Possible methods to apply after completion of training.

10. Evaluation after the programme has ended

References and resources

1. Quotation from *Mindshift: Strategic Dialogue for Breakthrough Thinking* by Juanita Brown and Sherrin Bennett:
2. *Medical education: beware the hidden curriculum*. Mahood SC. http://www.ncbi.nlm.nih.gov/pmc/articles/PMC3173411/ Can Fam Physician. 2011; 57: 983–985. [PMC free article] PubMed

The Hidden Curriculum: Exposing the Unintended Lessons of Medical Education. Monitoring Editor: Alexander Muacevic and John R Adler Laura Hopkins, Lana Saciragic, Joanna Kim, and Glenn Posner. Cureus. 2016 Oct; 8(10): e845. doi: 10.7759/cureus. 845

4. *The Reflective Practitioner* by Donald Schön, 1983
5. *Kirkpatrick's Four Levels of Training Evaluation* by James D Fitzpatrick. These ideas are also well summarised in a Wikipedia entry here: https://en.wikipedia.org/wiki/Donald_Kirkpatrick
6. Beth Leech describes questioning from a journalistic and anthropological perspective in this interesting article https://dornsife.usc.edu/assets/sites/298/docs/interviewing_techniques_asking_questions.pdf

1// EVALUATION DURING THE SESSION

In this section several simple techniques are described that will help educators evaluate a session while it is still going on.

“The Professor must not only teach, but be capable of inspiring a love of learning.”
Robert Saundby, 1898

What Fitzpatrick evaluation level is this method aimed at?

Techniques include assessment of learning points and continued problems, and summarisation. Observation by colleagues can also be a useful way to evaluate during a session and is covered in EVALUATE Observations by colleagues.

These approaches will help to illuminate **Fitzpatrick's levels 1 and 2**: the participants' responses to the education and the subsequent learning points. Changes in behaviour cannot be evaluated directly within the session. However, asking participants to reflect on and share their intended changes in behaviour as a result of the session, will help educators to evaluate whether their intended learning outcomes have been achieved. Reflection on behaviour change also reinforces that learning must be applied in action, if it is truly to be effective.

There is a parallel here, between evaluation during and at the end of sessions, and the "closing" part of a consultation, when action plans are reviewed and consolidated. Building in evaluative reflection, during every session, becomes part of the structure of an educational encounter, reinforcing learning points and raising participants' self-awareness

What are these methods most useful for?

These methods are best used to monitor and evaluate what is happening educationally in real time, during the session. Thinking about the model of educational sessions described in the introduction to the EVALUATE section, (see page 5), there are two aspects that need to be evaluated continuously by the educator, making changes as needed "on the hoof", as it were. These are, firstly, monitoring the relationships in the room and secondly, the structure of the session and progress towards its overall aims.

For the educator evaluating in real time provides:

- **Immediate feedback** so that changes can be acted on straight away.
- **Information** about what participants have learned.
- **Rapid identification** of any misconceptions or difficulties that participants may have.
- **Improved relationships** with participants because attention is paid to their progress during the session.

Some of the techniques that can be used have been described in the earlier sections of this manual. Their specific use for evaluation is outlined here.

For the participants evaluating in real time provides:

- **Immediate reflection** on learning which improves self-assessment skills.
- **Opportunities to improve their understanding** and develop critical thinking about what they are learning.
- **Improved retention** of learning because evaluation tends to reinforce what is important.
- **Improved relationships** within the group and reduced isolation especially if group sizes are large.
- **Demonstration of the educator's support** and commitment to participants' success.

Methods to evaluate during a session

One minute learning summary.

At the end of the session the learning needs agreed at the start of the session (see ENGAGE Establishing learning needs at the outset) can be reviewed. As the educator goes through the list, members of the group can be asked to summarise what they have learned about that issue. Alternatively, every participant can be asked to write down three things they learned, and three things they intend to do differently before the next session, (see also EVALUATE Reviewing the last session). One person can be asked to produce a summary for the whole group, as has already been described, (see ENERGISE making a learning summary).

Most muddled moments.

Using a pause, pair, square, share approach ask participants to spend a moment considering what their "Most Muddled Moments" were during the session. This can give valuable feedback to the educator, so that they can identify which aspects may need better teaching methods or more time. This approach can also help to reinforce to participants that identifying remaining learning needs is not a manifestation of failure, but rather the key to successful learning.

Snowball/pause pair square share.

These methods have been described elsewhere, (see EVALUATE Snowball evaluation and also ENERGISE Making questions effective). Such approaches can be very useful in highlighting key learning points, key behaviours that need to change and key areas that still need work. Asking the right questions is crucial and the underlying principles have been covered in the introduction to the EVALUATE section.

Ideas bring and buy

(See ENRICH Making rounds effective). This method is not discussed further here.

Using line ups

(See ENERGISE Using line ups to explore ideas). Line ups can also be used for evaluation. The first question might be of the form "how important do you think the things learned today are for your future work?", as before asking participants to line up, arranging themselves in order of how important they believe the learning to be. Encourage participants to discuss why they have put themselves in a particular position. What would change their position such that the content of today's sessions became less important or more important?

Follow this up by asking "how confident are you that you can make changes in what you do at work in the light of today's learning?" Again follow up with "what would make changes easier to do/what would help you to change/ what hinders you from making changes? How could that be tackled?"

Here is a further link between consultation skills and education skills: asking patients about how they rate the importance of a behaviour change, followed up by assessing their confidence that they can make such a change ("Scaling" answers from 1 to 10), is a key consultation skill for encouraging behaviour change.

Observation from an education colleague

See EVALUATE Observations by colleagues for details.

It can be seen from this list that the educator has many opportunities to evaluate a session while it is actually happening. The ability to do this, and to act on the feedback in real time, is one of the higher order skills that educators can bring to clinical training.

Working with another colleague can greatly enrich this, if resources permit, so that educators can rapidly assess how things are going, change tack or employ a different educational method to bring things back on track. This means being sensitive to clues about failure such as lack of participant engagement, sleepiness, bitter conflicts or simply an audience that feels like it might not return after the coffee break!

What are these methods less useful for?

These methods are essentially formative evaluations; they give educators information about how well the education is going. They are less useful for summative evaluations designed to determine whether specific end points or standards have been reached by participants. Because they take place in real time and during sessions, they are relatively less useful for Fitzpatrick level 3 (Behaviour), although could be used to assess participants' intent to change behaviours. These methods do not give any information about the outcomes in the workplace, for patients, clinicians or teams, (i.e. Fitzpatrick level 4).

Preparation

Most of these methods require little preparation except for the preparation of suitable questions. It is very likely that the right questions will emerge during the session, especially if the techniques of ENGAGE Hopes and fears and ENGAGE Establishing learning needs at the outset have been suitably employed. Educators could prepare sheets in advance listing the main learning point, or for the snowball evaluation methods, (see EVALUATE Snowball evaluation).

Set up with participants

Evaluation of progress towards the agreed learning goals can take place at any point in the session. However, if the educator decides to do this at the end, time must be set aside within the session for the reflection and discussion about what the key learning was. Otherwise educators risk losing the attention and interest of participants as they prepare to leave. It may seem that setting aside 15 minutes for discussion and evaluation is "wasting" limited education time. However, educators must balance this, against the benefits for themselves and for their participants, as outlined above. Valuing reflection and reinforcing key learning points, so that they are retained and acted upon, should be not seen as wasted time.

Debriefing or collation issues

For these direct methods, debriefing and collation happen within the session All that may be required is a flip chart to record ideas if the educator wishes to do that. Having one participant write a summary can be very motivating (see ENERGISE Making a learning summary). The educator can make brief notes for themselves at the end of the session to inform future planning and for any reflective portfolio they may keep for appraisal purposes.

Pitfalls

There are several possible methods outlined here. Clearly the educator must be selective in their use, choosing the method they feel is most appropriate. In any given session only one or two of these approaches need to be employed. It is probably worth becoming familiar with each method, trying it a few times before trying another, as educators have different approaches. It is very important to "walk the talk" about the importance of reflection and give these processes the time they need to be effective. While participants may be relieved that have no tick box forms to fill in, they will not be very well motivated if evaluation and reflection cause the session to run over.

How best to use the outcomes of this type of evaluation

The outcomes of this type of evaluation can be used during the session, to check progress towards goals, to reframe the time scale if one aspect is proving more difficult than expected and to get feedback on learning. The educator can use the feedback after the session, to inform planning of future sessions, according to the needs of participants. This type of immediate feedback is less likely to be useful for evaluating whole programmes or modules.

2// FEEDBACK FROM COLLEAGUES

This method of evaluation is directed, not to the participants, but to the *educator themselves*.

> “Remember that a teacher does not just need sufficient knowledge, skills and resources, but also the right attitudes and understanding of the overall context and cultural environment to be able to make the teaching relevant to the learner's needs.”
> Ruth Chambers, *Teaching Made Easy*

What Fitzpatrick evaluation level is this method aimed at?

A skilled observer will be able to comment on participants responses, and could possibly comment on their learning (if explicitly checked in the session using methods from EVALUATE Evaluation during the session). These observations would correspond to Fitzpatrick's levels 1 and 2 for the *participants*. However, if a colleague is present during the session the feedback they give will be much more usefully directed at the educator's skills and behaviours, which corresponds to Fitzpatrick's level 4 Results/Outcomes.

Educators continuously develop their educational skills, through reading, experience and training that can be obtained from conferences, meetings and discussions with educator colleagues. A reflective educator will want to know whether this translates into their practice with participants. A skilled observer can give immediate feedback on the educational activities in a session, enabling the educator to refine what they do even further. Remember, practice only makes permanent, feedback on practice is needed to "make perfect".

There is again a parallel between educational and consultation skills. One of the best ways to improve consultation skills is to review a video, or do a joint consultation, with a trusted and skilled colleague, using a suitable model and a suitable skills curriculum to compare what actually happened, with what is considered most skilful practice.

In the introduction to this section, a model of an educational session was proposed, see Resources, page 16. This framework can be used to evaluate the results/outcomes of the educator's professional development.

Evaluation information can also be sought from colleagues who supervise, mentor or teach participants in other settings. In General Practice, the Trainers form a useful pool of expertise and they will have useful feedback to give to General Practice educators via trainers meetings or workshops, and during practice visits (for accreditation purposes). In other specialities these opportunities may be less frequent. However, seeking the views of colleagues will always be a useful commentary on the educational provision.

What is this method most useful for?

This method is most useful for the educator to get feedback on their own educational skills. The main headings that could be considered correspond to the sections of this manual:

- How did the educator **ENGAGE** participants at the start?
- How did the educator **ENERGISE** participants with appropriate activities?
- How did the educator make use of any opportunities to **ENRICH** learning?
- How did the educator **EVALUATE** what was happening, during or after the session?

In addition there are two processes that run alongside, throughout the educational session:

- How did the educator **build relationships** with and between participants?
- How did the educator **structure the session** so that the aims, objectives and intermediate learning outcomes were met smoothly, and in the time available?

For any given session, it is probably best to concentrate in just one or two of these aspects. The educator may wish to get feedback on their use of a particular educational skill, (for example making a round of questioning effective, or enriching the session by involving a patient). Choosing which section to concentrate on, enables educators and observers to drill down and give feedback on specific skills.

Alternatively, the observer could give feedback on what skills were used to build effective relationships or how well the educator managed the flow and structure of the session overall.

Considering evaluation of the educators skills, using a formative feedback approach like this, can enhance the educator's development. It also gives observers specific things to look out for so that they will be able to give **SMART** (specific, measurable, achievable, realistic, timely) feedback, rather than generic non-specific praise.

By dividing up an educational session in this way, a reflective educator can themselves pick one aspect of the session to work on and reflect on. Educators can then experiment with different skills and approaches, to find out what works best for their group of participants.

What is this method is less useful for?

Direct observation from a skilled colleague whose task is to give the educator feedback can be hard to come by. Most skilled educators are busy delivering education themselves. Thus, it is likely that this kind of feedback will occur occasionally, rather than regularly. The observer can use a framework to inform the feedback, so that the educator gets the maximum benefit from the observation process. Therefore, this form of evaluation and feedback will not be used to evaluate a whole module or programme. Observation is not even likely to evaluate a whole session, because a focus on observing skills means that usually only a part of the session is likely to be considered.

Preparation

The educator must first find a skilled observer, so that they can discuss in advance what elements of the session the educator wishes to focus on, and the observer can prepare themselves to make notes on the specific skills employed. In a mentoring way, an observer can also discuss the implicit attitudes and values that the educator is promoting; how was the hidden curriculum delivered and what did it consist of?

The educator and observer also need to set aside some time after the session to discuss what happened, so that feedback can be digested and reflected upon. Then the educator can decide which skills they wish to develop in the future.

Set up with participants

Participants need to be introduced to any observer, if they are not already familiar with that person. If the educational sessions are jointly delivered by two educators anyway, the educators may quietly agree that one person will be observed by the other for one specific aspect of the session. Educators who are observing, can also agree with their colleague as to whether they will also seek the observations of participants, using techniques from EVALUATE Evaluation during the session.

In principle, and with the consent of participants, observers could use remote observation. This could be a video of the session, which should be deleted after feedback. Alternatively, the session could be live streamed to a remote location using video platforms such ZOOM or Google Hangouts, so that the observer need not be personally present at the session.

Debriefing or collation issues

All feedback needs to be given using the principles of good feedback and be SMART, (see above) and conducted with attention to the relationship between observer and educator. The observer can build trust by sticking to the process that has been agreed, giving specific positive feedback as well as exploring any elements that the educator may wish to develop further. Such feedback will provide excellent evidence for any educator appraisal process.

Pitfalls

Even a relatively short educational session is a complex mix of content, educational skills and relationships. All these elements contribute to the successful delivery of educational activities. Attempting to evaluate everything could easily overwhelm observer and educator alike. A specific focus is likely to be more effective. Being observed can be stressful at times and the observer has a responsibility to see the process as nurturing and developmental, not critical and undermining. Thus, good preparation and a supportive relationship is essential.

How best to use the outcomes of this type of evaluation

The outcomes of this approach are best used by the educator themselves to reflect on and further develop their educational skills. Reflection on their educational skills will of course be useful for any appraisal or reflective portfolio. Many educators learn from each other, so when a meeting, conference or appraisal discussion occurs, educators could share their experiences of being observed, and what they did with the feedback they obtained. Being available as a skilled observer and using the framework proposed here, offers opportunities for observers to improve their own educator skills

Resources

Model of an educational session

	Stage of the educational intervention	
Develop the relationship with the participants	ENGAGE at the start to get learners and teachers working together and to establish the relevant agenda for the process.	Attend to the structure of the educational programme and make this explicit to participants
	ENERGISE throughout the intervention using techniques that maintain interest.	
	ENRICH the experience by using varied techniques that enable working at different levels, exploring knowledge skills and attitudes.	
	EVALUATE effectiveness during the intervention and afterwards using techniques to promote reflection and improvement.	

3// PARTICIPANT DRIVEN METHODS

A small selection of methods is described here that harness the insight of participants to evaluate their own learning and that of their peers.

“Diffused knowledge immortalises itself.” James Mackintosh

What Fitzpatrick evaluation level are these methods aimed at?

A small selection of methods are described here that harness the insight of participants to evaluate their own learning and that of their peers. The aim is evaluate how effective the educator's intervention has been, by asking participants to assess their own learning and behaviour changes. Thus, Fitzpatrick's levels 2 and 3 (learning and behaviour) are being evaluated here.

Here is a selection of methods, educators can use these ideas as a springboard to develop their own approach.

Participant generated test questions

Ask pairs or small groups of participants to devise an examination type question about one aspect of the session and write it on a card/slip of paper. It may be helpful to assign different subject matter to different groups to ensure that not everyone asks the same question! Pass an envelope around for the questions to be collected in. Review them after the session.

The nature of the questions will help the educator to evaluate how well the material has been understood. Put the questions on a PowerPoint slide to be used as a warm up quiz for the next session. Participants can complete their answers privately (no need to do any formal marking).

The educator can then facilitate a discussion about the answers. This will reinforce learning as well as enabling evaluation by the educator as to whether key issues have been absorbed.

One-to-one meetings

If the educator has a process of one-to-one meetings with participants, a question about enhancing learning could be included in the discussion.

A drawback of this method is that some participants they may find it difficult to offer what they consider criticism face to face with the educator, see ENRICH One-to-one meetings.

Suggestion box

Give participants a card or piece of paper on which to record suggestions for improving the session they have just experienced. Leave a box or large envelope at the door for collection. This can be done formally, involving all participants when the educator wants feedback about a particular session. A suggestions box could be left there at every session if participants wish to comment at other times.

Educational review station

If doing a speed dating session, including a reflection station where participants are invited to reflect on the educational process, can provide some helpful evaluation for the educator also, (See ENRICH Enhanced educational speed dating).

Keep/change quadrants

Ask participants to use a sheet of A4,and divide it into four quadrants. Label the quadrants as follows:

- Top left, what aspects of the course are enhancing your learning?
- Top right, what could change or be improved to enhance learning on this course?
- Bottom left, what are you doing personally to enhance your learning on this course?
- Bottom right, what do you need to do personally to change or enhance your own learning?

Ask participants to make brief notes in each quadrant. The sheets can be collected and summarised if administrative time is available. Alternatively, a similar quadrant can be drawn on a flip chart, populated and discussed in the session. This method emphasises the shared responsibility that educators and participants have for successful learning (see Reference 1, page 19).

> “We live and learn, but sadly at different rates.” Alan Magid

What are these methods most useful for?

These methods encourage participants in self-assessment and can increase their self-awareness, (especially of their own learning progress). These methods also enable educators to understand what is actually being learned (as opposed to what educators think they are teaching), so that educators can modify their activities, as needed, to ensure optimal learning. The educator shows that they have a positive attitude to feedback and suggestions for change, while also having a clear "learner focused" approach.

Understanding what different participants gain from a session can assist planning of future sessions. The learning should be evaluated against the Intended Learning Outcomes that the educator had in mind. Did participants learn more or less than expected?

In addition, there is a powerful "hidden curriculum" message here. By seeking to evaluate their work and involve participants in this process, educators are demonstrating key attitudes; the importance of self-awareness, respect for participants and willingness to accept feedback with a view to change and improvement.

What are these methods less useful for?

While these methods may highlight areas that the educator may wish to improve on, specific strategies for improvement may not necessarily result. Sometimes participants can make very specific suggestions, which is helpful. More often they will recognise that there was a problem, "The session on ethics went on too long and was exhausting", without necessarily having a good solution. Clearly, the educator must deploy their educational skill, often in discussion with colleagues, to create effective educational strategies to overcome problems. Making the ethics session shorter, may not be the best way to make it less exhausting.

Preparation

It can save time and give more weight to the evaluations if the educator prepares appropriate cards/sheets/keep or change quadrants in advance. Where honest responses are sought, it can be helpful to try and preserve the privacy of individuals by gathering responses in a large envelope for example, or even by getting someone other than the educator to administer some of the evaluations.

Set up with participants

The methods are described above. The educator should explain the purpose of the activity; participants are being asked to participate in the evaluation so that the educator can establish how effective the educational activities are, so that areas requiring improvement can be identified and so that participants will get a better learning experience in the future. Explain exactly when and how the outcomes of the evaluation will be discussed with the group.

Debriefing or collation issues

Discussing the outcome of the evaluations is always important, but especially so when participants have generated the questions for assessment, or when the keep/change quadrant reveal their thoughts. Most of these methods are simple to collate and the outcomes can be discussed in real time in the session. The educator can outline how the results will be used, and indicate what kinds of development or changes are contemplated. The debriefing discussions also provide participants with many opportunities to learn from other participants: what do other people do that helps them? What are other people planning to change in order to enhance learning? Peer modelling can be more effective than instructions from an educator.

Pitfalls

When discussing the outcomes, the educator must be able to distinguish things that can reasonably be changed or developed and those that cannot. Sometimes educators face issues that cause difficulty but which cannot currently be altered. For example, rooms may be unsuitable in some way, the group size may be larger than is comfortable, and curricula are set by the Royal Colleges, not by the educator and so on. Being able to temper participants' desires for their education with realism about what is feasible, is a difficult art to master at times.

How best to use the outcomes of this type of evaluation

Results are best discussed with participants as soon as is feasible, ensuring that the whole group are aware of the collated issues where relevant. The results can also be used as part of an educators reflective practice, to be discussed at appraisal or combined with other information in reports and for course inspections or Royal College visits.

References

1. Material adapted from Helminski, L. and Koberna, S. (1995). Total quality in instruction: A systems approach. In H. V. Roberts (Ed.), *Academic initiatives in total quality for higher education* (pp 309–362). Milwaukee, WI: ASQC Quality Press.

4// ALL-PURPOSE QUESTIONNAIRES FOR FITZPATRICK LEVELS 1 AND 2

This evaluation method uses standard questionnaires with a mixture of open, directed questions and free text options

“A high quality portfolio of learning requires that the learner records not merely that they attended an event, but what they learned from it and how they plan to apply that learning.” Mark Cole

What Fitzpatrick evaluation level is this method aimed at?

These type of questionnaires are most usefully administered at the end of a module or one day course/single session. They are less suitable for evaluating longer programmes. There are specific examples given under the Resources section below. Such questionnaires tend to focus on Fitzpatrick's levels 1 and 2, i.e. What were participants' responses to the educational experience, and what did participants learn? Approaches to levels 3 and 4 are covered in EVALUATE End of Programme Fitzpatrick 3 and 4.

What this method most useful for?

All-purpose questionnaires are most useful when evaluating a specific session or short module, such as a residential course. Not every session needs to be evaluated every time it happens. When developing a new session, educators will need to evaluate whether the purpose of the session was achieved (against the proposed curriculum and compared to the expressed learning needs of participants expressed at the start of the session). Educators can also gain feedback about any improvements for future sessions. However, a well-designed session will not require repeated formal evaluation. Rather, the educator will elicit formative feedback during the session and perhaps at the start of the next session, to keep them on track.

What is this method is less useful for?

This method is less suitable for evaluating a whole programme or series of sessions, because it is rather focused. The examples given here do not address the Fitzpatrick levels of behaviour and outcomes (see EVALUATE End of Programme Fitzpatrick 3 and 4).

Preparation

Suitable questionnaires need to be prepared before the session and arrangements made for collation of the results.

Set Up with participants

The educator needs to explain the evaluation, which is needed to ensure that educational aims are met, so that the educator understands if any changes are needed for future sessions on this subject. The educator needs to allocate sufficient time for participants to read, reflect and complete the evaluation so that they do it properly and do not simply rush off having filled it in perfunctorily. A poorly reflected upon evaluation will not yield useful information (for educators or participants), and may result in comments like "I hate filling in these forms". The educator can pre-empt this, and get useful information, by explaining the purpose and encouraging reflection and recording of what has been learned. Referring back to the learning needs assessed at the outset of the session can be one way to help participants write down and reinforce their learning.

Debriefing or collation issues

In developing a new session, it may be most valuable for the educator simply to read all the evaluations and make notes on what changes they plan to the session to improve it next time. Discussing the findings with a fellow educator can be valuable, especially if they were able to observe the session. Administrative help to collate and report on such evaluations may be needed for inspection or appraisal purposes.

Pitfalls

Overdoing evaluation, or doing evaluations too frequently, risks making participants irritated and fatigued with the evaluation process. If that happens, they make not reflect properly, and simply rush to complete the questionnaire (in a desire to get away on time). Better fewer but better evaluations overall, is probably the way to go.

How best to use the outcomes of this type of evaluation

This type of evaluation is best used to fine tune the delivery of sessions, to ensure that the learning outcomes are aligned with participants expressed needs (what participants are most concerned about), and that outcomes are also aligned to the curriculum requirements, (what educators are most concerned about). In reviewing the answers, educators will be especially interested in those that confirm, (or refute) coverage of the formal curriculum, and which tend to support the implicit objectives of the informal or hidden curricula, (see General Introduction). A detailed report on the learning achieved in one session, with comments on how that may be improved, is likely to be far more interesting to any appraiser or programme inspection team, than many tick box evaluations, whose meaning may be difficult to discern.

RESOURCES

Sample questionnaires

Questionnaire 1 – a standard questionnaire for evaluating participants' responses (Fitzpatrick level 1) for a residential module

This questionnaire focuses on what was experienced by the participant, what they personally valued or found challenging and addresses any concerns they may have by providing a space for comment. It has a small focus on practical arrangements, but does not focus on whether participants "liked" the module or enjoyed it.

Residential courses (in General Practice training) often take place at the start of programmes. Suggestions for improvements to the module are not elicited in this evaluation because participants at this stage are less likely to have a clear understanding of the purpose of the residential, (to build rapport, relationships and begin the process of developing a community of practice) and are even less likely to have a clear understanding of methods to promote those aims, within professional education. If suggestions for improvement are requested they often take the form "more free time to go for walks" or "an abseiling course would have been nice". While these may be enjoyable additions, they are not likely to convince educational funding bodies that they directly contribute to the educational objectives of the course.

This is an illustration of how the evaluation questions need to be of the right construction, (open questions) and also used in a way that defines the scope of the enquiry (in this case Fitzpatrick's level 1, responses to the experience). The questions also embody the assumptions that experiences may be valued, but that it is also normal to have some challenging experiences, during educational activities. Thus, an evaluation like this can pave the way for participants to expect challenges that may take them outside their comfort zone.

In this example (see page 23) the reasons for asking the questions are added in *italics*. Educators can decide whether these reasons need to be on the form given to participants – it is not necessarily helpful.

Questionnaire 2 – an all-purpose questionnaire, to evaluate a specific session, emphasising participants learning outcomes (Fitzpatrick's level 2)

If the session has been set up using the methods from the ENGAGE section (Hopes and fears and Establishing learning needs at the outset) some evaluation will happen within the session, when the learning needs are reviewed at the end. Therefore any formal evaluation can focus on what learning participants have taken away from the session, and helps them to reflect on what the next steps might be. This can help educators get feedback on the effectiveness of the session and help them plan for future sessions.

In this example (see page 24) the reasons for asking the questions are added in *italics*. Educators can decide whether these reasons need to be on the form given to participants – it is not necessarily helpful.

Questionnaire 1 – a standard questionnaire for evaluating participants' responses (Fitzpatrick level 1) for a residential module

RESIDENTIAL COURSE EVALUATION

Date of course:

Please write a brief comment about:
LOCATION/PRACTICAL ARRANGEMENTS /ORGANISATION/ACCOMMODATION

(Emphasising a ***brief*** *comment on these practical arrangements indicates a willingness to receive feedback, but does not dwell on the "hotel" aspects of the residential. These issues are important, but not the main focus of the event.)*

What were the three **most important things you SAW** during the residential?

a.

b.

c.

(This question emphasises reflection on the participant's own experiences and responses to the event.)

List three **important things you HEARD** during the residential?

a.

b.

c.

(This question emphasises reflection on the participant's own experiences and responses to the event.)

What did you **VALUE most** about your experience?

(This question asks participants to reflect and make a judgement about what they value, what is important to them, and helps to demonstrate the educators concern for them as an individual)

What was the MOST CHALLENGING thing for you personally?

(This question recognises and normalises that education can be personally challenging, demonstrates the educators concern for the participant as an individual, and helps educators to identify any unexpected challenges. Educators will also glean what challenges occur and to for how many participants. For example, are there are many participants who are frightened to contribute to a group discussion? This aids planning of future events)

ANY OTHER COMMENTS/FEEDBACK/THOUGHTS/CONCERNS ABOUT THE RESIDENTIAL COURSE?

(The open nature of this question allows participants space to express concerns and any other comments, showing a willingness to hear things that may not have been said verbally in the group.)

Questionnaire 2 – **an all-purpose questionnaire, to evaluate a specific session, emphasising participants learning outcomes (Fitzpatrick's level 2)**

TITLE OF SESSION: **DATE:**

Please write your reflections on the session in response to the following questions. You can use these reflections on what you have learned as a guide to making your portfolio entry for today's session.

(This introduction raises the issue of reflection as an important educational process, and signals that participants may need to record their learning in an appraisal or training portfolio. This is an example of how the evaluation questions can incorporate assumptions about education, in this case that reflections, and recording reflections, are of value.)

At the start of the session, how were **learning needs discussed and identified**?

(This focuses attention on the discussion at the start when learning needs were talked through see ENGAGE Assessing learning needs at the outset)

How important were those learning needs in relation to your daily work?

(This helps the educator to ensure that subject matter is presented in a way that emphasises its relevance and importance; see ENGAGE Everything with a purpose)

Which of those learning needs did the **session address**?

What were your most important learning points from this session?

1.

2.

3.

Any other important learning?

(This question addresses the crucial issue of what was actually learned, rather than what the educator thinks they have been teaching.)

What **changes do you intend to make** to your practice as a result of this session?

1.

2.

3.

Any other changes?

(This question highlights that effective learning means change. It does not assess that change, but in signalling intent to change, helps to orientate the learner towards changes that need to be made in their daily work.)

When covering this subject matter in future, it would be better if …

(This invites suggestions for improvement or change in the session)

Any other comments or suggestions?

5// SNOWBALL EVALUATION

A Snowball Evaluation is a group based, rapid evaluation, using structured, formal steps to elicit, share and discuss the education.

“It is good to rub and polish our brains against that of others.” Montaingne

What Fitzpatrick evaluation level is this method aimed at?

This method can be used for more than one Fitzpatrick level (usually levels 1,2,3) For example, it could be used to evaluate participants' **responses** to an educational intervention and can just as easily be adapted to evaluate their key **learning** points or changes in their **behaviour** after training. It is similar to the "ideas bring and buy" described in ENRICH Making rounds effective.

If applied sometime after the educational intervention, this method can be a useful way to evaluate changes in behaviour as a result of learning. To use this method to evaluate outcomes, for example, effects on patients, systems or on participants stress or resilience levels, the questions would have to reflect the type of change to be considered. Examples of Snowball Evaluation sheets are given in the Resources section (Page 27).

What this method most useful for?

This method has two main uses. Firstly, by encouraging personal reflection and group discussions, it enables participants to focus in on the areas that the educator is particularly interested in. This could be the strengths and weaknesses of a particular session, what was learned, how learning was applied or what effects learning had overall. By using the "pause, pair, square, share" approach (see also ENERGISE Effective questions for groups), participants are also directly exposed to the thoughts and learning of others. This can highlight important messages from the education that some participants may have missed or undervalued. The process of evaluation thus becomes a potential way to extend and reinforce learning. The educator highlights the benefits of reflection both alone, and in discussion with others afterwards, so that reflection becomes a natural part of the learning process. This is so that participants increase their reflection skills, which are crucial for lifelong learning, by sharing and collating their views.

Secondly, this method enables educators to develop their understanding of the range of participants' views and experiences, fairly quickly and easily. Little collation work is needed afterwards, so that results can be discussed with participants at the time of the evaluation. Ideas and suggestions for improving the education will naturally follow. The educator can feed back their own thoughts to the group, explaining what changes might occur and why. When participants appreciate that evaluation is taken seriously, is not just "tick a box" and that change is likely to result, they become more committed to the evaluation process and to the process of reflection on their learning.

Relationships between participants and between participants and educator are strengthened through discussion and sharing of views, helping to further build a "Community of practice" (see General Introduction).

What is this method is less useful for?

This method occurs in real time, therefore it is less useful for evaluating the impact of training after the sessions have been completed, and participants have dispersed. One possible disadvantage, is that, if a small number of participants have very different views to the majority, this may not be clearly recognised in the final "group" outcome. If educators suspect that this may be the case, it can be worth alluding to this possibility in the debriefing, (see debriefing or collation issues, below).

As this method uses a significant period of time, it is not suitable for use after every session. It is best used for refining and evaluating new sessions, or groups of sessions on a related theme, or at the end of part of a programme, for example, at the end of a term. Does every session need to be evaluated every single time it is delivered?

Preparation

The educator must decide the focus of this evaluation before starting, perhaps by reflecting on which Fitzpatrick evaluation level they are most interested in finding out about. Having some pre prepared sheets (see Resources below) can help to make the process run smoothly.

Set up with participants

Explain the question to be discussed and ask participants to reflect silently, by themselves, as to their three most important thoughts. Then ask them to discuss these in pairs, coming up with a list that they both agree on, then in fours and finally in groups of eight to get a final list. Depending on the question, allow up to 5 minutes for each stage of the discussion and 10 to 20 minutes for whole group discussion/ debriefing at the end.

In a larger group, there may be several such "group of eight" sheets at the end. Depending on the size of the group, (and whether it naturally divides into groups of eight participants) the final sheet might be done by groups of six, combing three pairs together.

Debriefing or collation issues

Ask each group of eight/six to appoint a rapporteur to share their final thoughts with the whole group. The educator should keep these final sheets for their evaluation reports.

As each group shares their thoughts the educator can use this opportunity to ask:

- "How easy was it to get agreement on these points?"
- "Were there any sharply divergent views?"
- "Does anyone want to enter a dissenting note?"
- "What made that successful? What improvements would you suggest?"

Taking careful note of the answers can help the educator form a more nuanced view of the impact of the education they are evaluating. It is normal in post graduate education for different participants to gain different value from sessions. The educator delivers a range of educational methods, content and options, so that participants can pick up that which is most useful for themselves. Thus, it is inevitable that educators will not "please all of the people all of the time". Educators can make this explicit, while also valuing any negative feedback as an opportunity for reflection, so that they can develop and improve the educational offering for subsequent participants.

Pitfalls

This type of evaluation usually happens at the end of a session. At this point participants can be tired or may have to rush away to fulfil other commitments. This may mean that reflection is perfunctory, done speedily and therefore lacks usefulness. Educators need to plan for this and ensure that the evaluation happens at an appropriate time, scheduling adequate time for the reflective process, while still finishing the session punctually. If done well, this approach models and embeds reflection in the educational process, so that participants become more skilled in reflection, so that their lifelong learning will be more effective.

If educators are working with a stable group who work together regularly, a snowball evaluation of the previous session or term could provide a useful starting up/warm up exercise, and trigger reflections that have been enhanced by the passage of time. This can be especially useful for evaluating the "take home messages", i.e. what participants have retained weeks later. If participants cannot remember any take home learning points, the educator will get a valuable piece of feedback!

How best to use the outcomes of this type of evaluation

This evaluation lends itself to immediate discussion with the group, inviting suggestions about improvements, or comparing notes about what participants got most value from. Making notes on specific sessions and how they can be improved at the time, means that educators have helpful information to prepare them for next time. This can reduce planning time for future sessions, because any improvements needed have been noted when fresh in the memory.

RESOURCES

Here are two sample Snowball Evaluation sheets.

The first one is focused on the key learning points and activities during the session.

Title of session being evaluated (In this case "Developing skills in breaking bad news")
Fitzpatrick's level 2 – **learning**

REFLECTING ALONE		
What were the three most key learning points for you in this session?	Which activities during the session were most useful?	What improvements to this session could you suggest? ....
REFLECTING IN A PAIR		
What were the three most key learning points for you in this session?	Which activities during the session were most useful?	What improvements to this session could you suggest? ....
REFLECTING IN A FOUR		
What were the three most key learning points for you in this session?	Which activities during the session were most useful?	What improvements to this session could you suggest? ....
REFLECTING IN AN EIGHT		
What were the three most key learning points for you in this session?	Which activities during the session were most useful?	What improvements to this session could you suggest? ....

Title of Evaluation **(in this case Which programme speakers changed your behaviour in practice the most/the least?)** Fitzpatrick level 3 – **changes in behaviour**

REFLECTING ALONE	
Which three speakers changed your behaviour in practice the most? …………… …………… ……………	Which three speakers had the least effect on your behaviour in practice? …………… …………… ……………
REFLECTING IN A PAIR	
Which three speakers changed your behaviour in practice the most? …………… …………… ……………	Which three speakers had the least effect on your behaviour in practice? …………… …………… ……………
REFLECTING IN A FOUR	
Which three speakers changed your behaviour in practice the most? …………… …………… ……………	Which three speakers had the least effect on your behaviour in practice? …………… …………… ……………
REFLECTING IN AN EIGHT	
Which three speakers changed your behaviour in practice the most? …………… …………… ……………	Which three speakers had the least effect on your behaviour in practice? …………… …………… ……………

6// REVIEWING THE LAST SESSION

This method is aimed at considering the effect that education has had on behaviour in the workplace.

“Every defect is a treasure.” Japanese Quality Improvement slogan: finding defects offers important opportunities to improve what we do.

What Fitzpatrick evaluation level is this method aimed at?

This method corresponds to Fitzpatrick level 3, and will work best if the educator plans ahead. At the end of the previous week's session, ask participants to list their key learning points and any key changes they intend to make in their behaviour in the workplace. The week after, educators should refer back to the behaviours that participants intended to change and ask them to discuss what progress they made. Clearly, this evaluation approach will work best if the session in question contained skills, attitudes, values or knowledge which are readily and frequently applied. This could apply to almost any consultation skill, any clinical reasoning skill, and any session that aimed to improve ethical thinking, professionalism or resilience, for example.

What this method most useful for?

This method has two useful effects. It can give the educator rapid feedback about how effective the previous session was and whether it readily translated in behavioural changes in the workplace. This should help educators reflect critically on how their teaching is working so that they can use that information in planning similar sessions in the future. Furthermore, reflecting on what happened last time also links sessions, showing how they fit together into a systematic programme of learning so that participants understand how learning translates into to practice. The educator invites comment and reflection on what has gone before so that the discussion reinforces the learning in the minds of participants.

What is this method is less useful for?

This method is specific to the session from the very recent past. It will not work so well to evaluate a whole module or programme. If asked to reflect on a whole module or programme, participants may refer back to a variety of experiences in discussing behaviour change; the feedback will then lack the specificity that will enable to educator to act on it.

Preparation

The week before, the educator should ensure that participants identify and commit to making the changes in behaviour at work that the training has called for. Making notes on these, the educator should have them to hand in the following session. Then, appropriate questioning, and perhaps a pause/pair/share approach, can evaluate the degree to which participants were able to put their learning into action.

It can be helpful to signal that learning is going to be reviewed in this way, perhaps by indicating this in the programme, or asking the participant who does the learning summary to note this in the note they send to colleagues, (see ENGAGE Creating a learning summary).

The educator can also prepare by reflecting on how they themselves put the changes into action, when they were learning about the relevant skills. What helping factors/hindering factors do they remember? This may help them anticipate participants' reactions and have some suggestions to inspire continued effort. How much repetition and practice did it take to embed new skills? This can help educators guide the discussion and remain positive about the possibilities of change, even if participants are initially finding it difficult.

Set Up with participants

Ask participants to reflect on the key changes in behaviour that they were anticipating the week before, initially on their own, ("pause"). The educator can summarise the behaviour changes intended using the notes made the week before, so that the key changes are again reinforced with participants. Then ask participants to discuss their progress with a partner, ("pair"), focusing on what went well and also which things were difficult or did not seem to work. Then invite a general discussion with an open question like "what kinds of experiences have you been having with…."

It is likely that some participants will say that they did not succeed in using new learning. This is not necessarily a problem if the educator uses this information positively. Thank the participant for highlighting that behavioural change is not always easy and explore the problem. What did they try and why do they think it didn't work? Then invite comment from the rest of the group. Did everyone have the same experience? Has anyone got a different perspective or experience to share? How did others overcome these difficulties?

This approach shows acceptance of the participant's experience, so that they can comment on ways to improve the education that was delivered last time. Find out what would have helped them to translate classroom learning into behaviour at work. Effective education requires skills that many participants lack, so their suggestions for improvement may be limited. However, finding that a session did not work as effectively as hoped, can give great opportunities for the educator to reflect, seek alternative approaches or develop new educational skills.

Debriefing or collation issues

The information gleaned can be easily noted by the educator to aid planning for future sessions. It can be especially helpful to note what successful participants say about how the education helped them to succeed and change behaviour. Similarly, finding out what obstacles others encountered can also help the educator improve the training experience for next time. Making notes and referring back to them is crucial.

Pitfalls

This method is often best used for education about things that are common and frequently encountered so that participants are very likely to get a chance to implement a change in their daily work before the next session. If the educator is unsure about this, then this evaluation can be done a few weeks after the session in question, so that there will be time for opportunities to do things differently to occur.

How best to use the outcomes of this type of evaluation

The outcomes from this approach are best used to inform future planning and to identify any new skills the educator may need to develop.

The discussion can also be very helpful to reinforce learning amongst participants, so that new skills, or the effects of changing attitudes are reviewed. Weaker participants hear about the positive experiences that others may have, so that the idea of skills development is reinforced and there is a degree of "Role modelling". This modelling may be more powerful if it is a peer to peer process.

Without being explicit, the outcomes can be used to help to shift attitudes in weaker participants. The notion that new skills can be learned experientially and then applied in clinical practice rapidly, is sometimes lost on some participants. They may recognise knowledge deficits more readily than deficits in skills, or lack insight into their need to develop more helpful attitudes.

7// WORLD CAFÉ DISCUSSION

This method creates evaluation through discussion. It can be set up so that different tables address the different Fitzpatrick levels.

"Team members create new points of view through dialogue and discussion. They pool their information and examine it from various angles. Eventually, they integrate their diverse individual perspectives into a new collective perspective." Nanonka, the Knowledge Creating Company

What Fitzpatrick evaluation level is this method aimed at?

A World Café method is a simple, flexible and interesting way to promote large group discussions, using carefully chosen questions. Examples are given in the Resources section (page 34). The World Café approach aims to facilitate discussions by breaking larger groups into several small groups. Small groups gather round a table, with a specific question to discuss, and a large piece of paper to record thoughts and ideas. After a fixed period of time the groups break up and scatter to different tables, leaving one person behind to facilitate discussion with a new group of people, sharing what has gone before as a springboard to a further discussion. New thoughts and ideas are again recorded. Rounds continue until all participants have discussed questions at all the tables.

What is this method most useful for?

This method takes time, and this can be seen as an investment in developing group cohesion, developing reflection skills and in developing suggestions for improvements. As participants are encouraged to write or draw on the "tablecloth" it can be an interesting and enjoyable way to evaluate a programme, or term, of work.

A World Café approach can also be used for purposes other than evaluation. It can make a stimulating and interesting component of any training programme. The different tables can be set up with different tasks, or discussion questions that address different aspects of a subject. A World Café approach is suited to the discussion of challenging issues such as ethical problems, resource allocation, or for discussion of different aspects of a complex case study, (some examples are given in the Resources section below).

This method can be used when participants do not know each other well, or are meeting at long intervals. Ask participants to move between tables, so that they get to meet and engage with almost everyone in the group, so that the educational event gets off to a good start, with everyone participating.

What is this method less useful for?

This method is not suitable for evaluating single sessions, because it takes too much time. However, because it develops a collective perspective, it is useful for examining whole programmes, or modules.

This method will work better if participants are accustomed to small group working and discussion. If using it with participants who are used to very didactic educational methods, careful explanations and briefing will be needed. The educator should be available during discussions, to assist, facilitate or encourage discussion if a group seems to be struggling. This is usually indicated by silence, prolonged or recurrent laughter or other signs of "going off task".

Preparation

The educator using a World Café method for evaluation needs to prepare the room and the questions in advance.

The room needs to be set up as a "café", with enough tables and chairs for participants to sit in groups of no less than four and up to six people. Each table should be clearly labelled with a number or letter, and participants should be allocated to tables. Each table should have a "tablecloth" made of flip chart paper and have suitable pens of different colours available for participants to record thoughts/images. Educators may consider adding an optional "talking stick" (see ENGAGE Talking sticks).

Ideally participants will be told the order that they will visit the tables at the beginning of the café, (an example of how to do this can be found in the Resources section). If this is not done, then they should at least be randomly allocated to their first table, to ensure they do not just "sit with my friend".

Before the café, the educator decides what aspect of evaluation they are most keen to consider, and develops a suitable number of open, searching, debatable questions, one for each table.

Questions need to be open in format, (i.e. not answerable with a yes or no), so that they generate debate and discussion. Questions that begin with stems like "to what extent …" or "How would you rank the importance of …" can work well. In an evaluation context, the scope of the question at each individual table should address a clear Fitzpatrick level: is the discussion to be about *responses* to the education, or what was *learned*, or how *behaviour changed* as a result or what *effects* the educational had on outcomes for patients, professionals or teams? The question should be clearly written on a suitable pieces of paper and attached to the table.

Set up with participants

The total group of participants should be broken up into groups of four to six, and allocated to a "café table". Participants are then asked to discuss the question on the table (using a talking stick if needed) and to note their thoughts on the "tablecloth". Diagrams or drawings are also encouraged. Emphasise that talking together requires active listening, so that everyone contributes and issues are explored thoroughly. Encourage exploration of things that may be left unsaid initially, asking participants to comment on anything that "may have not been raised, or that people are reluctant to mention".

After a fixed period of time (say ten minutes in an evaluation context, more if complex cases are being discussed), participants disperse to other tables in the following way: one person remains behind at the table to chair the next discussion, the other members disperse to different tables, so that they do **not** move as a group, so that their **next** discussion will be with different participants.

At the end of the discussion, participants move again in the same way, leaving one member behind to chair, usually a different person each time. One person remains behind so that they can share what has already been discussed and build the discussion from there, perhaps being given some prompts to deeper discussion. The educator can open the second and subsequent rounds by asking questions participants to consider developing the discussion considering "how that happened", or "what assisted that process", or "what hindered it".

When all participants have visited all the tables/ questions, the process of "harvest" takes place. The educator invites silent reflection first, so that participants can reflect on what themes or patterns have emerged. Ask participants to consider anything that was left unsaid.

Then invite summaries and comments from the group, collating them on a central flipchart.

Debriefing or collation issues

This method collates results in real time, so that afterwards the educator need only ask their administration person to type up the results, which the educator can reflect or comment on if needed for reports or inspection purposes. It could be legitimate simply to record the outcomes photographically and use those images. The educator facilitates discussion in the "harvesting" process at the end by encouraging observation of themes or patterns, new insights, and asking if any major issues were omitted. This is so that there is not simply a rehash of what participants have already discussed. Educators can also ensure that there is some feedback from each groups "tablecloth".

Pitfalls

If the total group is very large, this can result in some chaotic milling about, as participants try to find a new table to go to, while also avoiding ending up with the same group that they started with. To avoid this, participants can be given a list specifying the order in which they will visit the tables. This needs to be prepared beforehand and each participant given a slip of paper with their table order on, (for example table A first, then C, then D, then B).

Discussions will be brief and inconsequential if the question is too closed, or is too narrow in scope. See EVALUATE Introduction for more information about asking good questions.

Skills to make this work even better

It can help discussions to go well if each table has an actual tablecloth, with flip chart paper on top, a few flowers in a pot (or even a jam jar if funds are tight), perhaps a few sweets or biscuits for people to share, and a selection of pens or other media to record ideas and discussions. The final group could be given a smaller sheet to highlight their "star finding", the key message they wish to take away.

Educators can also highlight how this is a *reflective* evaluation process: participants are invited to think about and discuss their learning. This reflection process can be transferred to relevant parts of training or appraisal portfolios. Participants usually enjoy talking about what they valued, or would like to see improved in a programme. Helping them to transfer this to their thinking and preparation for appraisal can help participants develop more positive attitudes towards reflection, and help them develop their reflective skills.

How best to use the outcomes of this type of evaluation

The discussions can help educators to identify areas where the education is "hitting the spot" and help to identify broad areas where more work needs to be done. For example, participants sometimes respond warmly and positively to training, but then cannot identify any change in behaviour or improvement in outcomes afterwards. Has that education fulfilled its purpose fully? Such findings may help the educator to plan relevant changes in their future sessions.

This evaluation method involves participants fully, so that educators can make good use of this to explore suggestions for improvement to the content, teaching methods or follow up of certain sessions, modules or programmes.

The "collective" view arrived at through this process creates helpful material for any reports or inspections required, or for the educators own CPD/Appraisals/reflections.

The impact on relationships

Using a World Café method can help develop good relationships amongst participants. The method ensures that conversations happen with a wide range of participants, which helps people to get to know each other better and increases engagement with the whole group. The educator puts in effort before the café, making tables look nice and developing good questions, so that a welcoming and pleasant atmosphere is created, so that participants can relax and share ideas freely. Some participants may not have felt very comfortable in their educational environments before and may really appreciate a sense of being cared for and that their welfare is seen as worthy of attention. These are powerful "hidden curriculum" issues which educators can plan for, so that the overall effect of the educational process is richer. This conveys the *educational values* of the training more clearly than words alone: actions speak louder than words.

References

1. The World Café: http://www.theworldcafe.com/key-concepts-resources/design-principles/

RESOURCES

Here is a sample table for allocating participants to tables. On arrival participants note down what order they will visit groups in. This example is for four groups. The same principle can apply if there are to be more participants. Educators could create more questions for more groups.

Participants name	First table	Second table	Third table	Fourth table
Ayesha	A	B	C	D
Brian	B	C	D	A
Chris	C	D	A	B
Dani	D	A	B	C
Edwina	A	B	C	D
Farah	B	C	D	A
George	C	D	A	B
Harriet	D	A	B	C
Ian	A	B	C	D
Jaya	B	C	D	A
Kush	C	D	A	B
Lin	D	A	B	C
Mo	A	B	C	D
Nicky	B	C	D	A
Oliver	C	D	A	B
Pat	D	A	B	C

Examples of questions for discussing complex issues, such as ethics

- Table A Discuss, with **real life examples you have encountered**, situations in which the clinician made the **patient's autonomy** the paramount consideration, above other ethical principles.
- Table B Discuss, **with real life examples you have encountered** situations in which **justice and fair allocation of resources** took precedence over autonomy/patient choice.
- Table C Discuss, with **real life examples you have encountered** situations where the **clinician's view of "beneficence"** differed from other people's views of what "beneficence" was (including the patient's own view, the carers view, and the views of other professionals).
- Table D Discuss, with **real life examples you have encountered** situations where the **clinician's view of harm ("maleficence")** might differ to the patient's point of view, (and also perhaps the carers view, and the views of other professionals)
- **Debriefing/"harvest" questions.**
  - What themes are emerging?
  - Which aspects of clinical care feature most often in your examples?
  - How can conflict between different people's views on ethical matters be managed most effectively?

These discussion points are open in construction, with no single or "correct" answer. The questions identify the scope of discussion (a particular ethical principle and participants own real life experiences) and imply certain assumptions (that the ethical terms are understood, that participants have had real experiences of ethical conflicts/resolutions).

Examples of discussion questions for evaluations

- **What were your experiences during the course like?** (Addressing Fitzpatrick's level 1 Responses). Follow up for the subsequent rounds could include:
  - How did that come about?
  - Any suggestions for changes in the course to improve this aspect?
- **What did you learn during the course?** (Addressing Fitzpatrick's level 2 learning). Follow up could include:
  - What helped that learning to happen?
  - Any suggestions for changes in the course to improve this aspect?
  - Did you learn anything that was not openly stated? (i.e. the hidden curriculum).
- **In what ways did your actions/behaviour at work change after the course?** (Addressing Fitzpatrick's level 3 Behaviour). Follow up questions for the subsequent rounds could include:
  - "How did you make those changes?
  - What helped or hindered that change in behaviour?
  - Any suggestions for changes in the course to improve this aspect?
- **What effects did the course have on you as an individual, on your patients, on your participation in the team at work?** (Addressing Fitzpatrick's level 4 Outcomes) Follow up questions for the subsequent rounds could include:
  - "How did you notice that effect?
  - What helped that along?
  - Any suggestions for changes in the course to improve this aspect?
- **Debriefing/"harvest" questions**
  - What themes are emerging about the education you are finding most enjoyable/interesting?
  - Most effective in helping you learn new skills?
  - Most effective in helping you to make changes in your workplace?
  - Which content has the biggest impact? Which learning methods have the biggest impact?
  - Is there any learning that has not been mentioned or that is not openly talked about?

8// END OF PROGRAMME FITZPATRICK LEVELS 3 AND 4

"The purpose of education is not to fill a bucket, but to light a fire." W.B. Yeats

What Fitzpatrick evaluation level is this method aimed at?

Evaluations during sessions, or at the end of a session, or reviewing last week's session, are all helpful for educators wanting to reflect on the immediate impact and learning that participants experience from their educational activities.

However, the ultimate aim of education is to develop the capacity for change in participants; the capacity to change their behaviour in the workplace and the capacity to change the outcomes or results for their patients, their colleagues, the systems they work in and for themselves. End of programme evaluations can be helpfully directed to Fitzpatrick level 3 and 4, by asking questions that specifically consider behaviour and outcomes, and that invite a higher level of reflection than a single word or tick box answer.

In order to know the value of a programme, the educator has to be clear about what value they were aiming to provide in the first place. To provoke an even deeper reflection, educators may also want participants to reflect on what *professional values* they developed as a result of their professional education.

The method suggested here, asks several "open directed" questions, addressing the desirable changes in behaviour and practice that the education has been directed towards. Deciding what is "most desirable" is not something the educator does in isolation. The subject matter covered and the outcomes to be evaluated will be a complex mixture derived from consideration of these themes:

- **The formal curriculum** – with limited time available, educators make choices about what to leave out and what to include.
- **The end point assessments** that participants are aiming for, influence the focus and selection of subject matter.
- **Participants expressed interests and wishes**
- **The hidden curriculum aims and objectives** considered by the educator to be of greatest importance.

Some possible examples, of suitable open directed questions, are given in the Resources section (page 39), together with examples of the free text answers which they generated, and a commentary on what educators might make of the evaluation comments.

What this method most useful for?

This approach is useful for evaluating a whole programme in a holistic way, aiming to get an overall sense of what is working well and what might need to be changed, developed or omitted in future programmes. Did the educator light any educational fires?

What is this method is less useful for?

This method is less useful for evaluating the impact of a single session or module within a programme. While participants often refer back to specific session, this is often because a particular sessions evoke strong and memorable emotions for some participants. While this should be taken note of, strongly positive or strongly negative emotional statements about session need to be understood in a context. Do all participants feel the same way? Does the outcome mean that the session needs to be omitted, or developed or that the educational method and the support given to participants needs to change? What weight should educators put on a few participants strong likes or dislikes compared the group as a whole?

Preparation

The educator needs to prepare question sheets in advance, one for each participant. The length and complexity of the questionnaire will influence how much time and energy is required for collation and subsequent reflections and discussions with colleagues. Educators will need to plan for this in advance by allocating dedicated time, (if they are to perform this task themselves) or designate some administration time from their course administrator if that is available. As with other evaluation methods, the educator can decide on what will be the most helpful focus. It may be too complex and yield too much information to try and evaluate everything about a programme, every year.

Set Up with participants

A thoughtful approach to evaluating a whole programme of study means that participants must be given adequate time to compete the questionnaire and reflect on what they wish to say. A dedicated section of the course programme needs to be allocated for evaluation. If the process is left to a hurried minute or two before everyone leaves, the quality of the feedback will reduce and the benefits of evaluation by participants will be lost. Allow 20 to 30 minutes.

Explain the purpose of your evaluation to participants and how the outcomes will be communicated to them, for example, in a follow up email. Explain what will happen next. Set out what reflections and discussions with colleagues will occur, who else will see the results of the evaluation, (for example senior staff, appraisers, inspection teams who come to review programmes) and how the results will be used to improve the programme.

It can help to give examples of how the current programme has been influenced by previous participants' feedback and comments. Giving specific examples of such changes, will increase participants' motivation to complete their responses. Getting a copy of the collated results with a commentary on what the educator intends to do with the results and any anticipated changes will also help to increase trust in the evaluation process.

Debriefing or collation issues

Questionnaires inevitably take time for collation, so that debriefing will normally be by follow up communication to course participants, perhaps in a summarising email. This message can have a copy of the collated results attached, and contain a summary of key findings and any anticipated changes. It may be helpful to be transparent about changes that cannot be made. There are often constraints about rooms, location, group sizes or course content that educators must acknowledge cannot be changed. If questions are worded well, they will address the aims of the programme overtly. Thus, the evaluation and reflection process can also help to reinforce learning.

Other approaches

A holistic evaluation (in the sense of understanding the "value" that participants ascribe to their educational programme) can also be gleaned by using methods from the ENRICH section of this manual. For example, ENRICH endings, ENRICH Artist in Residence and ENRICH creative writing could all be used with an evaluative focus.

Pitfalls

Asking good questions can be difficult. In trying to assess the impact of sessions educators may be tempted to ask about the most "memorable" session, for example. However, the most memorable session may the one the participant was most unhappy about, or could not see the point of at the time. It is better to think about the Fitzpatrick level in question and focus on behaviour or outcomes when devising questions.

Asking too many questions can also cause problems. Participants get tired, lose focus and become less engaged the longer the process takes. It is better to get good evaluations of a few areas, with actionable outcomes, than repetitive monosyllabic comments.

How best to use the outcomes of this type of evaluation

The collated comments will of course be of great interest to the educator or educator team involved and should allow for discussion about what went well and to what extent the aim of the programme were achieved. Sometimes hidden curriculum issues can be highlighted; for example, a participant who says "this is not what happens in real life is it?" This is valuable feedback for the educator who can use such information to address attitudinal issues, such as whether behaviour change in the workplace is anticipated as a result of training, in their next programme.

It can be helpful for the educator to write a short summary of the strengths and weaknesses of the programme as highlighted in the evaluation, with identified action points as needed for development in the future.

It can be even more helpful if such action points include any professional development the educator may need in order to advance their educational skills. This might be particularly relevant if the educator is concerned that "nothing can be done" about a particular difficulty. An attitude of helplessness towards difficulties, or one of "blaming the participants" may reflect a need for further development of educational skills. The educator may need to reflect on whether a different educational attitude or different educational values might help. For example, developing skills to become more learner centred, or in delivering difficult topics more effectively, or developing skills to teach attitudes and values, are all aspects of professional development for educators. Educational effectiveness can be learned.

RESOURCES

Here are some *possible* questions and some of the comments that resulted.

What have been the best things about Study Release Course this term?

- Not being in surgery – it breaks up the week/Giving us reflection time
- Finishing in good time/Christie cancer days – Free food and drink
- Enlightening experience /Confidence managing uncertainty – not just facts
- Getting to know cohorts and make friends/The course is fun!
- Confidence to deal with random unusual stuff/Reassuring everyone having similar experiences
- All in same boat/Bench marking/Working altogether central and south ☺
- We feel part of a team/Cohort/Protected learning environment
- Sharing experiences with each other/Chance to chair small group – improve leadership skills

Commentary

The educator can identify many positives here. Some participants clearly value working together in a community of practice. What does the approval of "finishing on time", "free food and drink" and "not being in surgery" tell us about potential hidden curriculum issues? Would it be better to ask "which parts of the course changed your behaviour at work the most?".

What things have changed your practice in some way?

Here are a selection of the responses that specifically referred to consultation skills.

- Picking apart words, phrases and skills practice" Yes and" instead of "Yes but"...
- Not 'any' questions but "what questions"
- Positive Language Especially when explaining/describing – for example, "I want to have a good listen to your chest".
- BATHE! Background, Affect, Trouble, Handling, and Empathy.
- "Skills rehearsal"
- Alcohol talk – explanation and planning, Focusing on language and phrasing of questions.

Commentary

There are some potentially specific changes in behaviour reported here, and clearly an increase in understanding of the importance of phrasing and language when consulting with patients. The educator still cannot be sure that these are being implemented or that patients or colleagues notice the difference. This illustrates that evaluating levels 3 and 4 can be quite difficult.

Which sessions on the SRC helped develop your "Professional artistry" (making judgements, room to be wrong, going beyond protocol, developing yourself, understanding self-regulation/professional regulation?)

This question aims to evaluate the professional values that participants have imbibed in the programme. The answers are given verbatim here.

- The SRC trip away. Great teamwork and personal feedback.
- POSSUM Conference. Managing Uncertainty. GMC
- POSSUM Conference, GMC
- WDYDWYDKWTD* Session. End of life session.
- Almost all.
- 'The Doctor' video sessions.
- Errors. CCG (final) ⇨ SWOT ⇨ Know yourself.
- Developing myself through thinking and assessing situations.
- Most sessions.
- Dealing with uncertainty. The film 'The Doctor' Wellbeing session.
- Ethics/assisted suicide. Managing uncertainty.
- I appreciate the value in right, wrong activation and this help with emotional resilience decision making and hope to develop this further.
- Live drug sessions.
- I this was more of a running theme throughout – both am sessions and small groups.
- Medical error, ethics assisted dying, Whitworth session.
- Residential trip, Artistic work.

**What do you do when you don't know what to do*

Commentary

Quite a wide range of sessions are mentioned here. When asked what they would omit, other participants mentioned some of these same sessions. This illustrates that in adult learning situations not everyone gets the same learning outcomes, and that is to be expected. Educators must then make judgements about how to weigh up different views of the same sessions.

9// USING KEY WORDS AND WORD CLOUDS

Sometimes an image or picture is worth a thousand words.

What Fitzpatrick evaluation level is this method aimed at?

This evaluation is a way to visualise participants' responses to the educational experience in a way that captures the information in an immediately appealing, visual way. Free text responses are turned into a "word cloud" or "wordle". There is no specific Fitzpatrick level aimed at, this is more a way of using an image to present results in a readily understandable form.

What this method most useful for?

This method can be used when evaluation information has been gathered in free text form. In many evaluations or surveys the most interesting and useful parts are the free text notes that participants add, so that inviting free text as the main way to obtain participants views gives rich material to work with (see EVALUATE Introduction for more details). The resulting "word clouds "can be useful for reflection, on the part of participants or educators. It can also be a useful way to show information visually to others, in reports or presentations. This may be appropriate, for example, when programmes are being inspected or evaluated and gives a "flavour" of what is happening in the education.

What is this method is less useful for?

This method gives a "broad brush" assessment of evaluation information. It is therefore less useful for detailed planning. Being rather global it is less useful for evaluating specific learning outcomes, nor specific behaviour changes or outcomes in practice.

Preparation

The educator decides what they are trying to evaluate and asks some questions that address that issue. For example, at the end of a residential the key questions could relate to how well participants feel they have been welcomed into and bonded with a group of their peers. At the end of a term, the key question may be what the most important sessions were, or what was learned most effectively, or questions that relate to the overall value that participants placed in their educational experiences.

The educator also can decide whether to give an evaluation form out as a paper copy, for collation afterwards, or whether to use an online system such as Survey Monkey. While the latter includes every participant, even if they are not present on the evaluation day, in practice online questionnaires also often fail to get responses from every eligible person. Depending on WIFI/ DATA availability and the willingness of participants to use online methods, it could be possible to use a Survey Monkey approach within the session.

Collation can be time consuming from paper copies, so the educator needs to allocate administration support time, where possible, to facilitate this. Software that creates the word cloud is available freely online (Reference 1).

Set Up with participants

The educator needs to explain the purpose of the evaluation and what the findings will be used for. This is normally to share views with other participants and to enable them to reflect on their experiences, so that when choosing educational activities in the future they will be able to identify the types of educational experience that have had the biggest impact on them, and choose to do similar types of education in the future. Explain how previous evaluations have resulted in changes to the programme, and that information from this evaluation will enable the educator to make relevant changes to the education on offer in the future.

Debriefing or collation issues

The software that converts text into word clouds is easy to use. Choices can be made about colours, fonts and shapes of the word cloud, to help support the underlying message.

Pitfalls

Sometimes free text generates a lot of words that do not convey content. The software removes obvious things like "the" or "and". However, educators should review the word list to remove words that are irrelevant, like "session" or combine words that have the same meanings such as relationship and relationships. This introduces a necessary subjective element to the word cloud. This does not negate the value, but is something to be aware of.

How best to use the outcomes of this type of evaluation

As suggested above, word clouds are not very nuanced but give an overall flavour. Therefore they are best used to give an "overall feeling" about the work that has been done, or to introduce a more detailed assessment of the outcomes. Word clouds make good title pages for presentations or reports. This type of image can also be used as an introduction to participants on the next course, to help indicate what value previous participants have gleaned from their education.

References and resources

1. Word clouds can be created using the Wordle website: http://www.wordle.net/ or from https://www.wordclouds.com
2. Here are two examples

Which five words indicate the *value* that the programme has had for you?

In this word cloud I have not removed repeated words like "support and supportive" or "education and educational". The educator can choose how to approach this.

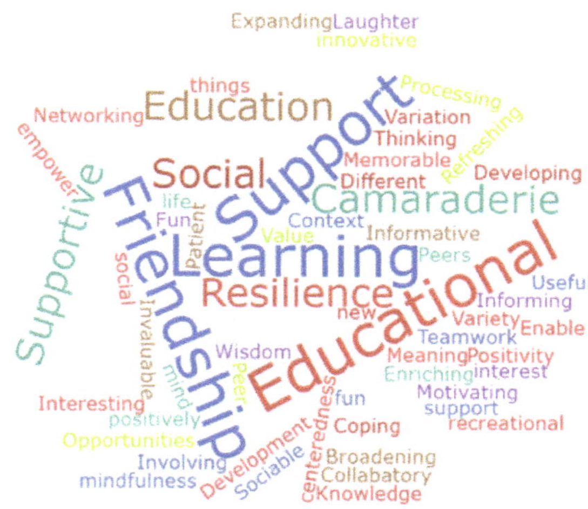

Here is another word cloud where the question was:

Which sessions on the SRC helped you to develop an understanding of "professional artistry" (i.e. concerned with making judgements, having room to be wrong, going beyond protocol, developing yourself, understanding self regulation/professional regulation?)

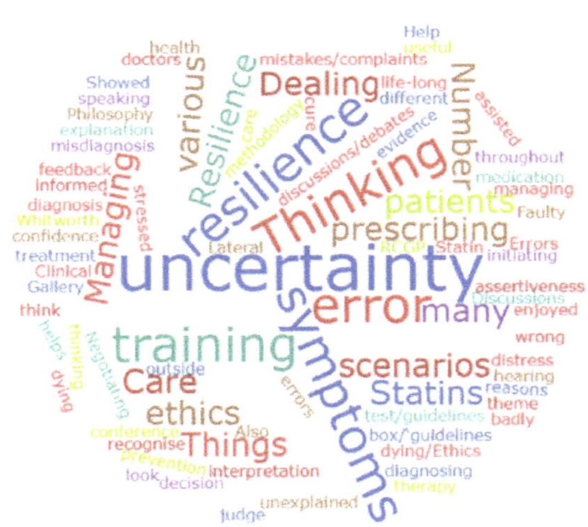

10// EVALUATION AFTER THE PROGRAMME HAS ENDED

"Do the difficult things while they are easy and do the great things while they are small. A journey of a thousand miles must begin with a single step." Lao Tzu

What Fitzpatrick evaluation level is this method aimed at?

Are training programmes truly the first step to life-long learning? The most important impact of education is also the most difficult to evaluate. Fitzpatrick's level 4 addresses the effects on outcomes in participants' professional work. This could include effects on patients, systems, teamwork, their own resilience or stress and their professional development in the long run. Not only are these difficult to evaluate once participants have left training to embark on the next stage of their careers, but also the final outcome is likely to be the result of many different aspects of training. This could include any formal programme, any mentoring or tutoring they have received, their own private study and individual experiences. Teasing out the effect of an educational intervention is likely to be rather complex.

There are two main ways of evaluating these longer term effects, asking the question "what difference did your educational activities make to your professional work long term?

The **formal** method is to attempt some kind of follow up evaluation, sending questionnaires to participants sometime after they have left the programme.

The second, **informal**, method is frankly biased, limited and totally subjective, although it may be the only feedback available. Educators will often meet their alumni in professional contexts long after they have left the programmes of study. Sometimes they spontaneously come and tell educators their thoughts on their programme. Sometimes educators have to be brave and ask them from their thoughts. It is very unlikely that the answers will be objective, unbiased or specific, measurable, achievable or timely. It is worth listening though, even simply as food for thought!

What this method most useful for?

Evaluating long after participants have left a programme of study is useful for getting the "long view" especially as regards wider issues of how the programme contributed to career development professional development or to the skills and values needed for successful clinical practice.

What is this method is less useful for?

This method is less suitable to consider individual sessions. It is unlikely that memory will be sufficiently accurate to give actionable detailed feedback on specific educational activities. It is far more likely to yield a broad brush picture. Attempting to evaluate courses a year or more after they are finished also has the serious drawback that it is very difficult to get responses from all the relevant participants. Many will have changed their contact details, be in another country, or be distracted by the demands of career and home, so that they do not respond. We all have too many inboxes to deal with anyway.

This means that caution must be taken when interpreting results.

Preparation

Anecdotal, spontaneous feedback, if an educator meets a participant years later, cannot really be prepared for; listen, try to make the most of the moment to ask any questions if you can.

If a formal evaluation is planned consider the questions carefully and keep them few in number. Identify what elements of Fitzpatrick levels 3 (behaviour) and 4 (results) it might be feasible to address. Posted questionnaires are fraught with difficulty because participants rarely provide any ongoing contact details. Electronic surveys sent by email such as "Survey Monkey" (Reference 1), also get low response rates. However, that may be the best that is feasible.

Ensure that the survey is to the point, while also allowing a space for free text comments, which are sometimes the most illuminating anyway.

Set Up with participants

If the educator decides to evaluate their programme sometime after it finishes, it will be worthwhile telling participants that this is planned, so that the educator can encourage them to participate, so that response rates improve. This will increase the value of the delayed evaluation. The beginning of the questionnaire may need a short paragraph of introduction about the purposes of the evaluation and what the educator intends to do with the results.

Debriefing or collation issues

As with other approaches, it is important to try and close the loop of this evaluation and feedback the findings to the participants, with a summary of findings and potential actions. This is also an opportunity to reflect on success and on the gratitude often displayed by alumni, who do appreciate the educational activities and support that they experienced in many cases. Clearly, the evaluation may also reveal problems with the course, difficulties in translating training into the workplace and this will be very helpful for the educator planning changes in educational activities.

One major problem with delayed evaluation is that responses are incomplete. Many participants will simply not reply. When reviewing the findings the educator will have to make judgments about how reliable the responses are, how representative they are, (of the whole group or of particular sub-sections of the group) and how realistic any suggested changes are.

Pitfalls

Evaluation taking place years or more after the education has finished will necessarily be partial, subject to all kinds of bias on the part of the memories of the participants and may not yield actionable findings. This might not be something to attempt regularly, unless the administrative support is sufficient to generate reports easily.

How best to use the outcomes of this type of evaluation.

The outcomes are likely to be broad, rather than detailed, giving a holistic feeling, rather than specific feedback to the educational activities. This can be good for morale if the feedback is good, but dispiriting if not. It takes time and effort to do this so educators must make a judgement about whether the outcomes will be really useful to them.

Before embarking on such a process it is probably worthwhile discussing with colleagues what the aims and objectives are and what to do with the findings. Positive findings could be very useful for feeding into inspection or appraisal processes. Having a clear analysis of any adverse findings and realistic plans for making changes will also be useful for any appraisal or inspection process.

References

1. Survey monkey – online survey creation tool: https://www.surveymonkey.co.uk

www.ingramcontent.com/pod-product-compliance
Lightning Source LLC
LaVergne TN
LVHW072119210926
848482LV00027B/701